An Introduction to Radiography

D1585596

For Elsevier:

Commissioning Editors: Dinah Thom; Claire Wilson
Development Editor: Catherine Jackson
Project Manager: Gail Wright
Senior Designer: George Ajayi
Illustrations Manager: Merlyn Harvey
Illustrators: Graeme Chambers; Chartwell Illustrators
Cartoonist: David Banks

An Introduction to Radiography

Edited by

Suzanne Easton MSc BSc PGCertED

Senior Lecturer, Faculty of Health and Social Care, University of the West of England, Bristol, UK

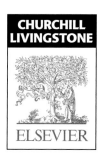

EDINBURGH   LONDON   NEW YORK   OXFORD   PHILADELPHIA   ST LOUIS   SYDNEY   TORONTO   2009

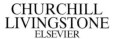

CHURCHILL
LIVINGSTONE
ELSEVIER

ISBN 978-0-443-10419-0

British Library Cataloguing in Publication Data
A catalogue record for this book is available from the British Library

Library of Congress Cataloging in Publication Data
A catalog record for this book is available from the Library of Congress

Notice
Neither the Publisher nor the Editor assumes any responsibility for any loss or injury and/or damage to persons or property arising out of or related to any use of the material contained in this book. It is the responsibility of the treating practitioner, relying on independent expertise and knowledge of the patient, to determine the best treatment and method of application for the patient.

The Publisher

Working together to grow
libraries in developing countries
www.elsevier.com | www.bookaid.org | www.sabre.org

ELSEVIER   BOOK AID International   Sabre Foundation

ELSEVIER   your source for books,
journals and multimedia
in the health sciences
www.elsevierhealth.com

Printed in China

The
Publisher's
policy is to use
**paper manufactured
from sustainable forests**

Contents

List of contributors

Sophia Beale
*Senior Lecturer – Diagnostic Imaging, Faculty
of Health and Social Care, London South Bank
University, London, UK*

Fiona Chamberlain IIPEM
*Senior Lecturer – Diagnostic Imaging, Faculty
of Health and Life Sciences, University of the West
of England, Bristol, UK*

Brian Channon
*Senior Lecturer (retired), Faculty of Health and
Life Sciences, University of the West of England,
Bristol, UK*

Karen Dunmall MSc(SRM)(Open) BSc(Hons) PGCert(HE)
DCR(R)
*Senior Lecturer – Diagnostic Imaging, Faculty
of Health and Life Sciences, University of the West
of England, Bristol, UK*

Sarah Fearn BSc MSc PGCert(HE)
*Senior Lecturer, Faculty of Health and Human
Sciences, University of Hertfordshire,
Hatfield, UK*

Stuart Grange MSc BSc(Hons) DCR(R) PGCert
*Senior Lecturer, Faculty of Health and Life Sciences,
University of the West of England, Bristol, UK*

Marc Griffiths MSc PGCert(HE) BSc(Hons) FHEA
*Subject Group Leader (Radiography), Faculty
of Health and Life Sciences, University of the West
of England, Bristol, UK*

Ken Holmes MSc TDCR DRI Cert CI
Senior Lecturer, University of Cumbria, Carlisle, UK

Vicki Major MSc DCR(R) DRI PGCert(HE)
*Senior Lecturer, London South Bank University; now
Clinical Lead – Nuclear Medicine and PETCT,
InHealth, High Wycombe, UK*

Simon Messer
*Senior Lecturer – Diagnostic Imaging, Faculty
of Health and Life Sciences, University of the West
of England, Bristol, UK*

Nick Oldnall
*Clinical Practice Developer (Imaging), Gloucestershire
Royal Hospital, Gloucester, UK*

Sally Perry MSc
*Senior Lecturer, Faculty of Health and Life Sciences,
University of the West of England, Bristol, UK*

Rita Phillips MSc DMU FAETC DCR
*Senior Lecturer – Diagnostic Imaging, Faculty
of Health and Life Sciences, University of the West
of England, Bristol, UK*

Aarthi Ramlaul
*Senior Lecturer, Faculty of Health and Human
Sciences, University of Hertfordshire,
Hatfield, UK*

Juliet C. Semple BSc(Hons) PGCert
*Superintendent III Radiographer (MRI),
Neuroradiology, John Radcliffe Hospital,
Oxford, UK*

Gillian Springett
Senior Lecturer – Radiotherapy (retired), Faculty of Health and Life Sciences, University of the West of England, Bristol, UK

Catriona Todd
Superintendent Radiographer, MRI Department – X-ray, Charing Cross Hospital, London, UK

Patti Ward MEd RT(R)
Professor/Clinical Coordinator, Health Sciences, Mesa State College, Grand Junction, Colorado, USA

Julie Woodley MSc TDCR HDCR FETC RT(R)
Senior Lecturer/Research Fellow, Faculty of Health and Life Sciences, University of the West of England, Bristol, UK

Acknowledgements

Sources of illustrations

Bowra J, McLaughlin R. Emergency ultrasound made easy. Edinburgh: Churchill Livingstone; 2006
Figs 17.1, 17.2

Bushong SC. Radiologic science for technologists: physics, biology and protection, 6th edn. St Louis: Mosby; 1997
Figs 12.8, 12.9, 12.19

Bushong SC. Radiologic science for technologists: physics, biology and protection, 8th edn. St Louis: Mosby; 2004
Figs 8.3, 8.4, 8.5, 9.3, 12.5, 15.7, 19.3

Canon Europe
Figs 11.6, 11.9, 11.10

Easton S. Practical radiography for veterinary nurses, 7th edn. Oxford: Butterworth-Heinemann; 2002
Fig. 12.10

Fauber T. Radiographic imaging and exposure, 2nd edn. St Louis: Mosby; 2004
Figs 8.1, 8.7, 9.1, 9.2, 10.1, 10.2, 10.3, 11.19, 12.1, 12.2, 12.11, 12.12, 12.14, 12.17

Graham D, et al. Principles of radiological physics, 5th edn. Edinburgh: Churchill Livingstone; 2007
Figs 6.9, 7.1, 7.2, 7.3, 7.4, 7.5, 7.6, 8.2, 8.6, 9.4, 12.7, 13.9, 14.8, 14.9, 16.1, 16.7, 19.4

Hardwick J, Gyll C. Radiography of children. Edinburgh: Churchill Livingstone; 2007
Figs 4.1, 4.2, 4.3, 4.4, 4.5, 4.6

Lee L, et al. Fundamentals of mammography, 2nd edn. Edinburgh: Churchill Livingstone; 2003
Figs 15.8, 15.9, 15.10B, 15.11, 15.17, 15.18, 15.19

Rothrock J. Alexander's care of the patient in surgery, 13th edn. St Louis: Mosby; 2007
Figs 15.3, 15.4

Toshiba
Figs 17.3, 17.4

Underwood JCE (ed). General and systematic pathology, 4th edn. Edinburgh: Churchill Livingstone; 2004
Figs 21.11, 21.24

University of Hertfordshire
Figs 20.11, 20.18

Waugh A, Grant A. Ross and Wilson Anatomy and physiology colouring and workbook, 2nd edn. Edinburgh: Churchill Livingstone; 2006
Figs 15.1, 20.2, 20.3, 20.4, 20.6, 20.7, 20.8, 20.11, 20.13, 20.14, 20.18, 20.19, 20.20, 20.21, 20.22, 20.23, 20.24, 20.25, 20.27

Xograph Healthcare Ltd
Fig. 11.2

Chapter 1

An introduction to ethics

Julie Woodley

KEY POINTS

- Ethics is a framework for the analysis and resolution of dilemmas and is loosely based on the concept of right and wrong.
- A dilemma may have an ethical component if it has a moral agent, a subject, an action and a consequence.
- There are a number of ethical theories that can be applied to an ethical dilemma.
- Radiographic practice involves a range of ethical considerations and decisions during the normal working day.

INTRODUCTION

The nature of the modern healthcare system means that ethical dilemmas commonly arise, and it is with this in mind that the following chapter will attempt to clarify our understanding of ethics and provide the reader with knowledge that may assist in the analysis and solution of some of the dilemmas likely to be encountered. These dilemmas may involve an individual patient or may have wider ranging societal consequences, as in the problem of whether patients should be given costly drugs or treatments at the expense of other services.

WHAT IS 'ETHICS'?

Ethics is defined as being 'the study of the moral value of human conduct',[1] and whilst this definition is useful the study of ethics has evolved from purely a philosophical pursuit into a branch of philosophy which has enormous implications for healthcare practice in general. It may therefore be useful to examine the fundamentals of the study of ethics in an attempt to examine its applicability to practice.

As Box 1.1 would suggest, ethics is not to be thought of as the musings of philosophers that have no real life applicability, nor should it be regarded as simply a matter of applying common sense. Ethics provides us with a framework by which we can analyse dilemmas and hopefully this structured scrutiny will subsequently lead us to be able to resolve the dilemma we may face.

WHAT IS AN ETHICAL DILEMMA?

Before we begin to examine the applicability of ethical analysis, it is essential that the exact nature of what essentially constitutes an ethical dilemma be understood, as opposed to being faced with choices that do not really have an ethical dimension to them. As previously stated, the study of ethics can be summarised as the analysis of what is right and/or what is wrong in any given situation and it also assists us with the concept of how we ought to act at any given time. We make

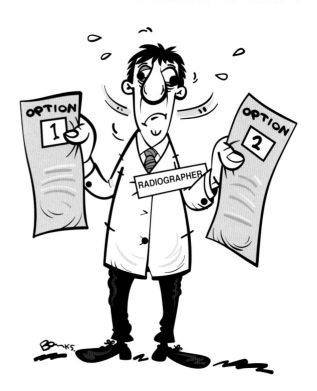

a lot of choices during daily life and not all of these choices necessarily have an ethical element involved with them. What we decide to wear, for example, is not normally of great moral concern. While an individual might inadvertently offend people with their terrible dress sense it would not necessarily be doing anyone any great harm, so as a result would not really be worthy of any kind of ethical/moral scrutiny or debate. If, however, this was taken a stage further and a T-shirt with a racist

---

Box 1.1 The fundamentals of ethics[2]

- Ethics is something that must be translatable into action. (It must work in real clinical practice.)
- Each one of us should think ethically and act in a moral way.
- Ethics is about individuals living and working in a community. (It is not just about 'me ' and 'mine'.)
- Individuals not only have specific rights but also duties/obligations towards others.

- We as healthcare workers have special obligations or duties as laid down in our professional code of conduct.
- Clinical practice, ethical analysis and moral action cannot be practised in isolation from one another. (Ethics is a necessary part of good clinical practice.)

slogan worn, this could truly offend many individuals as they quite rightly would regard individuals from another race as being worthy of their consideration. In other words individuals, or indeed communities, matter and we should consider their feelings, whereas choosing to wear black or purple is not really of any great concern to individuals or society in general. Box 1.2 demonstrates that for a dilemma to have an ethical dimension it should encompass the following elements: 1) a moral agent; 2) a subject; 3) an action and 4) a consequence.[3] All these elements have to be present before the dilemma can be defined as having an ethical dimension afforded to it.

To further qualify this statement there are also further conditions. First, the moral agent is someone who is assumed to be rational and capable of moral reasoning; then the subject must be worthy of moral consideration; the action could be good or bad, and the consequence should be of concern. Now, before readers start worrying that they have inadvertently picked up the hard core philosophy book that they leave around when trying to impress their brainy university mates, the author would just like to give an example in order to bring some clarity: If we choose to analyse a widely recognised dilemma, such as euthanasia, it soon becomes apparent that this subject more than fulfils the criteria, which results in it being arguably one of the most complex ethical dilemmas in modern medicine. In this case the moral agent is the physician who is in possession of a moral code and who can be regarded as rational. The subject (the patient) is a human being and therefore is afforded the status of being worthy of moral concern. The action is that their life is shortened by the actions of the physician, and the consequence is that they die. It is easy therefore to see that this dilemma has massive ethical perspectives.

Once we have ascertained that our dilemma has some ethical element we need to investigate the tools we have at our disposal in order to analyse and potentially come up with a solution or solutions to the problem.

BASIS OF MORAL REASONING

This analysis of ethical problems can alternatively be termed 'moral reasoning'. Here we can look at a problem and apply our moral and/or professional values to it. We can then decide what is the right option or course of action to take. We are all in possession of our own moral code (in other words, what we perceive as being right and wrong) and it is this code that we sometimes consult when deliberating about an issue. There has been much debate regarding our moral/ethical development;[4] however, it would seem that our moral reasoning capabilities may be influenced by a complex mixture of internal and external factors.

Box 1.2   Elements of an ethical dilemma[3]

Moral agent

- This is the person (or persons) carrying out the action. They should be in possession of moral values and should be rational. (So young children or those with mental illness may not be held morally accountable for their actions.)

Action

- This is the act that is carried out upon the subject. This act can be purposeful but can also be an omission.

Subject

- This is someone or something that is worthy of moral consideration (usually one or more human beings, but the status of fetuses and animals can also fall into this category).

Consequence

- In many dilemmas the consequence has a negative aspect but moral dilemmas can have good outcomes and still be morally questionable.

Box 1.3   Basis of moral reasoning

Conscience

- An action may feel 'wrong'. You may not at first be able to analyse this feeling but instinct would suggest that there is a problem.

Peer pressure

- It is very difficult to stand up for what you feel is right when others disagree. It may be easier to just go along with the group view.

Tradition

- Moral values may stem from tradition. A good example is marriage, which was widely regarded as the norm; but over the years other options, such as living together, have become socially acceptable.

Religion

- Many religions provide very clear frameworks to instruct us how to behave if we are to be regarded as a 'good' person. Some of these teachings may, however, be regarded as out of date in modern society.

Education

- Being educated means you can be more informed and thus in possession of more information that will assist you to decide what is right or wrong.

Life experiences

- Your values may change once you have actually experienced something; e.g. parenthood or nursing a terminally ill relative.

All the elements mentioned in Box 1.3 serve to provide us with our own set of values. These values may change as we mature or gain 'life experience' but they may also be supplemented by additional rules or values that come when we adopt a professional role.

THE MAIN ETHICAL THEORIES

In an attempt to evaluate the exact nature of human values, philosophers have proposed various theories in order to give more structure to the process of moral reasoning. Many of the theories that can be applied to ethical analysis come from a particular philosophical perspective. These theories can then be translated into principles by which we would wish to live and then further extrapolated into rules which should govern our judgements and in turn our actions. For example, in principle we would like to live a healthy life, so legislation is drawn up requiring authorities to provide basic healthcare provision for their population. These authorities then make judgements as to how that provision should be constructed and then ultimately delivered.

To help the individuals to make such decisions it may be helpful to provide a frame of reference on which to structure their deliberations. It is at this point that we may consult various ethical theories.

DEONTOLOGY

Immanuel Kant,[5] who was a philosopher in the 18th century, first proposed this theory, based on the idea of rights and duties. He hypothesised that:

- Each of us had a set of duties towards our fellow man.
- We should not treat a fellow human being as a means to an end and, indeed, we should treat others how we ourselves would wish to be treated.
- Certain acts were intrinsically right or wrong (for example he believed killing could not be condoned under any circumstances).
- Rules produced by any community should be rational and universally applicable.
- The rightness of actions should not be judged by their consequences.

Applying this theory, it would be widely accepted that we have a duty of care towards our patients and it would seem sensible that we should carry out that duty in a fair and just manner; i.e. treat all patients with equal regard. The main problem with this theory was how we could construct rules that could be applied universally; in other words, in every circumstance. So although we would like to treat all our patients equally it would seem very unfair to not give priority to those most in need. It would also not seem at all rational to ignore the consequences of our actions, even if they were well intended.

CONSEQUENTIALISM

Later on, in the 19th century, John Stuart Mill and Jeremy Bentham[6] went on to develop a theory by which the value of any action was based solely upon the end result or consequence. They termed this theory 'utilitarianism' and argued that certain utilities should be maximised if an act was to be performed. Their main utility was happiness and they believed that the aim of all human endeavour should be to strive towards 'The greatest happiness of the greatest number'. They believed that:

- All acts should be judged upon their consequences.
- Happiness and well-being should be maximised for the greatest number.

The problem with this theory was that it was highly subjective and often discriminated against the individual. For example, a radiological department with £10 000 to spend might be faced with the dilemma of whether to allocate this funding to either an angiography suite or a chest room. Utilitarianism would suggest that it would provide more benefit if it were awarded to the chest room, as it could potentially affect far more people's well-being than if it was put towards the more expensive procedures carried out in an angiography suite. That may on the face of it seem fair, but you might not think so if you were a patient who then had to have highly invasive surgery because angioplasty could not be funded. This maximising happiness would effectively mean that cheaper treatments that benefited populations would always be chosen over expensive individual treatments, and as a result the

seriously ill would almost certainly be discriminated against in most cases.

THE FOUR PRINCIPLES APPROACH

The two aforementioned theories are indeed just that – theories – and much of the criticism levelled against them was that they had flaws when applied to real-world dilemmas. It was with this in mind that Beauchamp and Childress[7] attempted to develop a more user friendly and more easily applicable theory that we could apply in any given situation. They framed their arguments into what has been commonly termed 'the four principles approach', which is summarised in Box 1.4.

Again, this theory is not without its problems as, whilst it is fairly simple to analyse the dilemma under the four categories and devise possible solutions based on each of the principles, the theory gives us no guidance as to which of these principles should be given the highest weighting in the event of a conflict between them.

For example, if a patient came into your department asking to be treated only by a female radiographer, she would be exerting her autonomy in making that request. Normally this would not be an issue, but if on this occasion the section of the department was staffed purely by men, you would have a problem: by facilitating the request you would please the patient but delay her procedure

---

Box 1.4   The four principles approach[7]

Beneficence

- Always act in the best interests of the patient.

Non-maleficence

- Do not harm the patient in any way.

Autonomy

- Facilitate and honour the patient's wishes.

Justice

- Treat everyone with equal regard.

whilst you reallocated staff (causing possible harm) and you might also inconvenience the patients to whom the female radiographer was already attending. Also, would it be right and fair (justice) that one patient should be able to disrupt others just to exert her choice? The four principles approach does not really help us to decide whether there should be limits to the patient's autonomy or whether the justice aspect of this course of action should be given more credibility in the decision-making process. It is, however, very widely referred to within healthcare literature and, if nothing else, does assist us to begin to frame the debate and produce alternatives on our journey to a resolution.

NARRATIVE ETHICS

The example used to illustrate the previous point was missing one vital piece of information in that at no point were the reasons behind the patient's request explained, and this leads us on to a further ethical perspective, termed the narrative approach, in which the patient's story, narrative, values and emotions become important. The patient's request may have a religious basis or it may simply be that the patient would feel more comfortable with a female radiographer; but without taking these aspects into consideration it is very difficult to proceed and ultimately take the right course of action. Patients are all individuals and, as such, all come with their own values and narratives which must be respected if at all practicable.

VIRTUE ETHICS

In this branch proponents enquire about how should we live[8] rather than looking for instruction on how to act. The theory attempts to analyse what should be desirable qualities or virtues, such as honesty and truthfulness.

FEMINIST PERSPECTIVES

A further group of theories that would appear to have great relevance to healthcare are feminist perspectives towards ethical debate. These views challenge the traditionally male perspectives and apply a more feminine idea of care.

APPLYING ETHICS TO RADIOGRAPHIC PRACTICE

Any one of the previously mentioned theories or combinations thereof may assist us in our decision making process. Whilst this is useful, the fact that we have some form of professional status will bring a further set of values that should also be brought into the equation. Further assistance in how we should act can also be found in the fact that most professions have devised a code of ethics/conduct for their members. Such a code assists the professional in that it gives guidance on how to carry out professional duties and it gives the public some idea of what to expect from the professional under whose care they may find themselves. In other words, it gives guidance on how we should act if we want to be regarded as a 'good' professional.

STATEMENTS FOR PROFESSIONAL CONDUCT

Radiography's professional body, The College of Radiographers,[9] has over the years produced and adapted what it terms as statements of professional conduct in an attempt to clarify our professional role. So not only are we in possession of our own values, by entering into the radiography profession we agree to act in accordance with these statements (Box 1.5).

These statements are indeed based on ethical principles and it is quite easy to see where principles such as beneficence and non-maleficence have informed these statements, given that most are written for the benefit and protection of the patient or member of staff. There is also a strong deontological ideology in that there are many references to 'duty', so this would imply that the patient has the right to a reasonable standard of care. All professional codes could be criticised as being a little vague but their role is to provide guidance rather

Box 1.5   Statements for professional conduct (2004)[9]

Statement 1

Radiographers are ethically and legally obliged to protect the confidentiality and security of patient information acquired through their professional duties, except where there is a legal requirement to do otherwise.

Statement 2

Radiographers have a duty to work in a co-operative and collaborative manner with other professional staff and carers in the interests, and with the consent, of their patient(s) except where there is a legal requirement to do otherwise.

Statement 3

Radiographers have a duty of care towards patients they accept for imaging/treatment procedures.

Statement 4

Radiographers must report to an appropriate person and/or appropriate authority, any circumstances that may put patients or others at risk.

Statement 5

Radiographers must identify and acknowledge any limitations in their knowledge and competence.

Statement 6

Radiographers must maintain and strive to improve their professional knowledge and competence.

Statement 7

Radiographers must uphold and enhance the good standing and reputation of the profession.

Statement 8

Radiographers must act in such a manner as to justify public trust and confidence, upholding and serving both the public interests and the interests of patients.

Statement 9

Radiographers are legally responsible and accountable for the results of their professional actions caused by act, negligence, omission or injury.

Statement 10

Radiographers must ensure that they pay due regard to the way in which they accept remuneration for their services.

---

than being inflexible rules.[7] Further expansion of each statement can be found in the full document that the college has produced.[9]

HOW SHOULD WE START TO ANALYSE AN ETHICAL DILEMMA?

So, armed with the theories, principles and codes we can then attempt to apply them to the dilemmas with which we are presented and this analysis is best done in a systematic way. Indeed some authors have formulated very structured ways of analysing dilemmas, which are termed 'decision making models', and whilst many of these are useful in particular circumstances, one size does not fit all and

many people have criticised them as being too restrictive. It would be nice to create a computer program that would allow us to type in all our variables and it would then compute the right course of action but, sadly, the complexity of many situations would render this program of limited value. Instead, it may be helpful to logically work our way through a dilemma in a systematic way, applying a mixture of principles and professional codes as shown in Box 1.6.

Making these decisions is not always straightforward and the decision may become 'fluid' as all parties become more informed, or indeed they may reach a point where there is just too much information and a solution may seem impossible. It may be that in some cases all parties may have to choose

Box 1.6   Analysing ethical dilemmas

Step 1

- Recognise the dilemma – realising that there is a problem is the first step towards offering a solution. (This may sound obvious but being ethically aware is a skill that does need training and is not all just common sense.)

Step 2

- Gather information – this is necessary to be able to make an informed choice, either by the practitioners or indeed the patient or a collaboration between the two.

Step 3

- Generate alternatives – these should be based on rights, duties and the best consequences.

Step 4

- Evaluate alternatives – balance out the risks and the benefits and evaluate the 'rightness' or 'goodness' of any action.

Step 5

- Apply ethical principles – are the four principles (beneficence, non-maleficence, autonomy,

justice) applicable or can lessons be learnt from the patient's narrative (story) or by applying feminist perspectives?

Step 6

- Previous experience or similar cases – can anything be learnt from similar cases? Can you consult with an 'expert' or colleagues who may be able to provide useful insight? If in doubt, ask.

Step 7

- Come to a conclusion – the decision should be made with all the information you have available at that time.

Step 8

- Revisit your decision – do not dwell on the fact that your conclusion turned out, in hindsight, not to have been the best option, but feel secure in the fact that you made the best decision at the time.

Step 9

- Learn from your decision – can you take anything forward into your future practice?

the least bad option but as long as this choice is based on sound principles then it will be ethically sound.

CONCLUSION

Ethical analysis may not always give you one correct answer. The complexity of dilemmas in modern clinical practice often means that the right thing to do is not always straightforward and the individual may be faced with having to make very difficult decisions. What ethics does allow us to do, however, is be aware of those options in order for us to be able to make the best choice at any given time. If that choice ultimately turns out not to be the best one then at least the selection of that choice was based on sound principles

and would not be regarded as any breach of professional conduct.

References

1. Collins Essential English Dictionary, 2nd edn. Glasgow: Harpercollins; 2006. Ethics.
2. Stirrat GM. How to approach ethical issues – a brief guide. The Obstetrician & Gynaecologist 2003; 5:167–170.
3. Beauchamp TL, Childress JF. Principles of biomedical ethics, 5th edn. New York: Oxford University Press; 2001:15.
4. Kohlberg L. The stages of ethical development: from childhood through old age. Glasgow: Harpercollins; 1991.
5. Kant I. The moral law: groundwork of the metaphysics of morals. Oxford: Routledge Classics; 2005.
6. Bentham J, Mill JS. Utilitarianism and other essays. Harmondsworth, UK: Penguin Books; 1987.
7. Beauchamp TL, Childress JF. Principles of biomedical ethics, 5th edn. New York: Oxford University Press; 2001:67.

8. Crisp R, Slote MA. Virtue ethics (Oxford readings in philosophy). Oxford: Oxford University Press; 1997.
9. College of Radiographers. Statements of professional conduct. London: CoR; 2001.

Recommended reading

Beauchamp TL, Childress JF. Principles of biomedical ethics, 5th edn. New York: Oxford University Press; 2001.

Campbell A, Gillett G, Jones G. Medical ethics. Melbourne, Australia: Oxford University Press; 2005.

Although this text addresses ethical issues in a more philosophical way, it does analyse many of the common dilemmas that arise in healthcare.

Parker M, Dickenson D. The Cambridge medical ethics workbook: case studies, commentaries and activities. Cambridge, UK: Cambridge University Press; 2001.

This text allows the reader to investigate ethical principles as applied to cases based on medical practice.

Savulescu J, Hendrick J, Hope T. Medical ethics and the law. Edinburgh: Churchill Livingston; 2003.

A text with a very easily understood structure that covers most of the main themes. Whilst focussed on medicine, these are equally applicable to radiography.

Wilson BG. Ethics and basic law for medical imaging professionals. Philadelphia: FA Davis; 1997.

This is one of the few texts specifically aimed at radiographers. (It is in actual fact an American textbook aimed at imaging technologists, but much of it is directly applicable to radiographic practice as a whole.)

Towsley D, Cunningham E. Biomedical ethics for radiographers. London: Mosby; 1994.

Although this text is a little outdated, it is still a very good introductory text which is directly applicable to radiography.

Chapter **2**

The law at work

Simon Messer

KEY POINTS

- The majority of the law involved with the workplace is related to health and safety.
- There are a number of acts of parliament and regulations that form the principal legislation of which you must be aware when working in a hospital.
- Underpinning British health and safety law is the Health and Safety at Work etc. Act 1974, which sets out general duties for both the employer and the employee.
- The Ionising Radiation Regulations 1999 and Ionising Radiation (Medical Exposure) Regulations 2000 are of particular interest.

INTRODUCTION

Whilst working in the hospital environment there are a number of key documents detailing regulations and acts of parliament that ensure the safety of the employee and the public as well as ensuring the safe function of the hospital for the employer.

The full text of each act or regulation is available on the Internet and the links are provided at the end of this chapter. You are strongly advised to read the actual regulations, using the sections below as guidance. This applies especially to those relating to ionising radiation.

THE HEALTH AND SAFETY AT WORK ETC. ACT 1974

The Health and Safety at Work etc. Act 1974 (HSWA) is the most important British health and safety law and is applicable to nearly every work activity. It is a huge document and its objective is to provide protection for people at work and for the general public. It does this by setting out general duties for both the employer and the employee. Failure to comply with these duties constitutes a criminal offence and both employers and employees can be prosecuted. It also provides the basis under which other health and safety regulations are enabled, the following of which are particularly relevant to radiographic work:

- Management of Health and Safety at Work Regulations 1999
- Ionising Radiations Regulations 1999 (IRR99) and the Ionising Radiations (Medical Exposure) Regulations 2000 [IR(ME)R], both of which are fundamental to radiographic practice.
- Reporting of Injuries, Diseases and Dangerous Occurrences Regulations 1995
- Manual Handling Operations Regulations 1992
- Personal Protective Equipment at Work Regulations 1992
- Control of Substances Hazardous to Health Regulations (COSHH)

GENERAL DUTIES OF EMPLOYERS

Section 2(1) of the Act places a general duty on the employer:

To ensure so far as is reasonably practicable, the health, safety and welfare at work of all his employees[1]

To achieve this, the employer is required to:

- provide and maintain safe equipment and safe methods of working (systems of work)
- provide safe arrangements for the storage, movement and use of materials
- give employees adequate instruction, training, supervision and information
- provide and maintain a safe workplace, including safe entrances and exits
- provide and maintain a safe working environment and adequate welfare facilities.

Employers are also required to ensure that people *not* in their employment, but who may be affected by their business activities, are not exposed to risks to their health and safety. This is particularly relevant to the hospital setting where public access is high.

GENERAL DUTIES OF EMPLOYEES

Employees have a number of duties and responsibilities. These include:

- to take reasonable care to ensure the health and safety of yourself and others, including the patient and members of the public
- to adhere to the systems of work specific to the department you are working in and report any hazards
- to cooperate with the employer, or anyone else, in complying health and safety legislation.

Sections 7 and 8 of the Act should be key to daily working practices. Section 7 of the Act states:

It shall be the duty of every employee while at work to take reasonable care for the health and safety of himself and of other persons who may be affected by his acts or omissions at work.[1]

Section 8 of the Act states:

No person shall intentionally or recklessly interfere with or misuse anything provided in the interests of health, safety or welfare in pursuance of any of the relevant statutory provisions.[1]

Failure to comply with either section 7 or section 8 may result in a summary conviction and a fine not exceeding £5000!

NO COST TO EMPLOYEES

Provision is made under the Act whereby 'no employer shall charge any employee in respect of anything done or provided in pursuance of any specific requirement of the relevant statutory provisions'.[1]

THE MANAGEMENT OF HEALTH AND SAFETY AT WORK REGULATIONS 1999

Whilst these regulations are not directly applicable to you as an employee, they are fundamental to all health and safety law and deal with an aspect which you will certainly be involved with; namely, risk assessment.

Under section 3 of these regulations, the employer is required to undertake 'suitable and sufficient assessment of the risks to health and safety' to which their employees are exposed while they are at work.[2]

Where a risk has been identified, the employer must then implement preventative or protective measures to avoid or minimise that risk. This is usually in the form of a thorough risk assessment.

THE IONISING RADIATIONS REGULATIONS 1999 (IRR99)

These regulations deal with the health and safety of those working with ionising radiation and are policed by the Health and Safety Executive (HSE). It is essential, as a radiation worker, that you are completely familiar with these regulations and you should therefore read them in their published form.

PART 1 INTERPRETATION AND GENERAL

The first section provides, amongst other things, definitions of terms such as 'dose rate'.

PART II GENERAL PRINCIPLES AND PROCEDURES

This is an important section and deals with the need for risk assessment, the principle of restricting

exposure to employees and the provision of personal protective equipment. It also covers the maintenance and examination of engineering controls, dose limitation and the need for contingency plans in the event of a reasonably foreseeable radiation accident.

PART III ARRANGEMENTS FOR THE MANAGEMENT OF RADIATION PROTECTION

This section deals with:

- the appointment and role of the Radiation Protection Advisor (RPA), whose main responsibility is to advise the employer and ensure these regulations are complied with
- the provision of information, instruction and training to employees working with ionising radiation
- the need for cooperation between employers.

PART IV DESIGNATED AREAS

The requirements for the designation and monitoring of controlled or supervised areas are detailed here, together with the need for Local Rules and the appointment of a Radiation Protection Supervisor (RPS). The RPS's job is to ensure compliance with these regulations with respect to any work carried out in areas identified in the Local Rules. The RPS also has a role under the Ionising Radiations (Medical Exposure) Regulations 2000 as detailed below.

PART V CLASSIFICATION AND MONITORING OF PERSONS

This section deals with classified workers who are defined as any employee who is 'likely to receive an effective dose in excess of 6 mSv per year or an equivalent dose which exceeds three-tenths of any relevant dose limit'.[3] It also covers dose assessment and recording, medical surveillance and requirements in the event of an overexposure.

PART VI ARRANGEMENTS FOR THE CONTROL OF RADIOACTIVE SUBSTANCES, ARTICLES AND EQUIPMENT

This section deals with radioactive materials, their storage and transport and the need for accurate record keeping. There is also a requirement to notify the HSE in the event of certain occurrences including the spillage of a radioactive substance, which would give rise to a 'significant contamination'.[3] It also deals with installation, maintenance and quality assurance of equipment used for medical imaging.

PART VII DUTIES OF EMPLOYEES AND MISCELLANEOUS

The important part of this final section details the duties of the employee (you). In summary, these duties include:

- not to expose oneself or any one else to more ionising radiation than is reasonably necessary for the purposes of work
- to use personal protective equipment (PPE), such as lead rubber aprons, where provided
- to report equipment defects
- to look after PPE
- to comply with the employer's dose monitoring and any request regarding medical surveillance.

THE IONISING RADIATIONS (MEDICAL EXPOSURE) REGULATIONS 2000 [IR(ME)R]

These regulations deal with the safe and effective use of ionising radiation used in clinical practice and they underpin all medical exposures.[4] They are policed by the Department of Health. It is essential that you are completely familiar with these regulations.

The regulations impose duties on those responsible for administrating ionising radiation to protect people undergoing medical exposure. This would include:

- medical diagnosis
- treatment

- occupational health surveillance
- health screening
- medical research
- medicolegal procedures.

IR(ME)R DUTY HOLDERS

There are four identified duty holders, whose responsibility it is to enforce these regulations:

- Employer ('Legal person')
- Referrer
- Practitioner
- Operator.

The employer

The employer has to provide a written framework of procedures for medical exposures and ensure that they are complied with by the practitioner, operator and him/herself and must also ensure that written protocols are in place for every type of standard radiological practice for each piece of equipment.

The employer also has to establish:

- recommendations concerning referral criteria, including radiation doses, and make sure that these are available to the referrer
- quality assurance programmes for standard operating procedures
- diagnostic reference levels for radiodiagnostic examinations, having regard to European diagnostic reference levels where available
- dose constraints for research where no direct medical benefit for the individual is expected from the exposure.

The employer must ensure that every practitioner and operator is adequately trained and undertakes continuing education and training after qualification. This must include training related to the use of new clinical techniques and the relevant radiation protection requirements.

The referrer

The 'referrer' is defined as being:

a registered health care professional who is entitled in accordance with the employer's procedures to refer individuals for medical exposure to a practitioner; 'registered health care professional' means a person who is a member of a profession regulated by a body mentioned in section 25(3) of the National Health Service Reform and Health Care Professions Act 2002.[5]

There is a legal requirement on the referrer to identify the patient fully and to supply sufficient clinical information for the request to be justified by the practitioner. A history and clinical examination of the patient is *essential* prior to any request for radiographs.

Essentials of an X-ray request

- Unique identification of the patient.
- Clinical information to justify the requested exposure.
- Unique identification of the referrer.
- If relevant, information on pregnancy or last menstrual period.

The practitioner

The 'practitioner' is defined as:

a health care professional who is entitled in accordance with the employer's procedures to take responsibility for an individual medical exposure.[5]

Practitioners must comply with employer's procedures. They are responsible for the justification and authorisation of individual exposures. The regulations require them to be adequately trained.

The operator

The 'operator' is:

Any person who is entitled, in accordance with the employer's procedures, to carry out all or part of the practical aspects associated with a radiographic examination.[4]

This is predominately the role that you will occupy. All operators must be adequately trained, not only to include professional qualifications but also in terms of suitable training on any new equipment or techniques.

ADMINISTRATIVE AND PROCEDURAL ASPECTS OF PATIENT PROTECTION

Justification

Before an exposure can take place, an IR(ME)R practitioner must justify it. For an exposure to be justified, the benefit to the patient from the diagnostic information obtained should outweigh the detriment of the exposure. The exposure would normally be expected to provide new information to aid the patient's management or prognosis. Under no circumstances can the routine radiography of 'new' patients prior to clinical examination be justified (Box 2.1).

Optimisation

For every X-ray exposure, the operator must ensure that doses arising from the exposure are kept 'as low as reasonably practicable' (ALARP) and consistent with the intended diagnostic purpose. This process is known as 'optimisation' and

---

Box 2.1   Considerations required to justify an exposure for a diagnostic examination

- The availability and findings of previous radiographs.
- The specific objectives of the exposure in relation to the history and examination of the patient.
- The total potential diagnostic benefit to the individual.

- The radiation risk associated with the radiographic examination.
- The efficacy, benefits and risk of available alternative techniques having the same objective but involving no, or less, exposure to ionising radiation.

relies heavily upon the professional competence and skill of the operator. So, while the operating procedures and protocols provide a framework, the operators should still use their skill and knowledge in deciding how best to perform individual exposures.

Where a standard protocol is followed, exposure factors do not need to be recorded. However, for non-standard exposures, the factors relevant to the patient dose should be recorded so that, if necessary, an estimation of the dose to the patient can be made at a later date (e.g. following an enquiry or complaint from a patient).

Clinical evaluation

The written procedures must ensure that a clinical evaluation of each X-ray is carried out and recorded. If it is known prior to exposure that no clinical evaluation will occur then the exposure is not justified and must not take place. Clinical evaluation does not necessarily entail a full radiology report but should show that each radiograph has been evaluated and also provide enough information so that it can be subject to a later audit.

Medicolegal and other third-party exposures

These are usually conducted for financial reasons rather than medical benefit. Consequently, the need for and usefulness of such examinations should be critically examined when assessing whether they are justified. The regulations recommend that the patient's written consent be obtained prior to such examinations taking place. Only a medical/dental practitioner can request such exposures.

Female patients of childbearing age

Regulation 6(1)(e) of IR(ME)R2000 prohibits the carrying out of a medical exposure of a female of child-bearing age without an enquiry as to whether she is pregnant. This is only relevant if the primary X-ray beam is likely to irradiate the pelvic area. If this is the case, the recommended course of action is as follows:

- The operator asks the patient whether she is, or might be, pregnant and records the response.
- If there is no possibility of pregnancy, the radiographic examination can proceed.
- If the patient is definitely, or probably, pregnant, the request should be referred back to the IR(ME)R practitioner to review the justification and decide whether to defer the investigation until after delivery.
- If the examination is undertaken, the fetal dose must be kept to a minimum consistent with the diagnostic purpose.
- Use a lead rubber apron.
- If the patient cannot exclude the possibility of pregnancy, she needs to be asked whether her menstrual period is overdue.
- If pregnancy cannot be excluded but her menstrual period is not overdue, the examination can proceed.
- If the period is overdue you should proceed as if the patient were pregnant.

'Excessive' exposure of patients

It is always possible that an incident may arise where a patient receives an exposure that is much greater than intended, either through equipment malfunction or operator error. If this happens, the regulations require the employer to make a preliminary investigation to confirm the incident and then notify the appropriate authority:

- HSE (equipment malfunction)
- IR(ME)R Inspectorate (clinical/operator error).

A detailed investigation must then be carried out to establish what happened and why, what doses were involved and what needs to be done to minimise the risk of a similar event in the future. The employer must retain the report of this investigation for at least 50 years! The Regulations require that exposed patients should be informed of the incident unless not doing so can be justified. It is a local decision on how, when and by whom the patient is notified, but the IR(ME)R practitioner and referring clinician should be involved.

It should be noted that patients who undergo a procedure that was not intended (as a result of mistaken identification for example), and thus exposed to a radiation dose, should be considered as having received an unintended dose. An investigation and notification to the IR(ME)R Inspectorate is required. It is therefore very important as an operator to ensure that you have the correct patient for the correct examination!

Radiation protection supervisor (RPS)

The RPS is appointed by the employer to help ensure compliance with IRR99, and in particular to supervise arrangements of Local Rules. Such a person must have received appropriate training and should be closely involved with radiography.

Radiation protection adviser (RPA)

The employer must appoint an RPA in writing. Their role is to give advice on any aspect of radiography, including:

- controls, design features, safety features and warning devices
- monitoring equipment
- risk assessment
- staff training
- the assessment and recording of radiation doses received by staff.

Medical physics expert (MPE)

An 'MPE' is:

a person who holds a science degree or its equivalent and who is experienced in the application of physics to the diagnostic and therapeutic uses of ionising radiation[4]

The role of the MPE is to give advice on such matters as the measurement and optimisation of patient dose. An RPA would be expected to be able either to act as the MPE or to suggest an appropriate person.

Diagnostic reference levels (DRLs)

The employer must consult with the MPE and adopt DRLs for local use, having regard to national/European DRLs where available. DRLs are defined in IR(ME)R as:

dose levels in radiodiagnostic practices for typical examinations for groups of standard-sized patients or standard phantoms for broadly defined types of equipment[4]

They are not normally expected to be exceeded without good reason. Where radiography is being carried out using doses consistently above the DRLs a thorough review of radiographic practice must be made by the employer, either to improve the current techniques or to justify their continued use.

Quality assurance (QA)

Both IRR99 and IR(ME)R2000 place clear, but different, responsibilities on the employer to establish and maintain quality assurance programmes in respect of radiography. The purpose of such QA is to ensure consistently adequate diagnostic information, whilst radiation doses to patients and staff are controlled to be as low as reasonably practicable. All necessary procedures must be in writing and should:

- identify who is responsible for implementation
- stipulate how often it (QA) should be undertaken
- detail what records need to be kept.

The essential procedures within a programme suited to radiography will relate to:

- image quality
- patient dose and X-ray equipment
- image production
- training
- audit.

Training

Staff engaged in any aspect of radiography must have received appropriate and adequate training commensurate with their duties so that they know:

- the risks to health created by exposure to X-rays
- the precautions that need to be taken
- the importance of complying with the medical, technical and administrative requirements of legislation.

Regulation 4(4) of IR(ME)R 2000 places a responsibility on the employer to ensure that every IR(ME)R practitioner and operator has received adequate and appropriate training and undertakes continuing education/training after qualification. An up-to-date record of training must be maintained and be available for inspection. It is also a requirement that other persons who are directly concerned with the radiography (a parent supporting a child for example) are given adequate information to ensure their health and safety.

Finally, female employees engaged in radiography must be informed of the possible risk to a fetus and of the importance of informing their employer, in writing, if they become aware that they are pregnant.

THE DATA PROTECTION ACT 1998

The Data Protection Act 1998 came into force on the 1st March 2000, replacing the previous 1984 Data Protection Act, and provides a set of rules for processing personal information (data).

The Act relates to 'personal data', which is defined as relating to a living person who can be identified from that data. This can take the form of automated/electronic records as well as manual/paper records held in a relevant filing system, including health records, and includes any expression of opinion about the individual.

The Act gives rights to individuals, defined as 'data subjects', about whom personal data is held and also places duties on 'data controllers' who record and use that information.

Obviously, within a healthcare setting, there is a vast amount of information held relating to patients, most of which (if not all) falls within the scope of the Act. It is essential, therefore, that you are aware of both your obligations under the Act and the patient's rights.

GENERAL PRINCIPLES

Schedule 1 details eight data protection principles, which need to be complied with. In summary, it states that all personal data shall be:

- fairly and lawfully processed (this includes the common law requirement of confidentiality)
- processed for specified and lawful purposes and not further processed in any manner incompatible with those purposes
- adequate, relevant and not excessive in relation to the purpose
- accurate and kept up to date
- not kept for longer than is necessary for the purpose
- processed in accordance with the data subject's rights under this Act
- secure against unlawful processing, accidental loss, destruction or damage
- not transferred to countries outside the European Economic Area without adequate protection.

Schedule 2 applies to all personal data and the first requirement is that the data subject has given their consent for processing. It also details a number of conditions, at least one of which must be met, under which the processing of the data can be classified as 'necessary'. The processing of 'sensitive personal data', which includes information about the individual's racial or ethnic origin, politics, religion, health, or sexual life, is dealt with in Schedule 3. Not only do the requirements of Schedule 2 have to be met for this type of data, but also more stringent conditions, one of which is that the data be used for 'medical purposes'.

RIGHTS OF DATA SUBJECTS

Individuals, or data subjects, have a number of rights, as detailed in Part 2 of the Act, which include:

- the right to be informed who their data controller is (NHS Trust for example) and for what purposes their data will be processed
- the right to prevent processing for the purposes of direct marketing or if the processing will cause them undue distress (there are, as ever, exceptions to this)
- the right to access their own personal data. This is one of the central aims of the Act and is achieved by applying to the data controller in writing and including a stipulated fee.

UNLAWFUL OBTAINING OF PERSONAL DATA

Section 55 of the Act makes it an offence to person to obtain *or disclose* personal data without the consent of the data controller. Anyone who suffers damage due to unauthorised disclosure of his or her personal information is eligible for compensation.

PATIENT CONFIDENTIALITY

The NHS has a confidentiality code of practice regarding patient data, which is underpinned by the Data Protection Act 1998 and ethical obligations of confidentiality.[6] Healthcare workers must be familiar with this essential document.

THE REPORTING OF INJURIES, DISEASES AND DANGEROUS OCCURRENCES REGULATIONS 1995 (RIDDOR)

Reporting accidents and ill health at work is a legal requirement. The information enables the authorities to identify where and how risks arise and to investigate serious accidents. The authorities can then advise on preventive action to reduce injury, ill health and accidental loss.

These regulations require the employer to notify the enforcing authority of any accident that results in or which could have resulted in death, injury or disease.

The regulations specify:

- the types of injury that must be reported immediately (e.g. death of an employee at work)
- the types of injury that must be reported within 10 days (e.g. accidents at work resulting in an employee being unable to work for more than three consecutive days – an 'over-3-day' injury)
- the types of occupational related diseases which must be reported
- incidents and conditions relating to flammable gases and LPG (propane and butane) which must be reported within 14 days

- types of incident with the potential for causing injury (Dangerous Occurrences) which must be reported immediately
- the requirements for keeping specific records.

THE MANUAL HANDLING OPERATIONS REGULATIONS 1992

Manual handling is defined as:

'An activity which involves lifting, lowering, carrying, pushing, pulling or supporting by hand or by bodily force'[7]

Manual handling is something that we all do every day. As a healthcare professional moving patients and equipment, you are even more susceptible to injury. In the year 2003/04, 10 040 'over-3-day' injuries to employees in the health services sector were reported under RIDDOR. Of these, 53% (5361) were a result of manual handling accidents.[8] It is essential, therefore, that you are aware of these regulations.

As far as health and safety legislation goes, these regulations are very simple and the substance is contained in one regulation:

- To *avoid* any manual handling operation which has risk of injury to the person performing the task.

Where this cannot be done, the employer has to undertake a risk assessment of all such operations and take appropriate steps to remove or reduce the risk of injury. The employer must then provide the employee with information about the task and appropriate training in handling techniques.

You, as an employee, have a legal duty to make full and proper use of any equipment or system of work the employer provides for manual handling and to inform your employer of any physical condition you might have that could affect your ability to do this (if you were pregnant, for example).

THE PERSONAL PROTECTIVE EQUIPMENT AT WORK REGULATIONS 1992

Personal protective equipment (PPE) relates to equipment designed to be worn or held by workers to protect them against one or more identified hazards. PPE should only be used when risks cannot be avoided or adequately reduced by technical means or safe systems of work.

The employer must:

- conduct a risk assessment
- select appropriate and suitable PPE that fits the worker
- provide both the PPE (free of charge) and a suitable place in which to keep it
- ensure the PPE is maintained in clean and good working order
- provide training for workers on its use and care.

As an employee, you must:

- ensure that all PPE provided is properly used in accordance with any training and instructions received in its use
- ensure that the PPE is returned to its correct place of storage after use
- report to the employer any loss of, or obvious defect in, that PPE.

THE CONTROL OF SUBSTANCES HAZARDOUS TO HEALTH REGULATIONS (COSHH)

The aim of these regulations is to prevent any disease arising from the use of chemicals and other hazardous materials in the workplace. These include substances used in work, such as adhesives and solvents, substances created by work activity (e.g. dust and fumes), naturally occurring substances and biological agents.[9] You might question the relevance to radiographic practice until you consider that even in today's environment of computerised/digital radiography, there are still photographic chemicals used in some areas of the department and these are regulated by COSHH.

The regulations place a number of duties on the employer:

- Assess the risk involved, including the route of entry into the body. No work may be carried out with that substance until the assessment has been completed.
- Decide what precautions are needed to prevent or control the exposure. (As ever with health

and safety, the emphasis should be on prevention rather than control.)
- Ensure that the control measures are used and properly maintained.
- Monitor the exposure in the environment.
- Conduct health surveillance of employees where necessary.
- Provide employees with adequate information and training.
- Ensure there are adequate measures in place in case of an 'accident, incident or emergency'.

As the employee, you have a duty under section 8 to make full and proper use of any control measure or system of work provided by the employer. Additionally, you have a responsibility to ensure anything you use under COSHH is returned afterwards to its proper place and, if defective, to report it to your employer.[10]

References

1. The Health and Safety at Work etc. Act 1974. London: HMSO.
2. Health and Safety Commission. Management of health and safety at work: approved code of practice. London: HMSO; 2000.
3. The Ionising Radiations Regulations 1999. (SI 1999/3232). London: HMSO.
4. The Ionising Radiation (Medical Exposure) Regulations 2000 (SI 2000/1059). London: HMSO.
5. The Ionising Radiation (Medical Exposure) (Amendment) Regulations 2006 (SI 2006/2523). London: HMSO.
6. Department of Health. Confidentiality: NHS code of practice. London: DoH Publications; 2003.
7. Health and Safety Executive. Manual handling: Manual Handling Operations Regulations, 1992 – guidance on regulations. London: HMSO; 1992.
8. Health and Safety Executive. Injuries and ill health in health services. Online. Available: http://www.hse.gov.uk/statistics/industry/healthservices.htm 2005
9. Health and Safety Executive. COSHH: A brief guide to the Regulations. What you need to know about the Control of Substances Hazardous to Health Regulations 2002 (COSHH). Sudbury, UK: HSE Books; 2004/5
10. The Control of Substances Hazardous to Health Regulations 2002 (SI 2002/2677). London: HMSO.

Recommended reading

The Ionising Radiations Regulations 1999 (SI 1999/3232). London: HMSO.

This document provides all of the regulations to ensure health and safety guidelines are followed and implemented when using ionising radiation.

The Ionising Radiation (Medical Exposure) Regulations 2000 (SI 2000/1059). London: HMSO.

This document provides the regulations, which ensure the safe and effective use of ionising radiation in clinical practice.

Websites

The Health and Safety at Work etc. Act 1974
http://www.healthandsafety.co.uk/haswa.htm

The Management of Health and Safety at Work Regulations 1999
http://www.opsi.gov.uk/si/si1999/19993242.htm

The Ionising Radiation Regulations 1999
http://www.opsi.gov.uk/si/si1999/19993232.htm

The Ionising Radiations (Medical Exposure) Regulations 2000 [IR(ME)R]
http://www.opsi.gov.uk/si/si2000/20001059.htm

The Ionising Radiation (Medical Exposure) (Amendment) Regulations 2006
http://www.opsi.gov.uk/si/si2006/20062523.htm

The Data Protection Act 1998
http://www.dh.gov.uk/PolicyAndGuidance/Information Policy/PatientConfidentialityAndCaldicottGuardians/fs/en

The Reporting of Injuries Diseases and Dangerous Occurrences Regulations 1995 (RIDDOR)
http://www.opsi.gov.uk/si/si1995/Uksi_19953163_en_1.htm

The Manual Handling Operations Regulations 1992
http://www.opsi.gov.uk/si/si1992/Uksi_19922793_en_1.htm

The Control of Substances Hazardous to Health Regulations (COSHH)
http://www.opsi.gov.uk/si/si2002/20022677.htm#3

Chapter **3**

Communication

Gillian Springett and Karen Dunmall

KEY POINTS

■ Communication has three key components – verbal communication, non-verbal communication and active listening.
■ Effective communication is essential in the provision of quality patient care.
■ Effective communication may be hindered by the environment, language barriers, physiological problems preventing the patient from communicating effectively and psychological issues.
■ Interprofessional working involves communication between all individuals involved in the care of a patient.
■ Interprofessional working encourages the care of patients from all aspects at all times, enhancing the patients' perception of their care.

INTRODUCTION

Communication is an everyday word in contemporary society and yet it encompasses a variety of complex behaviours that are often difficult to categorise. A basic definition is the process of information transfer, which can be an indicator of:

• emotional state
• physical state
• knowledge and instructions.

Humans communicate by using language, which may be divided into two separate parts – verbal and non-verbal – performed consciously or unconsciously, each with its own function but often intrinsically bound to the other. Written communication in radiography is primarily the use of investigation request cards and case notes. With the advent of a computerised imaging system there is an increasing reliance on electronic forms of communication.

EFFECTIVE COMMUNICATION

Effective communication is at the heart of quality health care. In radiography a considerable part of the working day is spent relating to others. Given the technical nature of radiography it is possible that practitioners may misjudge the amount of time spent in face-to-face contact and seriously underestimate the effect their own behaviours may have on the way the service users respond to and perceive the care received.

Effective communication significantly improves health outcomes by:

- improving the satisfaction of both patient and practitioner
- improving patient concordance with treatment regimes
- decreasing the anxiety and distress felt by patients
- encouraging speedier recovery from invasive surgical procedures.

Department of Health policies and the National Institute for Health and Clinical Excellence (NICE) all stress the importance of empowering users and the need to achieve a 'patient-centred focus' in all aspects of the health service. Most patients will trust that imaging practitioners will have the correct knowledge and skills to operate the equipment and produce optimal images (unless their actions and behaviour signal otherwise!). It is often the practitioner's interpersonal behaviours that the patient will consider when asked to assess the quality of the care received.

Learning to communicate effectively should be valued as a core clinical skill for all healthcare practitioners if service provision is to have a user orientation.

Much of the research over the past three decades suggests that when healthcare professionals use appropriate levels of eye contact, nods and gestures whilst maintaining an open posture they are regarded as more interested, empathetic and warm by their patients. Patient satisfaction, understanding and resultant concordance with the requirements of their healthcare interventions can improve when practitioners have displayed supportive, empathetic non-verbal behaviours.

Therefore, it is important that we are aware that non-verbal behaviours can serve to reinforce, regulate, qualify or replace verbal communication and show our patients and colleagues we are genuinely interested in them as individuals, however short our interactions may be.

Effective communication is essential in the interaction between staff and patients in order to maintain radiographic quality. By communicating effectively a patient's voluntary and involuntary movements can be minimised, thus reducing the need for repeat imaging and thereby complying with the IRM(E)R regulations (2000).

Remember:
Imaging may be one of the first investigations patients undergo as part of their health care. The experience patients have whilst in the imaging department may influence their future perception of their care and healthcare practitioners overall.

BARRIERS TO EFFECTIVE COMMUNICATION

There are many barriers to effective communication and they can be categorised as environmental, language, physiological or psychological.

1. Environmental:
   - privacy of room
   - temperature
   - light

- darkness of room (may inhibit non-verbal communication)
- equipment.

2. Language:
   - not having a common language
   - using colloquial phrases or professional, unfamiliar jargon
   - inappropriate expressions
   - patronising approach
   - lack of clarity.

3. Physiological:
   - ill health
   - pain
   - sensory impairment
   - level of consciousness
   - hunger
   - need to use the toilet
   - poor oral hygiene making speech uncomfortable or impossible.

4. Psychological:
   - embarrassment over personal health issues
   - mental health competency
   - anger
   - fear
   - low self-esteem
   - loss of dignity
   - loss of privacy
   - institutionalisation (loss of independence)
   - invasion of personal space.

VERBAL COMMUNICATION

Verbal communication is the language of facts and information. It is likely to be used in the giving and receiving of knowledge and instructions but remains inseparable from non-verbal behaviours.

The verbal use of words, phrases and sentences includes the prosodic (intonation, rhythm, pausing) and also paralinguistic systems (the vocal utterance of sounds, e.g. 'mmm', 'uh-huh').[1]

Within radiography there are many technical terms which patients may not understand; however, it is important for practitioners to be able to convey the information and instructions in a suitable manner. The effectiveness of a practitioner's communication will depend on the ability to use jargon-free and familiar language with patients.[2]

NON-VERBAL COMMUNICATION

Non-verbal communication displays our feelings and emotions and may demonstrate aspects of our personality and attitudes. It is often the unconscious expression of the 'truly human' part of us. Non-verbal signals have little or no meaning in themselves but they can acquire significance in particular contexts.

If effective communication is to occur, the non-verbal contribution to the interaction plays a critical role in the way messages are received and interpreted.

Consider the occasions you may have said something like: 'It's not what he said but the way he said it!' This implies a conflict between verbal and non-verbal communications and confusion in the interpretation. This may lead to an inappropriate response and/or behaviour. On the whole, non-verbal signals tend to be spontaneous, although of course if premeditated thought is given some behaviours can be 'stage-managed'. Non-verbal signals are often sent out and interpreted without conscious knowledge but the so-called 'body language' is often more representative of what the sender is trying to communicate than the spoken or written word.

EXAMPLES OF NON-VERBAL BEHAVIOURS

Facial expressions

The face can communicate:

- the degree of interest or liking of a person or a situation
- the degree of understanding of the signals (verbal and non-verbal) being received
- a range of emotional states ranging from happiness to despair
- an individual's feelings, whether the person wishes to display or try to conceal them
- a physiological response, e.g. sweating, flushing or pallor.

Facial expressions and eye contact can be used to start and sustain communication by showing interest in the individual and the conversation, but they can also be responsible for causing the cessation of an interaction.

The face can respond instantaneously, providing immediate feedback to others. This may be useful in certain situations where demonstrating empathy, concern and understanding to your patients is important. However, consider the messages that may be perceived if practitioners display uncontrolled, inappropriate facial expressions when faced with offensive body odours or unexpected, unpleasant visual information in the course of their work.

Emotional expression is under voluntary control and can be artificially manipulated, with the face demonstrating intensification or reduction of the emotion. In reality, trying to distinguish people's emotions from their facial expressions is often more difficult than we imagine because some people are capable of masking their true emotions. Social and cultural norms may distort expression of emotion (Fig. 3.1).

It is possible people may not actually know what their facial expressions are displaying but by showing you have 'listened to their non-verbal cues' you have given the patient, in a supportive way, an opportunity to confirm or deny any concerns.

However, it is important to remember that it is relatively easy to lie with the face – most people can fake anger or surprise with relative ease and patients are often astute enough to sense a false, frozen smile that is not genuine in nature!

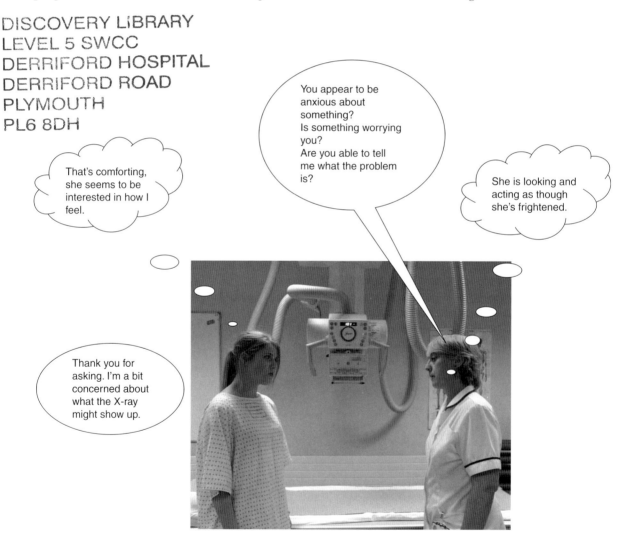

Figure 3.1 Non-verbal cues.

Eye contact

Eye contact can signal a desire to engage and communicate with another person. Others perceive gaze as a signal that they are liked.

The start of an interaction usually commences with a period of good eye contact but gaze may become averted. The speaker may look to see if the listener is being attentive or how the message is being received. If there is evidence that the listener is distracted, this may result in the speaker feeling uncomfortable and the interaction may falter.

Gaze can also be used to support the face in expressing emotions and attitudes. A strong gaze may indicate dominance or aggression but, alternatively, a person who avoids making eye contact may be viewed as submissive, ashamed, embarrassed, preoccupied or lacking in confidence and shy.

Having to interact with people who are partially hidden by facial garments, dark glasses and masks, or obscured by screens, may cause considerable discomfort.

People tend to avoid making eye contact when they do not wish to become involved or viewed as a 'volunteer'. This may be appropriate in some situations but can be a problem if practitioners use gaze aversion deliberately to dissuade interactions when they are busy, as this may signal a lack of interest. However, it is also important to remember there are some cultures and some contexts for which sustained eye contact may be inappropriate.

Gestures

Gestures may be used to:

- reinforce verbal communication by repeating, complementing or stressing the content of the message
- replace speech when verbal communication is not appropriate or when they may be the only way to communicate with an individual (e.g. where there is no shared common language or where someone has a severe hearing loss)
- act as regulators of the interaction, by demonstrating encouragement to continue, giving approval and showing understanding of what has been said (e.g. head nods)

- give useful indications of an individual's emotional state; for example clenched fists can indicate aggression.

Unintentional gestures are those which signal a personal reaction to what is going on. These include:

- face stroking
- hand over mouth
- clasping hands
- caressing hair
- polishing spectacles
- crossing legs
- shuffling papers.

Unintentional gestures can serve to relieve tension but they may also be very distracting and may send the message that attention has strayed!

Orientation and posture

Body posture is largely involuntary and can convey important social signals, such as feelings of friendliness or hostility. The way we position our bodies, arms and legs can signal our willingness to interact, our emotional status and perceived power. Similarly, if people are positioned so they cannot see our faces or make eye contact, this may affect their perception of our trustworthiness.

Remember, when you are positioning for a chest X-ray you are standing behind the patient, so consider what impact this has on the effectiveness of your communication (Fig. 3.2).

Appearance

This is included as an important dimension of non-verbal communication as many aspects are under personal control and can be manipulated. Alteration of our appearance is probably related to self-preservation, signalling how we view ourselves and would like to be treated.

Consider the uniform you are required to wear: what message does this send about you and your role in the organisation? Uniforms can signal rank and status and carry with them expectations of knowledge, behaviour and experience. You are also representing the organisation when

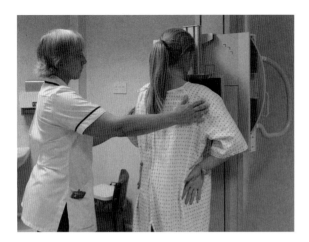

Figure 3.2 Positioning for a chest X-ray.

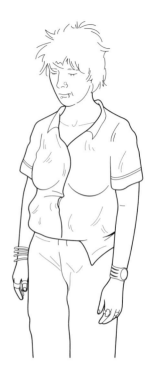

Figure 3.3 Inappropriate dress for a practitioner.

you put on your uniform, whatever your role and status within it.

Appearance can convey messages about an individual's attitude to others. Imagine arriving for work wearing a grubby, creased uniform! An unkempt appearance, dirty hair and nails, together with poor hygiene practices, may give the impression that your patients are not highly regarded or their needs respected (Fig. 3.3). Wearing inappropriate amounts of jewellery, perfume or make-up when you are working in a healthcare context may affect the trust patients place in your ability.

Touch

Touch is one of our five senses and is used to gather much information in life. Bodily contact is the most basic way that humans can convey their attitudes to another. When we are babies and children we tend to touch others by tickling, slapping, pinching, sucking or patting much more than we do as adults. As we mature we tend to reduce these behaviours as facial expressions and gestures take over the role served by touch.

Touch can communicate the following:

- Friendliness
- Concern, compassion
- Warmth and affection
- Tenderness
- Familiarity
- Encouragement
- Sexual interest and intimacy
- The nature of the relationship (and offer some cues to differences in status between individuals)
- Anxiety
- Aggression
- Nervousness
- The need to attract attention
- The importance of certain aspects of our message.

Many factors influence the meaning of touching behaviour and, of course, as part of your work in radiography you will be required to touch complete strangers when positioning them for their investigation. It is vital to reflect on the potential messages conveyed via your hands.

Although it may not be common practice in radiography, it is possible that if you shake hands when introducing yourself to the patient initially you may have 'broken the touch barrier' and this

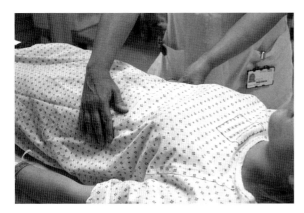

Figure 3.4 During the procedure.

makes further touching behaviour more acceptable to the patient (Fig. 3.4).

There has been much debate about the therapeutic use of touch in the healthcare environment. In Western societies the sexual connotations associated with its use are probably the biggest obstacle to the beneficial application of touch. Although a potentially powerful way of conveying an empathetic response to another individual's situation, the role of touch is very complicated. It should be used sparingly, giving careful thought to the potential for misinterpretation, especially given the cultural, social and gender variations of acceptability.

During the course of your work, for example if the patient is upset and it seems appropriate to demonstrate empathetic support by using touch, it is preferable to confine this to a light placement of your hand on their shoulder or upper arm. It is also important to monitor the recipient's non-verbal response to this gesture and if there are any signs of discomfort then it is probably pertinent to remove your hand.

Paralanguage

Voice quality should be considered as an important aspect of non-verbal communication. The vocal cues which may be used by people to make judgements about others are: volume, tone, pitch, clarity, pace and speech disturbances.

- Soft volume – associated with sadness or affection.

- Low volume – low pitch and slow pace may signal sadness or boredom.
- Moderate volume – associated with happiness or pleasantness.
- Loud volume – associated with confidence or dominance, which together with a high pitch and a clipped clarity may signal anger or impatience.
- Fast pace of speech – may suggest animation, surprise or anger.
- Flat, thin breathy voice – may suggest anxiety, depression or sickness.
- A sharp voice – might be perceived as complaining.

Utterances such as 'ums' and 'er' may be viewed as pause fillers, but the use of too many can signal boredom or lack of knowledge and confidence.

Proximity

Interpersonal proximity simply means the space between two people. There are four key zones:

- Public
- Social
- Personal
- Intimate

As part of radiographic work it is essential to invade the personal space of the patient, even working in the intimate zone at times. Healthcare practitioners are 'allowed' to breach these personal space conventions by the nature of their job but this is a privilege which would not normally be permitted. That patients may be embarrassed or nervous may be for no other reason than that their personal space has been invaded (Fig. 3.5).

Listening

Listening is fundamental to everyday basic communication; it is something we all do when we are interested or concerned about a person. One of the highest compliments we can pay to another is to give our full attention by actively listening. Sadly, although a primary skill in

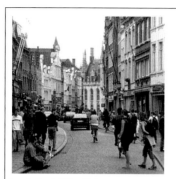

Public zone

(8 feet + or 2.44 m+)

This is the distance associated with public figures and public occasions. Public figures when addressing an audience are often situated on a stage, or will usually stand apart from the group

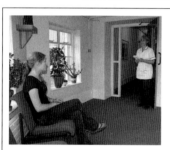

Social zone

(4–8 feet, 1.2–2.44 m)

This is the distance at which our day-to-day important relationships are conducted and the distance at which we are most comfortable when engaging with strangers or for formal interactions. A loud voice is usually required

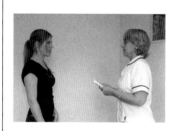

Personal zone

(18 inches – 4 feet, 0.45–1.2 m)

This is the distance people usually refer to when they talk about their 'personal space'. At this distance people can touch each other but are sufficiently far apart to see the individual properly. Invasion of someone's perceived personal space causes anxiety, especially when the individual who feels violated can not escape. Problems sometimes arise when people of different culture, who may have differing concepts of personal space, engage in conversation

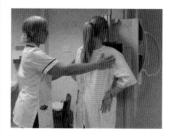

Intimate zone

(0–18 inches – 0–0.45 m)

People usually only allow intimate friends or relatives to come this close. At this distance bodily contact is easy, each person can smell and feel the others breath, plus body heat and odours

Figure 3.5 Proximity zones.

communication, it is probably the least exercised activity!

What people look for when determining whether they have been listened to is not another's ability to reiterate their words (they are not looking for a 'tape-recorder') but some demonstration that the other person has understood their physical, psychological and emotion messages as well. An empathetic response requires active listening.

Empathy means:

- seeing the problem from the patient's perspective – 'being with the patient' and
- communicating that understanding back to the person in a sensitive, supportive way.

Empathy should not be confused with sympathy, which is a feeling of pity. Whilst some of us can demonstrate empathy more naturally than others it is a skill that can be learnt and incorporated into our style of interaction so that, ultimately, it becomes a genuine response. Self-disclosure can be useful in some situations to show you have a good understanding of what the person is experiencing, but it is important to ensure that you do not make the person feel their own experience is not important.

Using 'active listening' (Fig. 3.6) and empathy can help your interactions by:

- showing a person you have understood and care. People are more likely to enjoy interacting with you and may open up more
- helping to clarify if you have understood and allowing the patient to correct any misunderstandings
- helping the patient feel that you are genuine, accepting and non-judgemental
- helping the patient to feel safe to talk about emotions, fears or concerns and perhaps helping you move the interaction towards more intimate, sensitive issues if required
- helping reduce your irritation with others – if we understand fully, we are more likely to forgive!

It may also help to reduce your prejudices and stereotypical assumptions about others.

To become an effective listener:
Active listening requires the listener to make a concentrated effort to attend not only to the verbal communication but also to any non-verbal messages and then to provide feedback to the speaker, using both forms of communication, to show that full attention is being given.

THE PRACTICAL APPLICATION OF VERBAL AND NON-VERBAL COMMUNICATION IN DIAGNOSTIC IMAGING

The spoken word is very important in radiography as it gives information and permits an exchange between individuals, but, as shown above, it must be linked integrally with non-verbal communication.

The patient's journey through the department can be divided into three parts:

1. Receiving the patient in the department.
2. Conversing and interacting with the patient during the examination.
3. Giving instructions to the patient on completion of the examination.

RECEIVING THE PATIENT

This initial stage of an examination consists of greeting and identifying the patient and conversing in a general manner to put her at ease. A member of the clerical or radiographic staff may carry out the greeting of the patient on entering the department (Fig. 3.7).

Reflect on how we refer to patients in discussions with colleagues. It is impersonal and disrespectful to label a patient as 'a chest in waiting area 3', for example.

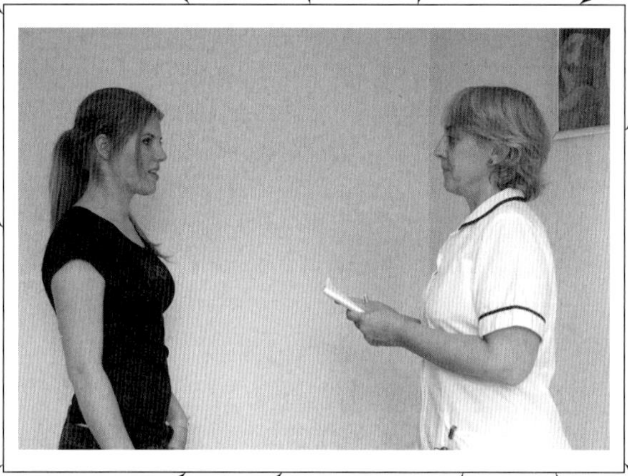

Position yourself at the same level (or below) as the person. Where possible, try to avoid standing over and looking down at the person (may be intimidating and suggests an authoritarian approach)

Adopt an open posture (if we cross arms and legs, this may become a barrier which signals an unwillingness to engage fully with another)

Look at the person; face them squarely (implies you are willing to listen). Echo the speaker's posture, if possible

Concentrate on what the speaker is saying rather than the problem

Maintain good eye contact (but learn to recognise the situations where breaking eye contact briefly may actually be supportive of the person. Consider cultural norms)

Listen not only to the speaker's words but also to the non-verbal messages which may help to convey information about the person's attitude or emotional state

Maintain a relaxed attitude. This will help to create the right pace needed for you to be able to listen and respond effectively. Try to keep calm even if you don't feel calm!

Check out with the speaker the messages you have received this way are correct and what the speaker wishes to transmit

Consider your own non-verbal communication. (Remember: your facial expressions, tone, pitch of voice, gestures and posture can convey messages both good and bad!)

Learn to tolerate and be comfortable with silences

Try to avoid being judgemental as you listen, especially if the speaker is introducing things which may be contrary to your own beliefs and values

Notice what you are feeling or imagine how you might feel in a similar situation. This can help your understanding and empathy but remember it is the patient's experience, feelings, concern, not yours

Try to listen with undivided attention (not easy in a healthcare environment!), do not interrupt and avoid asking too many questions. Be encouraging by using head nods and pause fillers such as, 'Hmmm', 'Yes, I see'

Figure 3.6 Active listening.

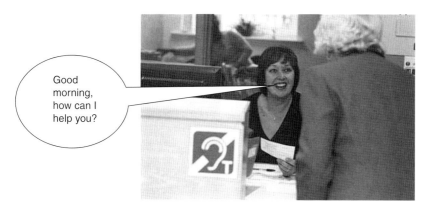

Figure 3.7 Clerical staff receiving the patient.

Greeting the patient

First impressions

One of the first things that we see in the waiting area is a patient sitting or standing. Within the space of a few minutes most of us will have come to a conclusion regarding the nature, character, status and disposition of that individual based on their physical appearance. It is essential that this assessment is neither judgemental nor prejudiced. If we are making assessments of our patients, their emotions and possible responses based on their non-verbal communication, it is very likely they are carrying out a similar assessment of our technical skills, caring nature and trustworthiness based on these aspects of our behaviour.

It is vital to gain a patient's trust in the first few interactions; therefore the member of staff should be correctly attired and maintain a social distance whilst establishing eye contact (Fig. 3.8). Remember also, when calling patients from a waiting area, that speaking too close to a person may appear intrusive; too far away can seem very cold, impersonal and unfeeling. The patient should be called by title and family name, for example Mrs. Smith. If there is more than one person with the same name then it may be necessary to use a first name to clarify the patient's identification. It is important not to shout from the doorway of the X-ray room or down a corridor as this can breach the patient's confidentiality. It may also be necessary to assist the patient to stand or walk, or she may be in a wheelchair and unable to move independently.

Although there may be time constraints for each examination, never assume that a patient requires assistance to move. A verbal confirmation from the patient establishing her personal needs is vital. If the patient declines assistance, be wary of demonstrating any inappropriate non-verbal communication that indicates impatience.

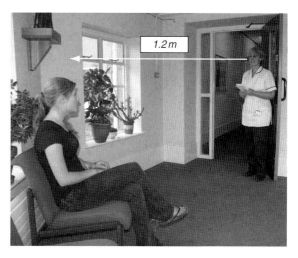

Figure 3.8 Greeting the patient in the waiting room.

Confidential questioning

Any confidential questions required for identification of the patient (name, age, address) must be asked with due consideration to the patient's right to privacy, e.g. in a changing cubicle (Fig. 3.9). There are usually signs in the waiting areas to remind female patients that if there is a possibility of pregnancy they should report it to a radiographer. However, to exclude pregnancy, female patients may also need to be asked about their menstrual cycle. The practitioner will now be working within the patient's 'personal space' and should be aware of some people's anxiety related to this.

Preparing the patient prior to the examination

Asking someone to undress can be embarrassing to members of the opposite sex or different age groups and therefore this must be carried out with sensitivity (Fig. 3.10). The instructions must be precise so that the patient does not get confused and anxious, but should not be delivered in a 'military style'. Conversely, communicating in a reticent manner can give the impression of unreliability and lack of confidence, which may introduce a barrier to the interaction. The patient must also be given instructions on what to do when ready. It is essential that the patient is not asked to wait in public areas in a state of undress where she may feel uncomfortable.

Preparing the room prior to the examination

Always prepare the X-ray room and equipment prior to carrying out the examination (Fig. 3.11). Consider the nature of the environment in which you work. Although as you become more experienced you may not perceive the technology as being anything other than 'a means to an end', for many of your patients their visit may be their only experience of diagnostic imaging. For some, the equipment and procedures can lead to considerable anxiety. Fear of possible pain and of the unknown, as well as apprehension of what the results may reveal, can add to a patient's stress. Using good observational skills to monitor your patient's non-verbal behaviours can help determine her needs during the procedure. Pre-procedure information about the investigation is helpful, but supportive interaction between staff and patient during the procedures can facilitate a significant decrease in anxiety levels.

INTERACTING WITH THE PATIENT DURING THE EXAMINATION

A patient entering the X-ray room may find the equipment quite daunting so the practitioner must realise that the patient may not be actively listening to instructions (Fig. 3.12). Therefore, it is essential to use gestures as well as words to

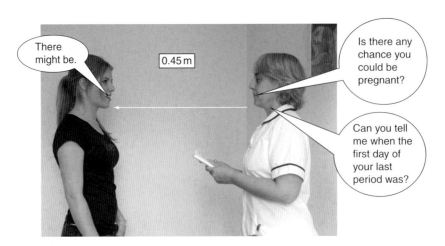

Figure 3.9 Checking personal information in a confidential area.

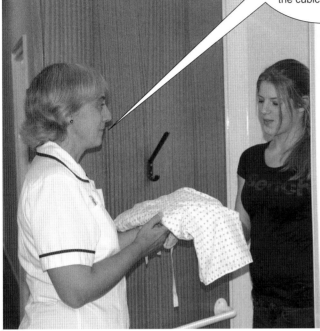

Figure 3.10 Asking the patient to put a hospital gown on.

indicate what is required. It is also necessary to use plain language and not technical jargon.

The practitioner will now be working within the 'intimate zone' so it is important to fully inform the patient, before commencing the procedure, about exactly what you will need to do in terms of touching her body and what actions are needed from her in order to obtain an optimal image. By inviting the patient to position herself wherever possible, any embarrassment associated with your touch can be reduced (Fig. 3.13).

Positioning the patient it is an ideal opportunity to make her feel at ease with general conversation. During early days of learning clinical skills it is possible that the technical aspects of positioning equipment and patient may overshadow the use of effective communication. Giving clear explanations of what is required is unlikely to take any longer than trying to manipulate an uninformed, rigid, anxious or embarrassed patient into the optimal position for the image capture. The patient may also need instructions on breathing techniques (e.g. halted inspiration/ expiration). A practice of the required technique before the exposure often saves errors and

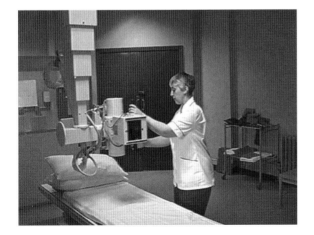

Figure 3.11 Preparing the room prior to the examination.

Figure 3.12 In the X-ray room.

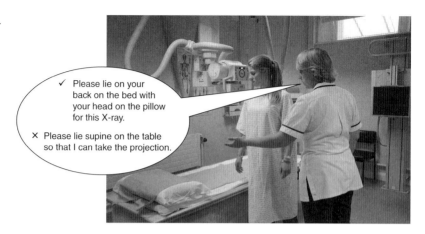

Figure 3.13 Positioning the patient.

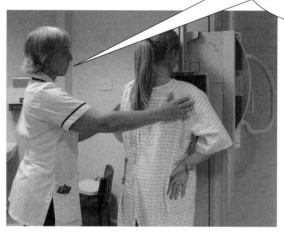

possible repeat images being required due to movement unsharpness.

INSTRUCTING THE PATIENT AFTER THE EXAMINATION

After the examination the patient will be required to wait (possibly remaining in the gown) until the image has been processed and checked for quality and technical suitability. When the checking of the image is complete the patient should be instructed on the process by which they can obtain the results of the examination (Fig. 3.14).

It is not within the remit of a student, assistant practitioner or practitioner to inform the patient of the diagnosis resulting from the image taken. However, the patient will inevitably ask and the

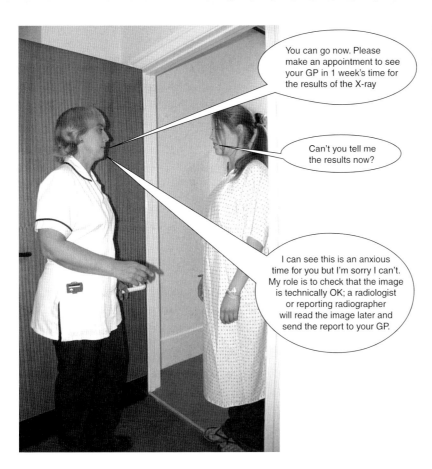

Figure 3.14 Giving instructions to the patient on completion of the examination.

response to this type of request can be difficult to deal with, especially if you are aware that there was an abnormality on the image. It is advisable to say that you cannot give details because the image will be looked at by a radiologist/reporting radiographer later. Do not feign ignorance of what the image shows because, as the patient will assume you have some knowledge of the human body, she might infer that you are lying. In this instance, your facial expression needs to match what you are saying.

DEALING WITH DIFFICULT OR AGGRESSIVE PATIENTS

In 1999 the Department of Health launched a policy of 'zero tolerance' towards intimidation and violence shown to NHS staff members by the general public in the healthcare setting. It should be remembered that all patients have the potential to be aggressive or difficult, not only the inebriated or the overtly psychologically disturbed. The key to diffusing the situation is to become proactive rather than reactive in the reduction of triggers for the unwanted behaviours.

The type of 'welcome' received by the patient on arrival in the department can defuse potentially difficult situations.[3] There are many reasons for escalating aggressive behaviour including:

- delays resulting from machine breakdown or staff illness. There are, however, times during major accidents when waiting times for non-urgent cases increase – from experience, these rarely result in anger when the situation is explained.

- a practitioner refusing to image a patient due to an incorrect request card (which falls under the IR(ME)R justification protocols).
- the waiting area environment being overcrowded and noisy. It would seem that this becomes even more annoying and irritating with the addition of children.
- patient anxiety about the outcome of the diagnostic tests resulting in misinterpretation of the communication from the practitioner.

The method of reduction appears simple; however, life is not perfect and strategies must be put in place to deal with the aggression demonstrated:

1. If the waiting times for examinations have increased ensure the patients are kept informed of the potential delay. Remember – if you promise a delay of 15 minutes and it is 30 minutes then they will be disheartened; promise the opposite and patients will feel better for the early resolution. A sign indicating the delay is not always suitable because some individuals may appear to queue jump for examinations requiring different equipment.
2. Be observant. When collecting patients from the waiting area ensure that any non-verbal indications of agitation are monitored and acted on before the behaviour escalates into aggression.
3. Use verbal and non-verbal behaviours to alleviate confrontation. Never stand arms folded, raising your voice; a quiet open posture will be far more successful. Also acknowledge the 'feeling' not the 'behaviour'; e.g. 'I can see you are annoyed, angry, etc. What can I do to alleviate the problem?' Speak in a quiet manner, shouting will only serve to lose the argument.[3]
4. Ensure that you do not place yourself in a location so that your exit from an escalating aggressive situation is blocked.
5. If the aggression cannot be de-escalated it is imperative that you remove yourself to a safe location and call for assistance.

INTERPROFESSIONAL WORKING

Your practice will show that there are many other healthcare disciplines with which an imaging practitioner may have a working relationship, and almost every user who seeks medical care interacts with more than one health professional. For some patients, the needs arising from their diagnosis require complex interprofessional collaboration. Problems with interpersonal communication across the different health or social care settings can have a profound impact on the user's experience of care.

The NHS modernisation agenda emphasises the importance of collaborative and partnership working at all levels of the organisation. The Department of Health promote the inclusion of the service user as an active member of the healthcare team.

Headrick et al[4] suggest the following barriers to interprofessional collaboration:

- differences in history and culture
- historical inter- and intraprofessional rivalry
- differences in ideology, jargon and language
- different professional routines
- varying levels of education, preparation, qualifications and status
- fears of diluted professional identity
- differences in accountability, clinical responsibility, salary and rewards.

A multidisciplinary healthcare team is no different to any other group in society. According to Tuckman[5] a team passes through various stages (forming, storming and norming) until it reaches a performing stage and a possible phase of adjourning. During the formation there will be the inevitable vying for position and conflict of ideas until the group settles down and performs the required task.

Headrick et al [4] highlight that improvements in health outcome are likely to occur if relevant practitioners (and users) are brought together to share knowledge and experiences as a means to agree what improvements are needed. These agreed goals can be tested in practice and are more likely to result in measurable improvements for patients than concentrating on what appear on the surface to be irreconcilable professional differences.

Quality teamwork and effective interprofessional collaboration share many characteristics:

- Goals or objectives are shared; there is an attainable and evolving, motivating vision with clear direction.
- Member roles and responsibilities are clear and known with responsibility for success shared among members.
- Atmosphere is respectful; mutual support is provided.
- Conflict is acknowledged and examined.
- The team is task orientated; the task is achievable.
- Authority and accountability structures are clear.
- Communication and information sharing is regular and routine.
- An enabling, supportive environment with access to required resources is provided.

Technological advances and the need for cost containment, whilst delivering improved quality and responsiveness of service provision to meet the demands of users, has meant that many NHS staff have had to adapt to changes in skill mix within their discipline. Health reforms have resulted in the adjustment of staff roles and the introduction of new roles or new types of workers, such as Assistant Practitioners.

If we are to provide a quality service for our users, especially at this time of NHS modernisation, it is important that we work hard to minimise the possible impact of interprofessional barriers. One of the major keys to effective collaboration and teamwork is effective interprofessional communication. If high quality care is to be offered by health and social care practitioners, communication must be viewed as a skill, which requires constant attention from each individual.

References

1. Ellis A, Beattie G. The psychology of language and communication. Hove, UK: Lawrence Erlbaum; 1986.
2. Minardi H, Riley M. Communication in health care: a skills based approach. Oxford: Butterworth-Heinemann; 1997.
3. Keane P. How to...de-escalate potentially aggressive interactions with patients. Synergy 2006;(Dec):8–10.
4. Headrick LA. Wilcock PM, Batalden PB. Interprofessional working and continuing medical education. BMJ 1998; 316(7133):771–774.
5. Tuckman BW. Developmental sequence in small groups. Psychol Bull 1965; 63:384–389.

Recommended reading

Barrett G, Sellman D, Thomas J. Interprofessional working in health and social care. Professional perspectives. Basingstoke, UK: Palgrave Macmillan; 2005.

This book provides an overview of the roles and perspectives of different health professionals and also includes the police and probation service. It explores the rationale behind interprofessional working, providing case studies which enable the reader to see how the underpinning knowledge relates and is integrated into practice.

Burnard P. Effective communication skills for health professionals. Cheltenham, UK: Nelson Thornes; 1997.

This book explores practical ways to improve communication between health professionals and the user groups, as well as between colleagues within teams. It covers communication skills required within different areas of work. There are self-assessment sections, which assist the reader in identifying personal areas that are strengths and those in need of development. It sets out to cover simple methods to enhance effective communication and shows the barriers that can exist and how to overcome them.

Chapter **4**

Patient care

Sarah Fearn

KEY POINTS

- Every patient is individual; no two persons react in the same way to a given situation.
- Prescriptive guidance with regards to patient care is not appropriate. There is no magic formula when caring for patients and skill must be developed in assessing and adapting to the needs of patients on an individual basis.
- In addition to caring for the patient, it is important to consider the needs of those accompanying the patient, such as friends, relatives or carers.

INTRODUCTION

Patients, no matter who they are or why they are attending hospital, are affected emotionally and physically by illness and pain. Whilst every patient is unique and will cope in their own way, this chapter examines aspects of patient care for a variety of patient groups from paediatrics and the elderly to those involved with trauma or with mental health problems.

When reading the chapter consider that issues discussed in the context of a specific patient group may also be relevant to other patients. For example, visual impairment is most common amongst the elderly population; however, the guidance given regarding this can equally be applied to all visually impaired patients, regardless of age.

ASSESSING THE PATIENT

It is difficult to care for a patient appropriately without first assessing their needs, and anticipating these as early as possible ensures a more pleasant patient experience. When assessing a patient's needs, the following questions may be helpful:

Who is the patient?

- What is his age? (This will often affect the approach taken to his care.)
- Does he have special needs, such as a hearing impairment or a learning disability?
- What is his level of understanding?
- What is his level of mobility?
- Are there any cultural or religious issues to consider?

Why is he here?

- Is the examination routine or is the patient symptomatic? (This may influence the patient's feelings and anxiety levels and also his behaviour.)

What examination is being undertaken?

- How long is the patient likely to be in the department?
- How invasive is the procedure?
- Are detailed explanations required?
- What aftercare will be needed?

PAEDIATRICS

Paediatrics range from the neonate to the young adult and each age presents a different challenge. A child in the hospital environment is faced with strange sights, smells and sounds which can be very frightening. The experience of visiting or staying in hospital may affect subsequent visits, and fears may be carried into adult life. Ensuring a child is as comfortable as possible is therefore essential. Before examining each age group, there are several general points to consider.

GENERAL ISSUES

Preparation

Prior to the child attending for examination:

- Preparation of the child and parent or guardian is extremely important.
- Play has an important role in helping a child relax and, although not always available, the use of a play specialist can help in preparing a child for a potentially distressing situation.[1]
- Child friendly leaflets (Fig. 4.1) can help explain information to a child using simple language and pictures.
- Remember that in order for the parents to prepare a child for an examination, they also need to understand clearly what is involved.

Once the child has arrived in the department:

- Ensure the waiting area and examination room are a pleasant temperature.
- Ensure all equipment is ready and a preliminary exposure is set to minimise the time the child spends in the room.
- Ensure help is readily available before bringing the child into the room.
- Think carefully how the examination will be carried out, having age-appropriate toys and distractions ready.

Is it our turn next Mummy?

It is inevitable that children will sometimes have to wait before an examination; however a child-friendly environment is likely to encourage a child to feel at ease.[2]

- Where possible a separate waiting area for paediatrics can have several benefits:
  - It is less stressful for parents who do not have to worry about other patients.
  - The child can be more easily distracted with toys and books whilst waiting.
  - A quieter area, avoiding the hustle and bustle of a busy waiting area, can help calm the child prior to his examination.

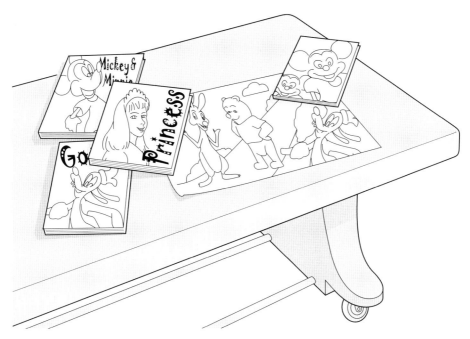

Figure 4.1 Child friendly leaflets.

- Keep waiting times to a minimum to avoid children becoming restless.
- Keep time spent in the examination room to a minimum.

Dealing with parents and guardians

Parents are often extremely anxious and it can be as much of a challenge caring for them as for the child. Remember that anxiety can result in an overprotective parent who may be more irritable and less patient than usual. When dealing with the parent:

- Plenty of reassurance is often needed, although be careful not to falsely reassure.
- Remain patient and calm at all times and ensure you are firm yet polite.
- Do not separate the parent and child unless absolutely necessary; use discretion with the older child.

- Involve parents in the care of the child, informing them what you are doing and why. This helps to make them feel more in control.
- Remember that parents know their children extremely well and will often be able to communicate with them more effectively than a stranger. Utilise this when providing explanations or instructions or if a child needs distraction.

In the past there have been many approaches to keeping children still for radiographic examinations, some of which today are considered inappropriate. Restraining a child should be the last resort. It is preferable to take time to build a rapport with the child in order to gain his trust. If the child is unable to keep still on his own, consider that the presence of a familiar face may be comforting enough to achieve this; for example sitting the child on a parent's lap.

Lastly, it may seem obvious but never leave a baby or toddler unattended, not even for a second. Even if a baby does not appear to be on the move, it only takes a moment for a him to roll over when your back is turned and this could result in serious injury, especially if he falls from a height.

AGE-SPECIFIC ISSUES

Having considered the general issues, paediatrics have been grouped into the following five age ranges:

- Neonate
- Older baby or toddler
- Pre-school child
- Primary school child
- Older child and young adult

Guidance is provided on how to deal with the issues and challenges associated with each age group, although it must be remembered that each child is unique and will develop at his own pace.

The neonate

Babies up to the age of one month are termed neonates (Fig. 4.2). These babies are most commonly encountered on the Special Care Baby Unit (SCBU), although remember that not all neonates requiring imaging are admitted to hospital.

- The neonate will be more likely to remain settled if they are warm and comfortable.

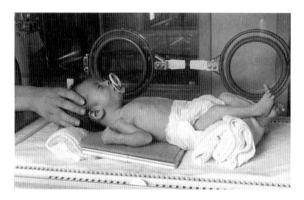

Figure 4.2 The neonate.

Maintaining warmth is important as the neonate loses heat very quickly; therefore, if he must be undressed, ensure that this is for as short a time as possible

- Always minimise movement of the baby, as this is unsettling
- Ensure all examinations are performed quickly and efficiently

Consider that parents of the neonate:

- may be shocked at the early arrival or the poor health of their baby and may need time to adjust
- are likely to be extremely anxious and this may cause changes in behaviour
- are likely to be protective of their child.

With regards to the mother, she may have had a traumatic birth and hormone levels are likely to affect her behaviour.

When dealing with the neonate on SCBU:

- Always seek permission from SCBU staff and wait for their assistance before beginning any examination.
- The neonate will often have numerous lines and tubes connected to him and care should be taken not to dislodge these.
- Minimise handling of the neonate as this can affect oxygen saturation levels.
- Avoid leaving the incubator open for any length of time so as to maintain warmth, and use hand holes where possible.
- Infection control is important:
  - Disposable gloves and apron should be worn and changed between patients.
  - X-ray equipment such as cassettes should be covered and cleaned.
  - Hands should be washed before and after contact with each baby.

The older baby or toddler

Although young babies tend not to mind who picks them up, as they become more aware of the world around them they begin to become upset if separated from their parent (Fig. 4.3). It is important, therefore, to ensure a familiar person remains with them throughout their examination.

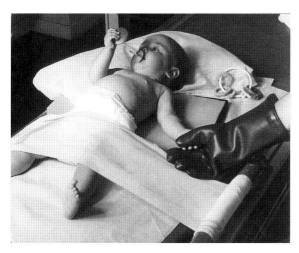

Figure 4.3 The older baby.

Although restraint should be considered a last resort, it is vital to remember that babies are unlikely to keep still unless they are sleeping. Holding of the baby by the parent or guardian is preferable to the use of restraining devices such as Bucky bands. In such a scenario, radiation safety is essential and the appropriate guidelines for holding patients should be followed. Older toddlers understand a significant amount and so techniques other than physical restraint may prove effective.

- If the child is old enough to understand then take time to build a rapport with the child in order to gain his trust.
- The presence of a familiar face may be comforting enough to achieve cooperation; for example sitting the child on a parent's lap.[3]
- Distracting a child with a toy, or playing a game may be all that is needed to keep a child still.[4]

Keeping a baby or toddler as comfortable as possible prior to and during the examination is essential.

- A dummy or favourite toy may comfort the child and provide familiarity.
- Do not place baby on a cold surface; instead cover with a sheet.
- Do not undress a child unnecessarily as he can feel vulnerable when undressed and may also become cold.

- Where possible, ensure the baby is not hungry, as a hungry baby is likely to be unsettled.

The preschool child

Once a child has reached preschool age (3 years and above; Fig. 4.4), his ability to communicate and understand has developed sufficiently to now be aware of his surroundings. Often at this age the hospital environment can seem very frightening and the child is still likely to need his parent present. The need for restraining a child becomes less necessary and time should be spent adequately preparing the child and gaining his trust and cooperation.

- When speaking to young children, use simple language. You may wish to elaborate when speaking to the parent but be careful not to exclude the child in conversation.
- To increase cooperation, always explain why you or the parent or child has to do something.
- Repeat instructions or explanations where necessary, always checking that you have been understood. This may be achieved by demonstrating what is required. Using a teddy or doll or even the parent (without exposing) can also help allay fears.

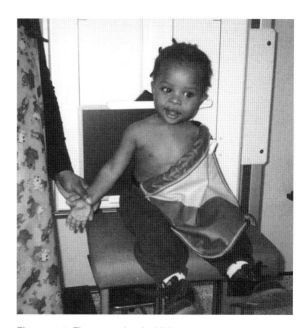

Figure 4.4 The pre-school child.

- Always be honest with a child. If something is likely to hurt then do not tell the child that it will not. This may result in broken trust which is difficult to restore.
- Remember that a child who is anxious may regress in age and explanations should be tailored to this.
- Even a young child can get embarrassed when undressed; therefore always consider the child's privacy, whatever his age.
- Consider using rewards such as stickers and certificates to motivate the child into cooperating.

The primary school child

Whilst it should become easier to gain cooperation, a child at this age will also be more aware of what is happening to him and distraction may not be as easy (Fig. 4.5). It is important not to treat the child like a baby, as if he is incapable of understanding, but neither is it acceptable to treat him as a little adult. Finding this balance can often be challenging, especially as different children develop at a different pace. Older children often like to feel independent and offering choices can help them to feel less vulnerable. Do bear in mind, however, that offering too many choices can also be overwhelming.

The older child and young adult

As children get older and head towards adulthood they naturally become more independent and may wish to make their own choices with regards to their care. There is no set age at which a patient can take responsibility for their own

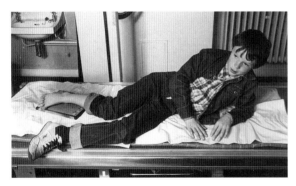

Figure 4.5 The primary school child.

treatment or care and if a child below the age of 16 is deemed as having sufficient understanding and intelligence, then they may be allowed to determine themselves whether or not they undergo hospital procedures. This is termed 'Gillick competence'.[5] Whilst parents of older children may still wish to accompany their child for an examination, discretion may be needed at times. For example, asking a teenage girl about pregnancy.

NON-ACCIDENTAL INJURY

Non-accidental injury (NAI) can be 'physical or mental injury, sexual abuse, negligence or maltreatment of a child'.[1] Where this is suspected, the child is likely to undergo a skeletal survey. Whilst skeletal surveys for NAI should be performed by two experienced radiographers, if asked to assist or care for the patient it is important to consider the following:

- Parents may be allowed to accompany the child; however, the need for the examination should have been explained to the parents by the paediatrician prior to any interactions with the imaging department.
- If a parent accompanies the child, staff should remain polite and non-judgemental. Remember that NAI has not been confirmed and is only suspected at this stage.
- Never leave the child unattended. Two members of staff should remain with the child at all times, to act as each other's witnesses.

THE ELDERLY PATIENT

With a continuing rise in the elderly population[6] it is inevitable that the number of elderly patients you will encounter is also on the increase. Just because a patient is elderly does not mean that they should be treated any differently. Older patients may feel vulnerable and worry about illness not just because of how it affects them personally but also how it may affect those that they care for, such as partners or pets. Many elderly patients have few visitors and may wish to talk at length to relieve their loneliness. In a busy department it can be difficult to devote this extra time; however, these patients may benefit significantly if they feel you have the time to listen.

Problems with mobility, sensory loss and dementia are perhaps the most common problems encountered with the older patient.

MOBILITY

Reduced mobility can mean anything from the patient confined to bed to the patient who is able to mobilise with a little help. The numerous causes range from loss of confidence following a fall to recovering from surgery.

Prior to the examination the following should be considered:

- Is the patient steady on his feet or able to stand still? Just because a patient has no obvious mobility problem does not mean that he will not require assistance.
- Patients with reduced mobility may need help changing, and therefore help should be offered.
- Choose the most appropriate examination room for the patient. For example, a larger room would be more suitable if it allows a bed to be more easily manoeuvred.
- If you foresee difficulties, ensure extra help is readily available.

Where the patient has a walking aid such as a frame or stick:

- Will the patient be able to let go of his walking aid if required? If this is necessary, ask the patient's permission before taking it away, returning the walking aid to the patient as soon as possible.

Where the patient is a wheelchair user:

- Consider why the patient is in a wheelchair and whether the wheelchair use is permanent or temporary (e.g. whilst they recover from surgery).
- Consider access to changing and toilet facilities. Always offer help and allow adequate time.

- Check with the user of a self-propelled wheelchair before pushing the chair. Some users may be offended if you push them when they can propel themselves.
- Do not presume that a wheelchair user cannot mobilise. It may be useful to ask the patient questions about his daily routine at home or on the ward to assess whether it is safe to get him out of the chair.
- If the patient is unable to mobilise and you must transfer the patient, ensure that moving and handling guidelines are followed and that equipment is used effectively and with training.

Where the patient is in bed:

- Consider why he is in bed and whether he can mobilise.
- Allow extra time with the patient and prepare the examination room in advance.
- Ensure you do not attempt to move a patient who is not allowed to mobilise; e.g. a patient who is postoperative.
- If the patient is unable to move himself then consider whether the patient can remain in the bed. If the patient cannot mobilise but must be transferred from the bed, always seek help, utilising moving and handling aids.

VISUAL IMPAIRMENT

Many patients suffer visual impairment, which may or may not be age related. The amount of help required will differ for each patient and may depend on the degree of visual impairment.

- Remember that many visually impaired patients remain independent and cope well with everyday life.
- Ensuring adequate lighting can often help a person to see more clearly.
- Do not remove a person's glasses unless absolutely necessary, and always return them to the patient promptly.
- If the patient requires guiding, do so slowly and carefully, avoiding obstacles and telling the patient where he is going.

- Always explain what you are doing or about to do: a person with poor sight will rely on your explanation.
- Always tell the patient if you leave the room, so that they do not feel isolated.

HEARING IMPAIRMENT

It can prove embarrassing for a patient to misunderstand due to poor hearing and patients will often not want to admit that they have not heard or understood. The following points should therefore be considered:

- Do not rely on simply calling the patient's name. It should not be assumed that no response means that the patient is not present. Look around the waiting room and collect the patient if necessary.
- Be extra careful when checking the identification of the patient. They may have mistaken another patient's name for their own, which could lead to an incorrect examination being performed.
- Reduce the level of background noise wherever possible. A patient with a hearing impairment may struggle when surrounded by high levels of background noise. A quieter environment may help.
- Do not remove hearing aids unless absolutely necessary and always return them to the patient as soon as possible.
- Use facial expressions and gestures to give visual clues as to what you are trying to communicate.
- Speak in close proximity to the patient, being careful not to invade his personal space.
- Raising your voice may help, but be careful never to shout. It will be obvious to the patient that you are doing so and this may be offensive.
- Speak clearly and slowly, allowing enough light for the patient to see you.
- Always face the patient when speaking, to allow them to lip read if they are able to do so.
- Consider using written instructions.

DEMENTIA AND ALZHEIMER'S DISEASE

It must be remembered that not all older people have memory problems or are senile, and we should not treat elderly patients as such; however, as people age, many undergo mental changes. Knowing how to deal with these patients effectively is essential. Dementia is a 'progressive deterioration in intellectual functioning',[7] affecting thinking, remembering and reasoning. Alzheimer's disease is the most common form of dementia and, in its early stages, forgetfulness and personality change are common features. As the disease progresses, it affects daily life more and more, reaching the stage where verbal communication is limited and the patient fails to recognise family members. It can be very distressing for friends and relatives to see someone they care about change in this way and they often need as much consideration and reassurance as the patient himself. When dealing with the patient with dementia:

- Treat the patient with respect, protecting his dignity and upholding his privacy.
- Comfort the patient, making him feel secure with plenty of reassurance.
- Consider the patient's friends and relatives, be approachable and show interest in their needs.
- Be patient. Confusion often requires instructions or explanations to be repeated several times before they are understood.
- Speak directly to the patient and do not be dismissive.
- Avoid changes of staff where possible to ensure consistency and to enable the building of trust.

OTHER ISSUES RELATING TO THE ELDERLY

Fragile skin

With age, skin becomes more fragile and susceptible to injury. This should be considered when assisting patients and extra care should be taken. Sharp edges, for example, can easily cause damage.

Falls

Falls are a major cause of disability and can lead to mortality in the elderly population.[8]

- Always consider that patients who are seemingly quite stable on their feet can suddenly lose balance and fall.
- If patients have previously fallen, they may also have a fear of falling, affecting their confidence in mobilising.
- Seek to prevent the risk of a patient falling by ensuring there are no potential hazards in the department, such as slippery floors or poor lighting.

Continence

Many elderly patients experience problems with control of bladder and/or bowel movements. This can lead to problems with hygiene and cross-infection. Patients suffering from incontinence of urine may have a urinary catheter and this should be considered. Where the patient has a urinary catheter:

- Be careful not to pull or catch the urinary catheter. Catheters are easily forgotten if attached to the patient's bed and may be tugged or pulled when transferring a patient.
- If a patient is in a wheelchair, ensure his catheter comes with him if he mobilises, and that it is positioned so that it does not pull.
- Patients with long-term urinary catheters often have a leg bag attached to their leg, which is then hidden under clothing. Consider this when asking a patient to undress for an examination as it may cause embarrassment if he has to wait with other patients.

MENTAL HEALTH PROBLEMS

At any one time, one in six adults suffers from a form of mental illness ranging from depression to schizophrenia.[9] Many patients will not require any special care, whilst others may prove challenging. Although the range of mental health problems is vast, here we consider three commonly encountered disorders. Note that dementia is discussed earlier in the chapter.

DELIRIUM/CONFUSION

This has many causes including medication, infection and head injury. Delirium has a sudden onset and is usually short lived, causing confusion, fluctuating awareness, short-term memory loss and disorientation.[7] When caring for these patients:

- Protect them from harm; never leave them unsupervised.
- Ensure quiet surroundings where possible, as noise can cause agitation.
- Speak in a calm voice, using simple language and be prepared to repeat instructions and explanations.
- Give plenty of reassurance, especially if they become embarrassed or ashamed of their behaviour.

SCHIZOPHRENIA

Patients with schizophrenia can have many symptoms, ranging from delusions and hallucinations to social withdrawal. Patients may be aggressive, struggle to make decisions and may exhibit strange behaviour and speech. When dealing with these patients:

- Avoid retaliating to the patients' behaviour, even if this appears socially unacceptable.
- Speak calmly and avoid being sharp or critical.
- Do not offer such patients too many choices or force them to make decisions by themselves.
- Neither agree or disagree with the patient's ideas.
- Consider the need to calm a potentially aggressive patient and bring a situation under control.
- Remember that friends or relatives may be distressed and may appear irritable or intolerant.

LEARNING DISABILITIES

A person with a learning disability has impaired intellectual and social functioning, and often has difficulty understanding, communicating and remembering new things.[8] These difficulties are present at birth or in early childhood but often continue into adult life. Patients with learning disabilities are not all the same and each patient will have different needs. Despite this, there are several general considerations when caring for these patients:

- Consider that it may be useful to involve a friend, carer or relative in the examination as she may know how best to gain cooperation from the patient.
- If the patient is accompanied by a friend, relative or carer, ensure you talk directly to the patient so he feels included.
- Talk to the patient using language appropriate for his level of understanding.
- Avoid asking the patient too many questions or providing too many choices.
- Be patient and be prepared to repeat instructions several times.
- A patient may respond to a demonstration of what is required rather than a verbal explanation.

THE TRAUMA OR EMERGENCY PATIENT

EMOTIONAL ISSUES

Emergency situations undoubtedly arouse emotions in both patients and relatives, often due to the suddenness with which events have taken place. You will encounter many patients and relatives who, due to a sudden illness or traumatic event, will exhibit high levels of anxiety and emotional stress, often causing them to behave in an uncharacteristic and apparently unreasonable manner. It is therefore important to consider how to deal effectively with them:

- Highly emotional patients may not be able to absorb information or follow instructions and so patience is required to ensure that they fully understand, even if this means repeating it several times.
- Patients and relatives often take their cues from the staff who care for them and therefore remaining calm and confident can help to reduce anxiety.

DEALING WITH AGGRESSION

Anger and aggression are common reactions following a traumatic event and can also be linked to alcohol or drug use. Knowing how to defuse a potentially violent or threatening situation is important in protecting yourself and others.

- Unrealistic expectations are often linked to aggressive behaviour and therefore good communication, especially with regards to waiting times, can help to remove the frustration which can lead to aggression. Minimising waiting times and providing a pleasant waiting area may also help.
- Consider that your body language and facial expressions, as well as the language you use, can affect a patient's behaviour. Speaking in a calm, non-confrontational voice with normal pitch and volume can help to keep the situation under control.[10] Do not be tempted to shout back at a patient as this will only provoke aggression.
- Do not leave yourself alone with a patient if you feel that your personal safety may be at risk. Always request the presence of another member of staff.
- Ensure that a patient does not come between you and your exit from a room. This allows for rapid escape should a patient become violent.

PATIENTS ON A TRAUMA TROLLEY

Patients will be encountered who are immobilised on a trolley (Fig. 4.6), often due to suspected spinal injury. When dealing with these patients:

- *Never* move the patient, unless given permission by medical staff.
- Ensure patients are aware of the importance of keeping still. Re-iterate this several times if necessary. Remember that it may be very frustrating for patients if they are either unable or not allowed to move.
- If a patient must be moved, then this must only be carried out with the assistance of the trauma team in a controlled manner; i.e. log rolling.

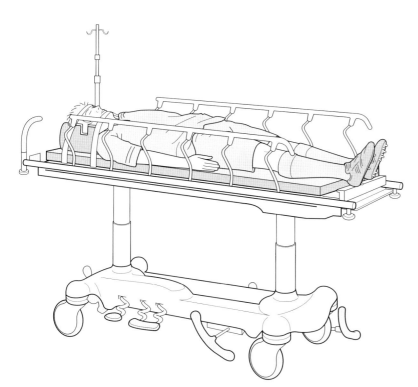

Figure 4.6 The immobilised patient.

- Always follow moving and handling guidelines.
- When talking to the patients, ensure that they can see you clearly and always explain carefully what you are doing.
- Avoid leaving the patient unattended where possible. Uncooperative patients may attempt to move or even remove themselves from the trolley and this could result in further injury.

PAIN

Trauma patients are often in a significant amount of pain and this can influence cooperation. Pain is an individual experience and, as such, the same injury can cause differing levels of pain. It is not therefore appropriate to judge pain level by the severity of an injury alone.

- Ensure that if necessary, and where possible, pain relief has been administered prior to the examination.
- Whilst movement should be minimised, there will be occasions when causing pain is

unavoidable and this should be explained to the patient.
- Reassure the patient and explain what you are doing and why.
- Be honest. If you are likely to cause pain, then tell the patient, explaining why it is necessary.

FRIENDS AND RELATIVES

When dealing with friends and relatives of the trauma or emergency patient:

- Reassure and care for them as well as the patient.
- Explain carefully to them what is happening and make them feel involved, being careful not to breach confidentiality.
- Use discretion as to whether they should accompany the patient for the examination. They may find the examination distressing, especially if they see the patient uncomfortable or in pain. Some patients, however, may be more cooperative if they can see a familiar face during an examination.

THE UNCONSCIOUS PATIENT

There are several considerations when caring for the unconscious patient:

- Ensure protocol is followed carefully when identifying the patient. Do not assume other staff have identified the patient.
- The patient is likely to have several lines, tubes and/or drains in situ:
  - Be very careful not to catch or pull these.
  - If moving the patient, be careful of tubes and drains attached to the bed or trolley.
  - Do not empty containers such as catheter bags without first seeking permission, as the contents may need measuring.
  - If the patient is being artificially ventilated, ensure that this is not accidentally disconnected. Ventilated patients should always be accompanied by the appropriate medical team and should never be left unattended.
- Whilst unconscious patients may not be able to communicate with you, they are often still aware of their surroundings[11] and therefore will benefit from physical contact and reassurance.
- Effective teamwork and communication are essential when caring for any patient, but never more so than where the patient is unconscious. Speed and efficiency are required to ensure risks to the patient are minimised.

References

1. Hardwick J, Gill C. Radiography of children: a guide to good practice. Edinburgh: Elsevier; 2004.
2. Drummond M, York C. Evaluating paediatric practice and care. Synergy 2001;(Feb):20–21.
3. Kurfis Stephens B, Barkey M, Hall H. Techniques to comfort children during stressful procedures. Accid Emerg Nurs 1999; 7:226–236.
4. Martin A, Salthouse. Imaging children: do's and don'ts. Synergy 1999;(Aug):11–13.
5. Dimond B. Legal aspects of radiography and radiology. Oxford: Blackwell; 2002.
6. Coni N, Nicholl C, Webster S, Wilson K. Lecture notes on geriatric medicine. Oxford: Blackwell; 2003.
7. Bauer B, Hill S. Mental health nursing: an introductory text. Philadelphia: WB Saunders; 2000:101.
8. Department of Health. Valuing people: a new strategy for learning disability for the 21st century. London: HMSO; 2001.
9. Department of Health. National service framework for mental health. London: HMSO; 1999.
10. Walsh M, Kent A. Accident and emergency nursing, 4th edn. Oxford: Butterworth Heinemann; 2001.
11. Rideout A. The unconscious patient. In: Toulson S, ed. Accid Emerg Nurs 2001:142–171.

Recommended reading

Culmer P. Chesneys' care of the patient in diagnostic radiography. Oxford: Blackwell; 1995.

The early chapters of this text provide guidance on general aspects of patient care; such as dealing with aggression and preparation of the patient. There is also a helpful chapter on working with trauma and acutely ill patients.

Gunn C, Jackson C. Guidelines on patient care in radiography, 2nd edn. Edinburgh: Churchill Livingstone; 1991.

Although now dated, this clearly written text covers all aspects of patient care. Focus is given to a variety of patient groups and guidance provided on patient psychology.

Hardwick J, Gill C. Radiography of children: a guide to good practice. Edinburgh: Elsevier; 2004.

Easy to read guidance on all aspects of paediatric radiography. Whilst focussing on radiographic technique, the more general aspects of paediatric patient care are comprehensive.

Chapter **5**

Clinical skills for preparation of the patient and clinical environment

Karen Dunmall

KEY POINTS

- Infection control is essential to ensure that the environment is safe and clean for patients and staff at all times.
- Aseptic techniques are utilised to minimise the risk of contamination during clinical procedures.
- Record keeping is needed to provide a continuation of care for the patients during their stay or treatment within the clinical environment where a number of professionals and individuals are involved at different times.

INTRODUCTION

Great importance must be put on the maintenance of a safe and clean clinical environment for the patients. Within the diagnostic imaging department it should be recognised that all patients have the potential to carry and transmit organisms. It has been shown that nosocomial infections (those occurring in a hospital setting) can be reduced considerably with the introduction of basic hygiene procedures.[1] In order to prevent the transfer of infections it is important to be aware of the specific organisms that can cause infection and the mode of transfer so that the cycle of replication can be disrupted.

DISEASES AND ORGANISMS

A disease is a condition causing symptoms of an illness, which occurs when cells or molecules within the body stop functioning properly. For example, a disease can be caused through aging, the effects of chemicals, or arise from gene mutation/alteration.

There are four main groups of pathogenic organism which can cause diseases, some of which are harmless to the host when sited in the correct place; for example there are organisms living in the bowel which cause infection when they enter the urinary or respiratory tracts.

BACTERIA

Bacteria are small unicellular organisms which are much smaller than a typical animal cell. There are many species of bacteria and they may be characterised in a number of ways, such as by shape (e.g. rod-like (bacilli) or spherical (cocci)). Within each species there are many different strains. Some bacteria are susceptible to treatment; however, there is an increase in the number of bacteria becoming resistant to drug treatments due to the overuse of antibiotics.

Examples of bacteria

- *Escherichia coli* 0157:H7 is one of hundreds of strains of *E. coli*, which can be found in human and animal gastrointestinal tracts.
- Staphylococcus has more than 20 species, including *Staphylococcus aureus* and *Staphylococcus epidermidis*, which can be found in the nose and on the skin of healthy individuals.

VIRUSES

Viruses are not cellular and exist as genetic material (RNA or DNA) enclosed in a protein coat.

Unlike bacteria, which replicate by a simple cell-division process, viruses require a cellular organism in which to reproduce. The genetic material invades the cell and hijacks the replication process. Antibiotics are ineffective against viruses; however, there are some antiviral agents (aciclovir) that prevent the virus from functioning normally, thus disrupting reproduction.

Examples of viruses

- Human immunodeficiency virus (HIV)
- Herpes simplex virus

FUNGI

Fungi can be found in soil, air and water and are in fact primitive plants. Some fungi live in and on humans in balance without causing illness; these include *Candida* and *Aspergillus* species. Conditions caused by the presence of fungi are called mycoses. It is usually the unbalanced propagation of a fungus that causes the illness. Some antibiotics are fungi that are beneficial in the treatment of bacterial infections, one example being penicillin.

Examples of fungi

- *Aspergillus fumigatus* can cause aspergillosis, which affects the respiratory system.
- Overgrowth of *Candida albicans* is known as candidiasis and can be found in the immunocompromised; it is also known as thrush.

PROTOZOA

Protozoa are unicellular microscopic animals. They can live in decaying matter, assisting with decomposition; however, when found in humans protozoa normally cause disease.

Examples of protozoa

- *Toxoplasma gondii* causes toxoplasmosis in humans.
- *Plasmodium* is responsible for causing malaria in humans.

CROSS-INFECTION

An infection occurs when other organisms, e.g. bacteria, viruses, fungi or protozoa, enter or come into contact with the body and multiply. The organisms can cause direct damage or prompt an immune response, which causes symptoms to manifest, e.g. fever.

Infections can be:

a. Acute – lasting 2–24 days, e.g. a common cold
b. Chronic – duration of months, years or lifetime, e.g. hepatitis

c. Latent – remaining hidden after the first manifestation, e.g. *Varicella zoster* (chickenpox).

The cross transfer of a pathogenic organism from one individual to another (cross-infection) can occur in the following ways:

- Direct contact between individuals or indirect contact involving an infected item, e.g. a toilet door handle.
- Transmission through bodily fluids, e.g. blood, urine or saliva.
- Transfer of organisms between the gut and mouth (the faecal–oral route).
- Through the air via droplets/particles containing pathogens, e.g. sneezing.
- By the use of contaminated non-sterile medical equipment.

Therefore, it is essential that the equipment, environment and healthcare professional are subject to varying levels of cleanliness dependent on the clinical requirement (Table 5.1). There are

Table 5.1   The purpose and contraindications of cleansing agents

Cleaning agents	Purpose in department	Contraindications for use
Chlorhexidine gluconate solution 2.5%	For cleansing the skin prior to a procedure	Not for hard surfaces
Chlorhexidine gluconate 0.015%, cetrimide 0.15% (e.g. Savlon/Tisept/Sterets)	Pre-injection Skin sterilisation Bottle tops	Not for hard surfaces or open wounds
Chlorhexidine gluconate solution 2.5% (e.g Hibiscrub)	Preoperative surgical hand disinfection Pre/postoperative skin antiseptic	None
Detergent, sanitiser, blue bleach powder (sodium hypochlorite)	For body fluids and spillages	Not for skin
Cleansing foam (e.g. Esemtan)	Antimicrobial deodorising foam	Not for hard surfaces, floors, etc.
Povidone iodine 7.5% (e.g. Videne antiseptic solution)	A rapid acting non-irritating aqueous iodine solution	For skin only. Not for hard surfaces, floors, etc.
Alcohol impregnated wipes	For hard surfaces and skin	Not for open wounds
Sodium chloride 0.9% solution	For skin and open wounds	None
'Decon'	For neutralising radioactive spills	None

three main levels of cleanliness that exist with regards to equipment and surfaces: clean, disinfected and sterilised.

CLEAN

Cleaning removes visible contamination (blood, faeces and the majority of microorganisms), normally using detergents. The process is designed to remove dirt and other materials from objects, surfaces or instruments. It can be done in water, with or without the inclusion of detergents. This is the first stage of removing contamination from the environment prior to disinfecting and sterilising.

DISINFECTED

Disinfecting reduces the number of microorganisms to a 'non-harmful' level by using chemical or heat treatment of items in contact with mucous membranes or bodily fluids. Spores are not usually destroyed. This process is halfway between cleaning and sterilising and a range of chemicals that inactivate most serious pathogens can be used. Immersing instruments in boiling water can ensure disinfection. In the case of floors, these will be mopped using chemical disinfectants, an example of which is chlorhexidine.

STERILISED

Sterilising removes and destroys all microorganisms, including spores. It is used on items that penetrate the skin or mucous membranes and enter sterile body areas.

The process involves:

- physical cleaning
- heat treatment
- ethylene oxide gas
- liquid, e.g. Cidex OPA.

Where possible, the CSSD (Central Sterile Supplies Department) should be used.

STERILE SUPPLIES PACKAGING

In order for the healthcare professional to know whether a set of instruments is sterile there are indicators on the outer packaging, which must be intact (Fig. 5.1).

Specialised tape will seal the package. Non heat treated CSSD tape will have diagonal white lines: heat treated and therefore sterile tape will have black diagonal lines. A label will also indicate the date and cycle number of sterilisation (Fig. 5.2).

IMAGING EQUIPMENT CLEANING

It is not practically possible to disinfect by immersion or sterilise large items of equipment such as an X-ray tube or table; however, measures can be employed to maintain a level of visual cleanliness. It is recommended that there should be changes of linen on X-ray table mattresses and a fresh gown for each patient after each examination. However, there are considerations of time and environmental issues to be considered so that the changing of the mattress linen after each patient could be replaced by the use of paper roll to cover the sheet, which must be fresh for each patient. The sheet must also be changed following an infectious patient or if soiling has occurred. Naturally, the sheet should also be changed at regular intervals; for example after a clinic session or daily, dependant on the patient throughput of the room.

The used gowns and bed linen must be collected and sent to the laundry in the appropriate coloured linen bag. A white plastic or terylene/polyester bag is used for routine linen that is not fouled or infected. Any linen which is heavily

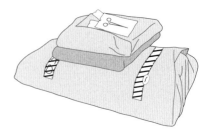

Figure 5.1 Sterile supplies packaging.

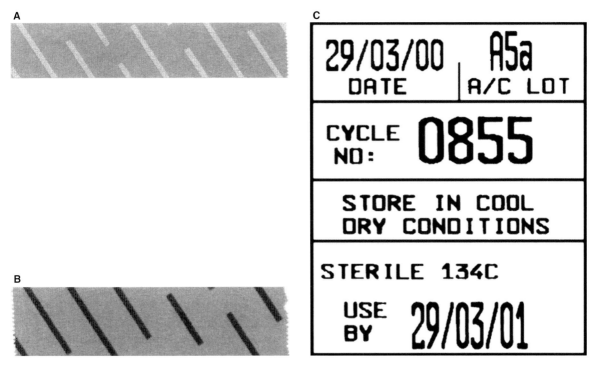

Figure 5.2 A Non-heat-treated Central Sterile Supplies Department (CSSD) tape. B Heat-treated CSSD tape. C Sterilisation information label.

soiled with blood, faeces, urine or other bodily fluids should be placed in a sealed red water-soluble bag covered with an outer red plastic or terylene/polyester bag.[2]

Research has shown up to one third of nosocomial infections may be prevented by adequate cleaning of hospital equipment.[3] Within the diagnostic imaging department the equipment most commonly in contact with the patient is an image receptor; that is, a cassette or digital device. These should be wiped clean after each patient using alcohol or bactericide impregnated wipes. There should also be a protocol in place for regular and frequent cleaning of all equipment within the X-ray room to reduce risk of infection. It is not only the patient contact surfaces which require regular cleaning but also those operated by the practitioner. The control panel and X-ray tube controls are also at risk of harbouring bacteria from the operator and contact with the patient and therefore would also benefit from frequent cleaning using alcohol or bactericide impregnated wipes.

In some situations, when a patient with a known infection requires imaging, it may be necessary to carry out a method similar to that of 'barrier nursing'. Barrier nursing is carried out to reduce the risk of cross-transfer of infection between staff and patients. A patient with a known infection (e.g. MRSA) should be imaged at the end of a session/day so as to give time for thorough cleaning of the area and to reduce contact with other patients in the department. It is necessary to have two practitioners in order to provide a 'clean' and 'dirty' person. The 'dirty' person who is dressed in gloves, apron and mask is responsible for positioning the patient and image receptor whilst the 'clean' person sets the exposure and manipulates the X-ray equipment, thus reducing the opportunity to transfer the infection.

PERSONAL HYGIENE

The following aspects of personal hygiene must be observed:

a) The laundry of uniforms, remote from household washing, at a temperature high enough to kill microorganisms.[4]
b) The tying back of hair and/or the wearing of a head covering to reduce the risk of contamination of wound sites or clinical areas.
c) The need for personal cleanliness, including regular baths and showers and abstention from wearing strong perfumes or aftershaves.
d) The covering of potential sites of infection (e.g. cuts, piercing sites) with clean waterproof dressings of a distinctive colour.
e) The limiting of jewellery to a gold wedding band to reduce possible sites of microbial habitation.
f) Regular hand washing between patient contacts.

HAND WASHING

There are three levels of hand washing (Fig. 5.3):

1. Social/routine hand washing

The purpose is to reduce the risk of transmission of microorganisms via the hands of staff. This should be carried out:

- on arrival and before leaving the duty area
- after performing bodily functions
- before and after contact with the patient/clinical environment
- before and after preparing and administering patient medication.

The procedure should be carried out using non-medicated soap or, for hands that appear clean, an alcohol rub can be used.

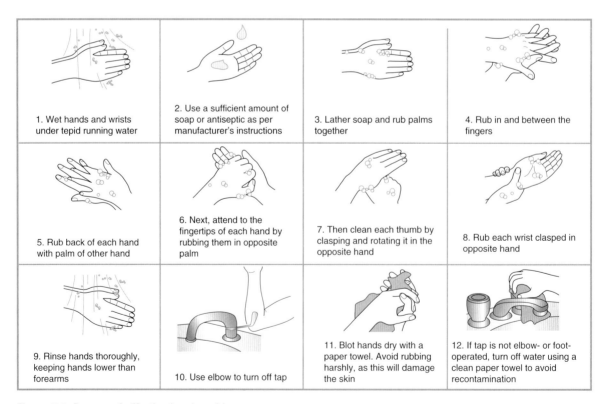

Figure 5.3 Process of effective hand washing.

2. Antiseptic/hygienic hand washing

The purpose of this method is also to reduce the risk of transmission of infection. This is known as a basic or 20 second hand wash. It involves washing with antiseptic followed by an alcohol rub, which will remove transient microorganisms and reduce residents.

3. Pre-surgical aseptic technique

The purpose of this is to minimise the transmission of microorganisms from or via the hands/forearms of staff to patients during surgical procedures. It is carried out before the surgical procedure starts and involves washing the hands and forearms for 5 minutes and then repeating the procedure for a further 3 minutes.

ASEPTIC TECHNIQUE

Many hospital procedures, including surgical operations, require the use of sterile equipment to prevent the introduction of organisms. They also require a sterile field, which can be defined as a region for work within which it is deemed to be sterile. All items and materials placed within the sterile field must also be sterile. The contamination of the field by air-borne bacteria is minimised by the flow of 'scrubbed' air; for example, in operating theatres.

Within an imaging department an aseptic technique may be required for dressing following the insertion of a drainage tube or during a specialised procedure such as a biopsy. Initially, in order to set up the sterile trolley it is necessary to carry out a basic hand wash. The trolley shelves should then be wiped down with a hard surface disinfectant before any items are placed on it. The individual setting up the trolley should then stock the trolley with the following, ensuring that the items are in date and sterile where appropriate (Fig. 5.4):

- Top shelf
  Sterile pack containing:
  – gallipot
  – cotton wool balls
  – forceps/tweezers
  – dressing pack with gauzes.
  Plus any sterile equipment required for procedure.
- Lower shelf
  Lotions for disinfecting skin.
  Selection of needles for local anaesthetic introduction.

A

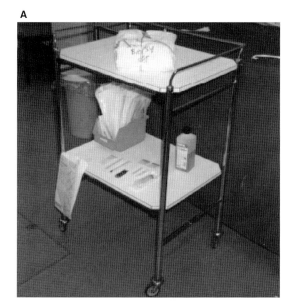

B

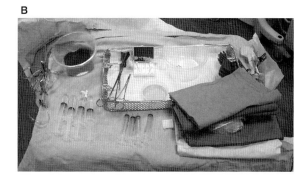

Figure 5.4 Sterile trolley prepared for a biopsy.

Selection of biopsy needles.
Scalpel blade.
Syringes.
Local anaesthetic, e.g. lidocaine.
Contrast medium (if appropriate).
Sharps bin (Fig. 5.5).

The sterile pack should only be opened immediately prior to the procedure and only the corners of the outer paper should be pulled back. The inner wrappings should only be removed or touched by an individual who has performed an aseptic hand wash and is wearing a pair of sterile gloves.

Following completion of the procedure all used objects should be either disposed of in the correct receptacle or returned to the sterile supplies department for re-sterilisation and re-issue (Table 5.2).

Extreme caution must be shown with any used 'sharp' items to avoid a needlestick injury. If an individual is pricked or cut by a needle or scalpel the following procedure should be followed:

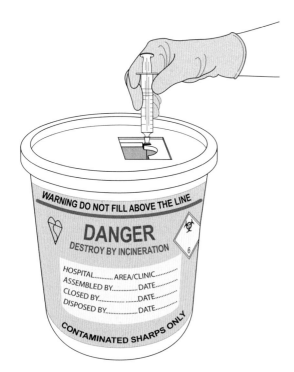

Figure 5.5 Sharps bin.

- Encourage the site to bleed, washing it simultaneously with soap and water.
- Apply a dressing.
- Dispose of the contaminated item in the sharps bin.
- Inform the person in charge of the area and Occupational Health.
- Complete the appropriate paperwork.

FLUOROSCOPIC EXAMINATION PREPARATION

Practitioners or radiologists usually perform fluoroscopic procedures with assistance to ensure that patient care is maintained to a high standard. The main examinations that take place in a fluoroscopy room are:

1. Contrast investigations of the gastrointestinal tract (e.g. barium enema, swallow/meal, follow-through).
2. Contrast investigations of the genitourinary tract (e.g. cystography).
3. Contrast investigations of the biliary tract (e.g. endoscopic retrograde cholangio pancreatography (ERCP).

PREPARATION FOR A BARIUM ENEMA

The patient is collected from the waiting area and, after checking her identity, is asked to change into an X-ray gown with the opening at the back. The patient should be asked to remove all clothes including underwear. Once the patient is dressed in a hospital gown a brief explanation of the procedure should be given to her. This must include a brief explanation of the examination including:

- the insertion of a tube into the rectum
- the running in of fluid and introduction of air
- the requirement for a small injection into the arm to relax the bowel
- the need to keep the fluid and air in the bowel

Table 5.2   Guidance for the safe disposal of waste

Type of waste	Containment	Ward/dept route of disposal	Hospital route of disposal	Comments
Sharps, including glass ampoules	Sharps bins – sealed and labelled with department title; no more than 2/3rds full	Via 'Eurobin' which must always be locked	Incineration	Responsibilities of producer to ensure initial disposal is safe
Contaminated/ blood/infected glassware	Sharps bins – sealed and labelled with department title; no more than 2/3rds full	Via 'Eurobin' which must always be locked	Incineration prior to landfill disposal	Responsibilities of producer to ensure initial disposal is safe
Clinical – not sharps; i.e. dressings etc.	Yellow bags – sealed and labelled with ward/dept	Via 'Eurobin' which must always be locked	Incineration	Responsibilities of producer to ensure initial disposal is safe
General waste (e.g. flowers)	Black bags – sealed when 2/3rds full	Placed in refuse store	Landfill disposal	
Cardboard	Boxes flattened, tied into manageable bundles	Placed in refuse store	Recycling	
Paper/tins/ glass	In recycling containers	Placed in refuse store	Recycling	
Confidential waste	In plastic bags	To be shredded, either on site or by specialist contractor, prior to recycling	Recycling	

- the need to turn around on the table following the instructions of the radiologist/ radiographer
- the length of the examination (approximately 30 minutes)
- the facility to have a shower and a private loo after the examination is finished.

There will need to be a check carried out as to whether the patient has any allergies to medication and, if the patient is of childbearing age, the possibility of pregnancy also requires establishing. It is important that any issues raised by the patient are referred to the radiographer/radiologist. To prepare the barium enema solution 700 cc of water is added to a barium sulphate powder, which is pre-packaged in a plastic 'giving set'. An enema tube is then added to the end of the tube and covered in a lubricating jelly ready for insertion into the rectum.

PREPARATION FOR A BARIUM MEAL/ SWALLOW

The patient is collected from the waiting area and after checking her identity she is asked to change into an X-ray gown with the opening at the back. The patient should be asked to remove all clothes, excluding her briefs. Once the patient is dressed in a hospital gown a brief explanation of the procedure should be given to her. This must include a brief explanation of the examination including:

- the requirement to drink the barium solution on request
- the need to also swallow some fizzy powder and keep the gas produced in the stomach
- the need to be able to turn around when standing and lying down within the X-ray equipment

- the possibility of an injection in the hand/arm to relax the stomach
- the length of the examination (approximately 15 minutes).

There will need to be a check carried out as to whether the patient has any allergies to medication and, if the patient is of childbearing age, the possibility of pregnancy also requires establishing. It is important that any issues raised by the patient are referred to the radiographer/radiologist. When the examination is complete it is important to remind the patient to drink plenty to reduce the possibility of blockage due to concretion of the barium.

PREPARATION FOR BARIUM FOLLOW-THROUGH

The preparation is similar to that of a barium meal or swallow, the difference being that the patient has a series of images taken at approximately 30-minute intervals to watch the transit of the barium. The patient is still required to swallow approximately 300 cc of barium sulphate solution with Maxolon (an accelerator to increase transit time through the bowel). All films taken should be shown to the practitioner or radiologist overseeing the procedure.

PREPARATION FOR CYSTOGRAPHY

The basic preparation is as above, the ID and pregnancy is checked and the patient changes into a gown with no underwear on. It is possible that the patient will already have a catheter inserted into the bladder but this is not always the case. The explanation to the patient should include the following:

- The information that the patient's bladder will be filled remotely from a container until the patient feels ready to urinate.
- The need to be able to urinate into a receptacle in order to see the functioning of the bladder.

At the end of the examination the patient may require a shower, as the contrast medium used can appear sticky.

PREPARATION FOR ERCP

In this examination it is necessary for a light sedative to be administered in order to ease the endoscopy and patients may therefore have brought someone to accompany them home. Patients need to remain in the hospital until the sedation has worn off (usually about 1–2 hours). The initial patient identification and LMP checking is as above and patients are required to undress and put on a hospital gown with only their briefs remaining. It is likely that throughout the examination a pulse oximeter will be placed on the tip of a finger in order to ensure that the blood oxygen level does not drop. Patients are unlikely to remember very much about the procedure because of the sedation but it is essential that their well-being is paramount during the procedure, including maintaining their dignity whilst on the X-ray table.

Following completion of the examination the patient should be placed in the recovery position on a trolley and should be accompanied until a satisfactory level of consciousness has been re-established.

SPECIALIST PROCEDURE PREPARATION

A range of specialist procedures are carried out within a diagnostic imaging department, from angiography to embolisation. The trolley setting should be adapted to the size required for the procedure. There are many different catheters that might be required during the course of the special procedure and the relevant one should be selected prior to its commencement (Fig. 5.6).

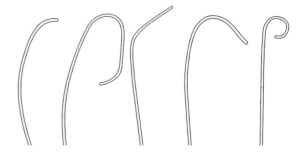

Figure 5.6 Selection of catheters used in specialised procedures.

The patient will probably be an inpatient due to the requirement for sedation and possible surgical intervention, dependant on the outcome of the procedure. In this instance, the patient's identification needs to be checked against the wristband as well as asked verbally. The special procedures require informed consent from the patient, which should be obtained by the practitioner or radiologist performing the examination. It is possible that postoperative observations of pulse; respiration, blood pressure and angiopuncture site will be required.

RECORD KEEPING

Records within a diagnostic imaging department can range from a request card to observation sheets and accident forms. Record keeping is an integral part of the healthcare professional's practice as identified by the Health Professionals Council 2003.[5]

In today's litigious society any record can be called upon during criminal procedures, Trust investigations and professional disciplinary investigations. The most common faults in record keeping are failure to document an incident or recording inaccurate accounts of events.[6]

There is a requirement to document all drugs administered; this includes all contrast and other drugs used during radiological examinations.

REQUEST CARD

This should detail (Fig. 5.7):

- Personal identification
  - For checking patient identification use open questions:
    'What is your name?'
    'What is your date of birth?'
- General practitioner details
  - This is mandatory information to identify the 'referrer' under IR(ME)R (see p. 14). It is also important that the GP who requested the examination receives the results.
- Pregnancy status
  - For women of childbearing age it is mandatory to ascertain pregnancy status when imaging the area between the diaphragm and knees.
- Clinical indications
  - This section should contain information related to the area and mechanism of injury in order for the request to be 'justified' under IR(ME)R.
- Investigation required
  - This section should contain information related to the diagnostic imaging procedure requested.
- Previous X-rays
  - This information is not mandatory, but preferable. All efforts must be made to ensure that duplicate examinations are not performed without 'justification'. All relevant reports must be viewed in the case of follow-up examinations to highlight any significant aspects of previous studies.
- Referrer's signature and date of referral
  - A valid signature is mandatory in order for the request to be 'justified' under IR(ME)R. In the case of electronically requested examinations the signatory has a password to ensure security. The date is essential to demonstrate that it is a current request.
- Operator's details
  - This information must include the details of the individual performing the examination and the incident dose given. It can also include any examination-relevant information.

CONTRAST MEDIUM INFORMATION RECORDED

- The batch number and expiry date of the contrast medium used.
- The type, quantity and strength of the contrast medium used.
- The name of the supervising clinician.
- The name of the administering clinician.
- Patient reaction to contrast medium.

\multicolumn{4}{c}{**DIAGNOSTIC IMAGING REQUEST (HOSPITAL)**}			

DIAGNOSTIC IMAGING REQUEST (HOSPITAL)

1	Hosp No. / Surname / Previous Surname / Forename / Address / Postcode / NHS No.		Date of Birth:
			Sex: M ☐ F ☐ / Pt. Tel. No.
			PATIENT I.D. LABEL IF AVAILABLE
2	Referral Source	Outpatient ☐ / Inpatient ☐ / Day Case ☐ / Ward Attender ☐	Ward/Dept _____	NHS: ☐ Private Patient: ☐ / Other:_____ / (Cat II/Other Human Source/Non-NHS Inst.)
		Hospital: / Other Source: / (i.e. P/P rooms)		
3	Transport	Walking ☐ Bed ☐ Chair ☐ Trolley ☐ Oxygen ☐ Mobile Exam ☐		
4	Pregnant?	Yes ☐ No ☐ Date of L.M.P.		
5	Clinical Problem			
6	Investigation requested			
7	Previous X-rays	Where? When?		
8	Consultant		Speciality	
9	Referring Doctor / Bleep Number / Signature			
10	Date			

FOR RADIOLOGY DEPARTMENT USE ONLY

Appointment:

Special Instructions:

Radiologist: Radiographer:

Figure 5.7 X-ray request card.

THE INCIDENT FORM

An incident form is completed in the case of an accident or dangerous occurrence.

Within the diagnostic imaging department the most likely events are:

- slips, trips and falls by a member of staff or patient
- a collision involving a piece of imaging equipment and a member of staff or patient
- a radiation incident caused by over-exposure or inappropriate exposure of a member of staff or patient
- a reaction to contrast medium.

In the event of any of the above occurring the relevant sections of the incident form should be completed and a copy sent to the Health and Safety Officer for audit purposes. Forms for documenting incidents and accidents within hospitals may differ between Trusts and departments.

References

1. Pittet D. Compliance with hand disinfection and its impact on hospital-acquired infections. J Hosp Infect 2000; 48:541–546.
2. NHS Executive. Hospital laundry arrangements for used and infected linen. HSG(95)18. London: NHS Executive; 1995.
3. Schabrun S, Chipcase L. Healthcare equipment as a source of nosocomial infection: a systematic review. J Hosp Infect 2006; 63:239–245.
4. Society and College of Radiographers. Health care associated infections (HCAIs): practical guidance and advice. Society and College of Radiographers; 2006.
5. Health Professionals Council. Standards for conduct, performance and ethics. London: Health Professionals Council; 2003.
6. Dimond B. Legal aspects of documentation. Exploring common deficiencies that occur in record keeping. Br J Nurs 2005; 14(10):568–571.

Recommended reading/bibliography

Ayliffe GA, Babb JR, Quoraishi AH. A test for hygienic hand disinfection. J Clin Pathol 1978; 31:923.

Culmer P. Chesneys' care of the patient in diagnostic radiography. Oxford: Blackwell; 1995.

This book is a revised and updated text which advocates a 'holistic approach to patient care' and covers the basic tenets of patient management for a range of imaging procedures.

Department of Health. The NHS healthcare cleaning manual. London: DoH Publications; 2004.

Lawrence JC. The bacteriology of burns. J Hosp Infect 1985; 6[Suppl B]:3.

Nicol M. Essential nursing skills. Edinburgh: Mosby; 2003.

This book sets out a wide range of clinical skills in a staged form and with easy to follow illustrations. It provides the foundation for working in the clinical setting.

Website

http://www.niaid.nih.gov/publications/microbes.htm

Chapter **6**

Procedures in radiography

Karen Dunmall

KEY POINTS

■ All patients follow a standardised pathway through the imaging department, coming in to contact with the same key areas regardless of their examination.

■ Patient privacy and comfort should be ensured at all times.

■ Mobile radiography provides a diagnostic service for patients who are unable to attend the X-ray department.

■ Mobile radiography introduces radiation safety issues which should be addressed during all examinations.

■ The use of contrast media enhances areas that may not be visualised during conventional examinations.

■ Contrast media are either barium or iodine based.

■ Some contrast media can cause undesirable side-effects in patients and all patients should be observed after the introduction of the contrast medium to ensure swift action in the event of a reaction.

INTRODUCTION

Radiology is an integral department within the hospital in that many inpatients are required to have at least one radiological examination in some form or another during their hospital stay. There are many other sources of referral for

Table 6.1 Referral sources and input in a diagnostic imaging department

Referring source	Diagnostic imaging input
Medical/ surgical	Departmental appendicular and axial skeletal radiography
	Departmental chest and abdominal radiography
	Mammography
	Dental
	Mobile ward radiography
	Departmental and theatre based fluoroscopic examinations
	Non ionic iodinated contrast studies
	Theatre based appendicular and axial skeletal radiography
	CT, MRI, US, RNI
Outpatients/GPs	Departmental appendicular and axial skeletal radiography
● Orthopaedic	Departmental chest and abdominal radiography
● ENT	Mammography
● Gynaecology	Dental
● Obstetrics	Departmental fluoroscopic examinations
● Oncology	Non ionic iodinated contrast studies
● Paediatric	CT, MRI, US, RNI
● Care of the elderly	
Accident and emergency	Departmental appendicular and axial skeletal radiography
	Departmental chest and abdominal radiography
	Mobile resuscitation unit radiography
	CT, MRI, US

CT, computed tomography; MRI, magnetic resonance imaging; RNI, radionuclide imaging; US, ultrasound

imaging examinations, ranging from outpatient clinics to accident and emergency departments (Table 6.1).

PATIENT PATHWAYS THROUGH THE IMAGING DEPARTMENT

(Figs 6.1 and 6.2)

RECEPTION DESK

This is most likely to be the first contact point that a patient or carer has with a diagnostic imaging department. It has been documented that patients should be given good quality information with regards to their care and be sufficiently informed before any medical examination takes place. It is therefore essential that the information process begins well. The reception team must be able to converse with the patients to ascertain their personal details; however, they must also be aware that there is the potential to be overheard by others. In some departments there is a line indicated by a stripe on the floor, indicating that only one patient should be at the desk at one time, whereas in other departments there may be a separate cubicle in which to ask personal details (Fig. 6.3). There are various notices informing patients of the no-smoking policy and zero tolerance of aggressive behaviour.

WAITING AREA

The patient will usually be directed to a sub-waiting area close to the X-ray room where their examination is to be carried out. In Figure 6.4 it can be seen that chairs have wipeable upholstery to reduce the risk of cross-infection. The chairs are also ranging in height and style to suit patients with mobility problems. A waiting area should be light and airy and have a selection of reading materials. The inclusion of wipeable toys may also be preferable in areas dealing with small children. It is important that if there is a delay due to unforeseen circumstances, the patients are aware of the time delay; this can often defuse difficult situations.

CHANGING CUBICLE

A changing cubicle should contain a bench or chair to sit on. There should be a supply of gowns to accommodate both male and female statures. The door should be lockable but with safety locks in case of emergencies and patients should not be placed in a cubicle for long periods of time.

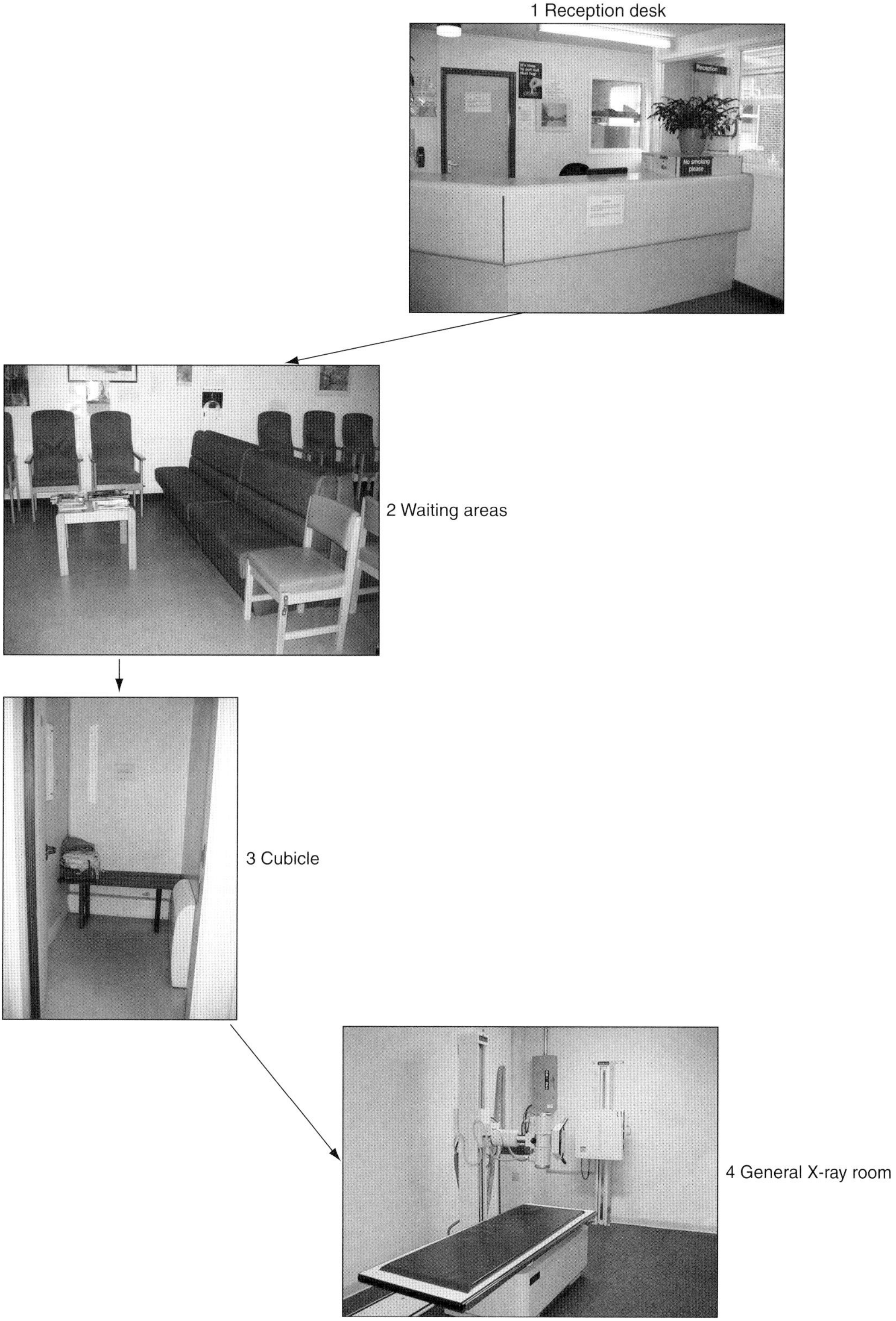

1 Reception desk

2 Waiting areas

3 Cubicle

4 General X-ray room

Figure 6.1 A patient's pathway through a diagnostic imaging department for routine appendicular, axial, chest and abdominal radiography.

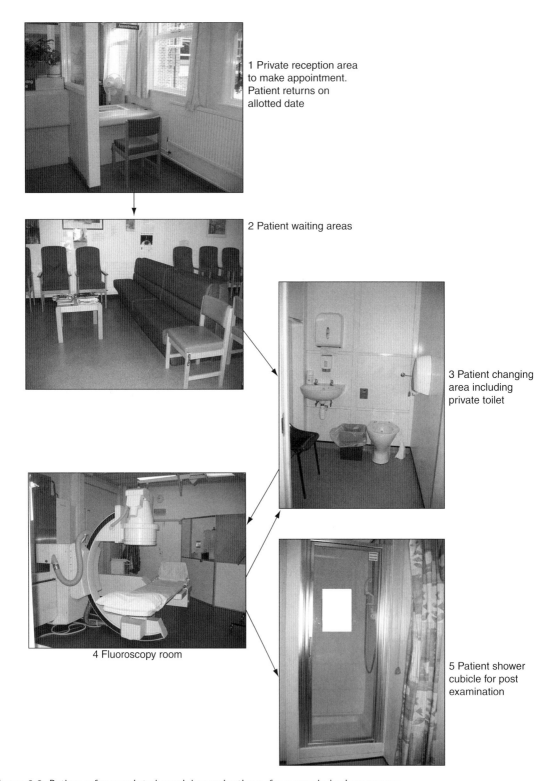

1 Private reception area to make appointment. Patient returns on allotted date

2 Patient waiting areas

3 Patient changing area including private toilet

4 Fluoroscopy room

5 Patient shower cubicle for post examination

Figure 6.2 Pathway for appointed special examinations; for example barium enema.

Main reception

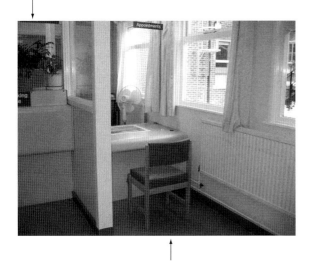

Private area

Figure 6.3 Reception desk with separate cubicle.

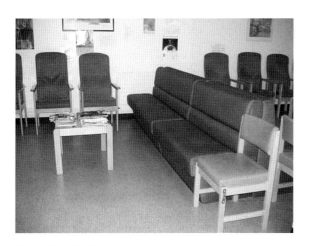

Figure 6.4 Waiting area.

Some hospitals provide baskets/lockers for the patient's clothes in order to reduce the risk of theft and also free up cubicles for a more rapid throughput of patients.

For certain examinations (e.g. barium enemas) where patients may need to access a toilet promptly after the examination, a cubicle with toilet and shower facilities should be used. An emergency cord is also essential in case a patient feels unwell (Fig. 6.5).

GENERAL X-RAY ROOM

In the X-ray room it is important to remember that to a member of the public, old or young, this room containing lots of big pieces of machinery may look rather frightening. Therefore, it is important to make the patient comfortable and at ease by giving instructions in simple non-jargon terms. For example, to most people a bed or couch is what you lie on, not a table, so be aware of potential confusion. Following the examination the patient should be asked to wait until the image is checked and then given information on when and how to get the results. Table 6.2 shows patient preparation and aftercare for some typical departmental examinations.

FLUOROSCOPY ROOM

The impression of this type of room is very similar to that of a general radiography room, but more high-tech. It is essential that the patient receives succinct instruction of what to do and is told in advance of any table or X-ray tube movements.

The patient is likely to spend more time in this room than in a general room. It will also be necessary for the patient to wait for any effects that the drugs or the examination may have had to wear off; for example the administration of a muscle relaxant (e.g. Buscopan or glucagon) may give blurred vision and therefore driving is not recommended until adequate vision has returned.

PATIENT SHOWER CUBICLE

In some examinations the end product of the examination might involve emptying the bladder whilst on the X-ray table or the leaking of contrast during the procedure. In either case patients usually feel as though they require a shower before getting dressed to remove traces of contrast medium. For this reason a shower cubicle may be provided in close proximity to the toilets and cubicles.

A

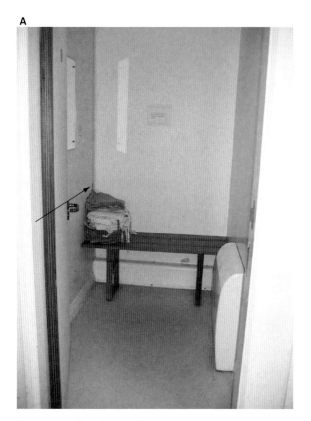

B

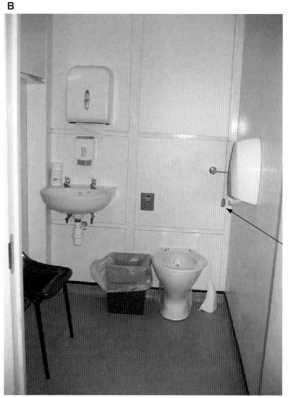

Figure 6.5 Changing facilities with emergency cords highlighted.

MOBILE RADIOGRAPHY

The imaging of a patient using equipment other than the static department-based equipment is commonly known as mobile or portable radiography. However, the term portable only relates to equipment that can be carried. Mobile radiography can be divided into two distinct types:

1) Mobile plain-film radiography using mobile X-ray equipment (Fig. 6.6).
2) Mobile fluoroscopy using a mobile image intensifier (Fig. 6.7).

PATIENT TYPES AND LOCATIONS FOR MOBILE RADIOGRAPHY

The patients who require mobile radiography are usually unable to come to the diagnostic imaging department due either to their condition or to the operating theatre environment required for the surgical procedure they are undergoing. The following areas within a hospital are likely to contain patients requiring mobile radiography:

1. Intensive therapy unit (ITU)
2. Coronary care unit (CCU)
3. High dependency unit (HDU)
4. Special care baby units (SCBU)
5. Neonatal intensive care units (NICU)
6. Isolation wards
7. Recovery wards
8. Resuscitation/major trauma units
9. Minor operating departments
10. Operating theatres (orthopaedic/general surgical)

The most common mobile procedures are:

- plain film imaging of the chest (in areas 1–8, above)

Table 6.2 Patient preparation and aftercare for some typical departmental examinations

Examination	Duration of examination	Special considerations	Dietary preparation	Drugs/contrast medium	After care	Results availability
Routine plain radiograph – abdomen, pelvis and femora	5–30 min	28-day rule for females of childbearing age Use gonadal shields	None	None	Transport arrangements. Instructions to make appointment for results	2 weeks
Routine plain radiograph – extremities, skull	5–30 min	Use radiation protection over gonads	None	None	Transport arrangements Instructions to make appointment for results	2 weeks
Barium enema	1 h	10-day rule for women of childbearing age Diabetic patients should be scheduled for the morning and can eat a light breakfast	Low fibre diet for 2 days and laxative to be taken a day before examination; clear fluids on day of examination	Barium sulphate solution; glucagon or Maxolon injection as muscle relaxant (IV)	Transport arrangements Escorted to bathroom to eliminate barium Shower facilities Maintain good fluid intake	2 weeks (GP) or at next hospital appointment
Small bowel meal	1 h	28-day rule for females of childbearing age	Low fibre diet 2 days before examination; laxative at 10 pm on evening prior to examination Diabetics need special advice	Barium sulphate solution with added Maxolon syrup as muscle relaxant	Transport arrangements Instructions to make appointment for results	2 weeks (GP) or at next hospital appointment

Continued

Table 6.2 Patient preparation and aftercare for some typical departmental examinations—cont'd

Examination	Duration of examination	Special considerations	Dietary preparation	Drugs/contrast medium	After care	Results availability
Barium swallow and meal	1 h	28-day rule (females of childbearing age)	Nil by mouth from midnight before the examination Diabetics need special advice	Barium sulphate solution, Carbex granules with effervescent lemon flavouring	Transport arrangements Instructions to make appointment for results	2 weeks (GP) or at next hospital appointment
Intravenous urograms	1 h	28-day rule for females of childbearing age Contraindications for adverse reactions to contrast medium	Low fibre diet for 2 days before the examination	Non ionic iodine based contrast (IV) injection	Transport arrangements Instructions to make appointment for results	2 weeks (GP) or at next hospital appointment
Venograms	1 h	28-day rule for females of childbearing age Contraindications for adverse reactions to contrast medium	None	Non-ionic iodine based contrast (IV) injection	Monitor and dress IV injection site Transport arrangements Instructions to make appointment for results	2 weeks (GP) or at next hospital appointment

IV, intravenous

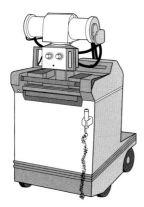

Figure 6.6 A mobile X-ray machine.

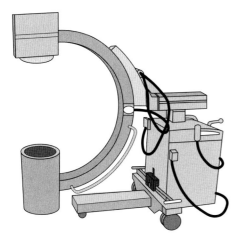

Figure 6.7 A mobile image intensifier.

- a plain film trauma series (cervical spine, chest, pelvis) and other appendicular/axial skeleton plain film imaging (resuscitation/major trauma units)
- mobile fluoroscopy of surgical procedures involving appendicular/axial skeleton, abdomen and chest (operating theatres and including pacemaker insertion in CCU).
  Orthopaedics:
  – hip pinning, screws and plates
  – femoral nailing
  – tibial nailing
  – open reduction internal fixation (ORIF) of fractures
  – closed manipulation and reduction of fractures.

General surgery:
– vascular studies
– urology studies
– endoscopic retrograde cholangio pancreatography (ERCP).

CONSIDERATIONS SPECIFIC TO MOBILE RADIOGRAPHY

There are four issues which must be considered when undertaking imaging outside the static department and which involve patients who may be unconscious or unable to cooperate:

1. Patient identification.
2. Radiation protection.
3. Health and safety.
4. Infection control.

PATIENT IDENTIFICATION

The request form for mobile plain film and fluoroscopy must be completed to the same standard as required for a department-based study. If the patient is to be anaesthetised then the identification and pregnancy status should ideally be determined before anaesthetic is administered; however, in the case of patients who are anaesthetised, the anaesthetist should check and confirm the information required. In cases of patients who are unconscious or unable to confirm their ID, the following should be used:

1. A wrist band.
2. Nurse/carer verification.

When needing to establish pregnancy status for the above types of patient, the referrer must complete the last menstrual period (LMP) details on the request card.

The identification of the image requires the patient's name, date of birth, sex and hospital number (according to the departmental protocol). Images acquired from mobile procedures should also include:

a) Time of examination (if not automatically recorded on image).
b) Source–object distance (SID, see p. 109).

c) Exposure values.
d) Patient position, e.g. erect/supine, anteroposterior.
e) Anatomical marker.

The adaptation of the technique, especially SID and exposure factors, can mask changes in patient condition varying with time or operator.

RADIATION PROTECTION [IR(ME)R]

When carrying out mobile imaging procedures using ionising radiation it is essential to establish a temporary controlled area and to ensure that there are sufficient numbers of lead equivalent aprons for all individuals who require one.

Wards and units

Radiation protection and safety can be achieved by using warning cones and placards in the vicinity of the mobile examination and also by using a verbal warning when imaging is occurring. It is difficult to restrict access to a whole ward which contains patients other than the one undergoing the examination. In this instance, the inverse square law is utilised to reduce the dose to individuals who cannot leave the area. All staff, patients and visitors should be asked to move as far away as possible from the patient under examination, but if this is not possible then lead-equivalent shielding should be used to afford protection. If a staff member or carer is required to give physical support to the patient they must wear a lead-equivalent apron and the details of exposure must be recorded in conjunction with the name of the 'holder'. The issue of immobilising patients is most pertinent in SCBU/NICU where the named nurse of several babies may be called upon to hold them in the case of serial imaging over the course of ventilation.

Theatre environment

Within an operating theatre it is possible to contain the area within the walls of a room. Only persons whose presence is absolutely essential remain in the theatre and there should be local rules to cover this. All essential people must wear lead-equivalent aprons during the time when radiation is being produced. The image intensifier should be operated using the pulsing mode whenever possible and stringent collimation should be applied. Lastly, the image intensifier should be positioned correctly before 'screening' begins, fluoroscopy should not be used to locate the area under examination. Monitoring of the theatre environment should be carried out on a routine basis using personal and area dose recorders. The image intensifier must be key operated to maintain the security of the unit.

HEALTH AND SAFETY

The health and safety issues of mobile radiography relate to:

- manual handling
- electrical safety
- trip hazards.

Manual handling

The mobile and image intensifiers must be stored in an area where they are easily reachable and do not block fire exits or corridors. A mobile machine may not be motorised and therefore should not be stored on an incline, which would require great force to remove it. When moving the mobile items it is also important to have assistance when manoeuvring the equipment through doors and corridors, as it is not always possible to see over the machine for on-coming 'traffic'. When leaving a piece of mobile equipment in place it is essential to ensure that all locks and brakes are on. If imaging an ill patient on a ward, it is preferable to remove the machine whilst returning to the department to process the image in case of the need for emergency resuscitation procedures.

Electrical safety

It must be remembered that X-rays are generated at high voltages and therefore electrical safety must be paramount. The units have special heavyweight plugs, which must only be plugged into a wall socket, not an extension cable. The environment may also have flammable gases being administered to patients (e.g. oxygen or anaesthetic gases); therefore all equipment must be earthed to prevent sparks. Care should also be taken in areas where water may be used to irrigate patients, such as in urology theatres; waterproof covers are used to prevent fluid entering the image intensifier.

Trip hazard

Mobile units have long cables to enable the machine to access areas remote to a socket, and the image intensifier is connected to the monitor via several leads. When positioning the mobile units care must be taken to keep any trailing cables from crossing main pathways, or a rubber mat should be placed over the cable to reduce the possibility of a trip hazard.

INFECTION CONTROL AND OPERATING THEATRE DRESS CODE

The mobile machines should be regularly cleaned to prevent cross-infection between wards, in the same way as equipment is cleaned following an infectious patient in the department.

In operating theatres and sterile environments there should be disposable sterile covers available for the X-ray tube head and intensifier sections of the mobile intensifier. The dress code in operating theatres serves two purposes:

1. Maintenance of hygiene and infection control.
2. Identification of staff.

Maintenance of hygiene and infection control

Microorganisms can be found on the skin, hair and clothing of everyone, without causing obvious infections to that individual. For the purpose of prevention of cross-infection, anyone entering an operating theatre is required to wear special clothing and head covering (Fig. 6.8).

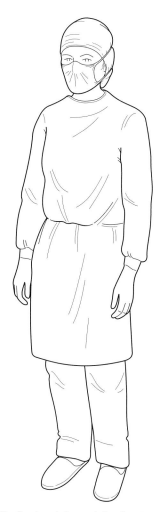

Figure 6.8 Professional dressed for theatre.

- Mask – this is optional for staff members not directly involved in the surgical procedure.
- Footwear – outdoor shoes must be exchanged for theatre footwear and stored separately. There is a need to be aware of hand hygiene when changing shoes.
- Headwear – disposable theatre caps are designed to cover hair and facial hair to reduce skin/hair particles being shed.
- Clothing – theatre clothing must only be worn whilst in the theatre environment and not during visits to other departments.
- Green drapes are also placed over the patient. Care must be taken not to de-sterilise the area by touching the sterile drapes.

USE OF CONTRAST MEDIUM

The contrast of an image is the difference in optical density between different tissues of the body. Body tissues attenuate the beam to different degrees dependent on many variables related to the number of electrons in the path of the incident X-ray photons. The number of electrons in the object is dependent on:

- the *proton number* of the tissue
- the *thickness* of the object being studied
- the *density* of the object being studied.

There is a naturally occurring contrast between bone and soft tissue due to the difference in proton numbers (bone $Z = 13.8$, soft tissue $Z = 7.4$); hence the outlines of the structures can be visualised. However, if the two organs have similar densities and proton numbers then it is not possible to distinguish them on a plain image; for example blood vessels within soft tissue organs.

The contrast of the blood vessel or the lumen of hollow structures can be increased by the introduction of a liquid with a higher average proton number, e.g. iodine or barium.

CONTRAST MEDIA TYPES

There are two main types of positive contrast agent:

1. Barium based.
2. Iodine based.

BARIUM SULPHATE SOLUTION

A suspension of large insoluble particles, which have good coating properties, is utilised in the visualisation of the lining of the gastrointestinal (GI) tract. Barium is used because it has a high proton number ($Z = 56$), is relatively cheap and inert. However, if barium sulphate permeates outside the GI tract it can be irritating to peritoneal membranes or cause pulmonary oedema in the lungs. Therefore, in cases of suspicion of perforation or aspiration, a water-soluble iodinated contrast is recommended.

Examples of barium sulphate used in diagnostic examinations

- Barium swallow: Baritop G 150% w/v 100 ml
- Barium meal: E-Z HD 250% w/v 135 ml + CO_2
- Barium follow-through: Baritop G 100% w/v 300 ml
- Small bowel enema: E-Z Paque 150 ml (+ gastrografin)
- Barium enema: Polibar 125% w/v 500 ml (+air)

IODINE BASED CONTRAST MEDIA

These are differentiated into ionic and non-ionic media containing iodine in solution.

Ionic contrast media

Ionic compounds dissociate into charged particles when the contrast enters into a solution (e.g. blood). An ionic contrast agent has an osmolarity approximately five times that of human plasma. The high osmolarity is associated with unwanted side-effects.

Examples of ionic contrast media

- Conray 280
- Conray 325
- Conray 420

The number refers to the iodine concentration in $mg\ ml^{-1}$

Non-ionic contrast media

Non-ionic contrast media do not dissociate into discharged particles when introduced into a solution. These media have low osmolarity and are more expensive than ionic contrast media. Non-ionic dimer contrast media tend to be reserved for patients undergoing vascular investigations and those at risk of reactions.

Examples of non-ionic contrast media

- Niopam 150, 200, 300, 340, 370 monomer
- Omnipaque 140, 180, 240, 300, 350 monomer
- Isovist 240, 300 dimer

Iodised oils

These are used infrequently in radiography, where water-soluble agents are contraindicated or when viscosity is required. Examinations include lymphoscintigraphy and sialography. This agent is not easily absorbed and in some circumstances it carries a risk of oil emboli. It is made of poppy seed oil.

Examples of iodised oils

- Lipiodol
- Myodil

Water-soluble iodine based contrast agents

These are used for imaging the GI tract and are characterised by an aniseed taste. They are recommended for use where there is a suspected leakage into pleural or peritoneal cavities.

Examples or water-soluble iodine based contrast media

- Gastrografin 370 mg ml^{-1}
- Gastromiro 300 mg ml^{-1}

CONTRAST MEDIA USAGE

ANGIOGRAPHY

This is defined as the investigation of blood vessels and can be divided into arteriography, venography and digital subtraction angiography.

- Arteriography: Contrast medium is introduced via a catheter into an artery, which then follows the natural flow of blood into the periphery of the body or organ.
- Venography: Conversely, contrast medium is introduced intravenously (IV) and follows the normal flow of blood returning to the heart.
- Digital subtraction angiography: A specialised type of angiography which utilises the computer hardware to subtract a precontrast image from a postcontrast image to leave the contrast filled vessels free from overlying structures.

INTRAVENOUS UROGRAPHY (IVU)

The rapid elimination properties of contrast media mean that the kidneys excrete it. Following an intravenous injection of contrast media into the median cubital vein a series of images of the urinary tract can be obtained.

BILIARY TRACT

The gall bladder can be visualised by the ingestion of contrast medium, which concentrates in the liver and collects in the gall bladder.

In percutaneous transhepatic cholangiography (PTC) the ducts are cannulated via a needle which passes through the skin and liver. In ERCP, the ducts are cannulated via the ampulla of Vater in the duodenum.

GASTROINTESTINAL TRACT

The upper GI tract is visualised by the ingestion of contrast media. The large colon is visualised by contrast medium introduced via the rectum.

OTHER EXAMINATIONS

There are a wide variety of examinations where contrast media can be used, e.g. in joint visualisation, salivary glands.

CONTRAST MEDIA SAFETY

There are many characteristics of contrast media that are responsible for causing reactions:

- Dose dependent adverse reactions due to the physiochemical effects of the contrast medium, e.g. osmolarity or electrical charge. Reaction is seen as heat, pain, vasodilation, cardiac depression or hypotension.
- Some reactions are almost independent of dose and concentration. These present as nausea and vomiting or allergy-like hypersensitivity reactions such as urticaria, bronchospasm or laryngospasm.
- Viscosity may cause pain due to the force needed to inject the contrast medium through a needle or catheter.
- The higher the osmolarity the more water is drawn into the solution from the tissues. The higher the osmotic pressure the poorer the tolerance, which is directly linked to heat and discomfort.
- Chemotoxicity. This refers to the mechanism responsible for causing toxic effects, such as histamine release. It is thought that some contrast media can cause histamine release from mast cells causing allergy-like reactions.

For clinical purposes reactions are divided into three categories:

1. Minor – flushing, nausea, vomiting, pruritus, mild rash, arm pain.
2. Moderate – more severe urticaria, facial oedema, hypotension, bronchospasm.
3. Severe – hyposensitive shock, laryngeal oedema, convulsions, respiratory and cardiac arrest.

EXAMINATION PREPARATION

For all examinations carried out in the diagnostic imaging department, preparation before the patient enters the room is essential. In the general X-ray room this may involve getting a cassette ready, selection of exposure factors and ensuring any positioning aids required are ready for use. In the fluoroscopy room preparation will be as for a general room but, in addition to this, the contrast medium will need preparation, as will the patient. A trolley may need to be set up for the examination and this should be sterile with all equipment laid out ready for use.

PREGNANCY CHECKS

For all radiographic examinations it is essential that a pregnancy check be carried out for all patients of reproductive age undergoing examinations of the abdominal area. These checks are divided into high dose and low dose examination checks, depending on the region and examination.

LOW DOSE EXAMINATIONS

Plain film abdomen, pelvis, lumbar/sacral spine may be undertaken within 28 days of the patient's LMP if the patient verifies that there is no possibility of pregnancy, also known as the '28-day rule'.

HIGH DOSE EXAMINATIONS

These examinations are defined as procedures that carry a potential fetal dose greater than 10 mGy

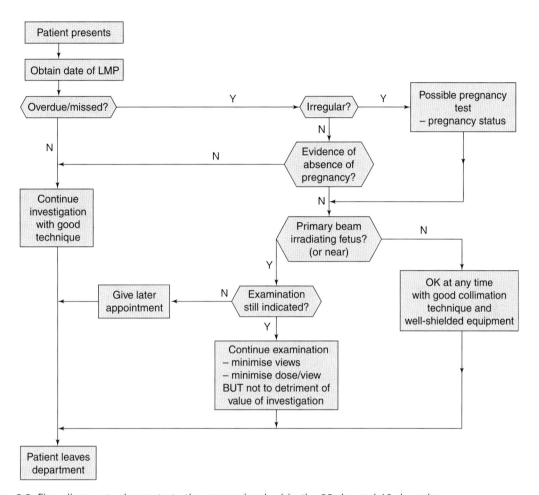

Figure 6.9 Flow diagram to demonstrate the process involved in the 28-day and 10-day rules.

(e.g. abdominal/pelvic CT, barium enema; see p. 84 for SI units commonly used in radiography). For these examinations patients should be booked an appointment within the first 10 days of the menstrual cycle, known as the '10-day rule'. However, the average length of the patient's menstrual cycle should be ascertained, as 10 days is an arbitrary figure for a 28-day cycle; 7 days is more applicable for a 21 day cycle (Fig. 6.9).

Recommended reading

Chapman S, Nakielny R. A guide to radiological procedures, 4th edn. Oxford: WB Saunders; 2001.

This publication provides details on how to carry out common procedures. It follows a standardised format throughout, ensuring the reader has the same depth of knowledge about all examinations.

Chapter **7**

Physics of radiography

Marc Griffiths and Ken Holmes

KEY POINTS

- In order to standardise the units of measurement used in science, the International System of Units (SI) was developed, which is derived from seven standard base units.
- Some of these units (e.g. length (metre), mass (kilogram), electric current (ampere)) represent the fundamental measurements underpinning the physics of radiography.
- From the standard base units, other SI units may be derived which are more applicable to radiography.
- All elements are composed of atoms.
- All atoms with exception of hydrogen have neutrons, protons and electrons.
- Elements may combine with other elements to form compounds.
- Some elements known as isotopes have atoms with varying numbers of neutrons.
- Electromagnetic radiation is a spectrum of energy levels containing a wide range of radiation types.
- The inverse square law determines the intensity of radiation reaching both the patient and the image receptor.

INTRODUCTION

It is essential that any practitioner operating within the realms of an imaging department and using ionising radiation has a sound knowledge base. In order to comprehend the various factors affecting the production of diagnostic images, there is a requirement to demonstrate an awareness of the fundamental definitions of classical physics and how these terms may be applied to radiography. An understanding of atomic structure, the electromagnetic spectrum, electricity, magnetism and the inverse square law are also essential principles that can be applied to radiography.

DEFINITIONS

Radiography involves the safe use of ionising radiation and the production of quality images. The process by which images are produced involves the conversion of energy from one form to another and the use of various specialised materials, such as the X-ray tube. The law of conservation of energy states that energy cannot be created or destroyed but merely changes from one form to another. Understanding this fundamental law is central to the basic knowledge base of a practitioner. Within the scope of basic physics there are numerous SI units and their definitions, and the practitioner must be aware of these base units.

SI BASE UNITS RELEVANT TO RADIOGRAPHIC PRACTICE

LENGTH

This is used to measure the size of an object or, in radiography, the distance between different aspects of the imaging system. The SI unit of length is the metre (m) and in radiography one of the most important length measurements is the distance between the X-ray tube focal spot and the imaging receptor. With the advent of digital imaging this distance has become known as the source–image distance (SID), but it is also still widely known as the focus–film distance (FFD). In terms of assessing image quality, the practitioner may wish to use a smaller unit of length, the millimetre (mm), for areas such as focal spot size calculations and image unsharpness. It is important to remember to convert all parameters into SI units before undertaking any calculations.

MASS

Matter is the fundamental material of which everything in the universe is made. Matter is composed of particles known as atoms and molecules. The SI unit of mass is the kilogram (kg). Different materials contain varying amounts of these particles and therefore vary in overall density, and this determines the characteristics of the overall exposure settings used by the practitioner. For example, lead is heavier than wood because it has more densely packed atoms.

ELECTRIC CURRENT

This is the movement of electrons flowing per unit time within a conductive material, such as copper. The SI unit of electric current is the ampere (A) and in diagnostic radiography this determines the quantity of electrons produced by the filament and hence the overall number of X-ray photons in the beam. The term milliamp (mA) is used in diagnostic radiography to express the tube current and is one thousandth of an ampere (10^{-3} A). The amount of electric charge flowing through an X-ray tube during an exposure is the sum of tube current (mA) and duration of the exposure time in seconds (s). This is expressed as mA s and in order to obtain a short exposure time (e.g. 0.03 s for a chest radiograph) the electric current (mA) needs to be suitably higher.

DERIVED SI UNITS RELEVANT TO RADIOGRAPHIC PRACTICE

Derived SI units result from a combination of the base units and some of them are used frequently in radiography. Practitioners are required to name them and define their values (Table 7.1). Some of these derived SI units are outlined below.

ENERGY

This may be a difficult concept to understand but fundamentally energy is the ability to do work. This may be demonstrated in radiography as potential

Table 7.1 Common SI units used in radiographic practice

Term and SI unit	Definition	Application to radiography
Energy (joule; J)	The ability to do work	Production of X-rays
Mass (kilogram; kg)	A measure of the number of atoms and molecules in a body	Important when determining the radiation dose to a patient
Gray (joules per kilogram; Gy)	The energy imparted to a body by ionising radiation	Unit of absorbed radiation dose measurement
Sievert (joules per kilogram, Sv)	The energy imparted to a body by ionising radiation multiplied by the quality factor	Unit of radiation dose equivalent, which takes biological factors into account
Power (joules per second)	The rate of doing work	Output of X-ray generator
Electric current (ampere; A)	The movement of electrons flowing per unit time	Quantity of electrons flowing per unit time
Electric charge (coulomb; C)	1 ampere flowing per second	Quantity of electrons flowing per second
Electrical potential (volt; V)	The force which moves electrons within a conductive material	Potential difference across an X-ray tube, acceleration of electrons and quality of X-ray beam
Frequency (hertz; Hz)	The number of cycles per second	Electromagnetic radiation

energy (PE), which is applied to the negative (cathode) and positive (anode) ends of an X-ray tube, subsequently causing the flow of electrons across the vacuum environment. This is kinetic energy (KE) and is subsequently converted into X-ray energy (photons) when the electrons interact with the anode material (tungsten atoms).

The potential difference between the cathode and anode of an X-ray tube is measured in kilovolts (kV). This determines the acceleration of electrons across the X-ray tube and hence the quality (penetrating power) of the X-ray beam.

POWER

This is the rate of doing work and is measured in joules per second ($J\,s^{-1}$) or watts (W). This unit is referred to in terms of the power output of diagnostic imaging equipment generators. For example a typical general X-ray room will have 50 kW generator to supply electric power to the X-ray equipment. However, a mobile X-ray unit may only have a 35 kW generator because the requirement to produce higher exposure values is less.

ATOMIC STRUCTURE

All matter consists of atoms and can be thought of as having a central nucleus surrounded by a cloud of particles called electrons (Fig. 7.1). The diameter of the nucleus is approximately 10^{-15} m.

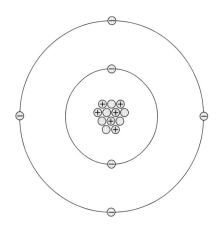

Figure 7.1 An atom with a central nucleus and orbiting electrons.

The nucleus contains a number of particles called protons and neutrons, together termed nucleons. Each nucleon is nearly 2000 times the mass of an electron. This means the mass of an atom is concentrated in its nucleus, around which the much lighter electrons orbit. If a nucleus were scaled up to the centre spot of a football pitch, the electrons would start orbiting around the perimeter of the pitch in their various orbits stretching out for several miles. This analogy demonstrates why X-rays may pass through a body of material unattenuated, as the X-ray photons may simply pass 'between' the electron orbits and totally miss the nucleus of an atom.

PROTON NUMBER

SYMBOL: Z

The proton number (Z), which is the number of protons in the nucleus of an atom (also known as its atomic number), determines the element. For example, a nucleus with just one proton is hydrogen (Z = 1); a nucleus with eight protons is oxygen (Z = 8) and one with 29 protons is copper. The names of all the different elements and their proton numbers can be found in the Periodic Table.

NUCLEON NUMBER

SYMBOL: A

The nucleon (or mass) number (A) of a nucleus is the total number of nucleons in the nucleus; that is, the number of protons plus the number of neutrons. If you subtract the proton number from the nucleon number you will end up with the number of neutrons in the nucleus. Tungsten is used as the anode material in an X-ray tube construction and has a nucleon number of 184 and a proton number of 74. This means tungsten has 74 protons and 110 neutrons in the nucleus of each atom.

ELECTRONS

Electrons are the small, light particles orbiting the nucleus of an atom. They are arranged in shells, called K, L, M, N, O and P. Normally, the number of electrons orbiting the nucleus equals the number of protons in the nucleus. An atom of oxygen, for example, has 8 electrons orbiting the central nucleus in the K shell (n = 2) and L shell (n = 6) (Fig. 7.2).

The number of electrons in each shell follows certain rules; for example, the maximum number in the K shell is 2; in the L shell, 8; and in the M shell, 18. However, the outermost shell (valence shell) may only hold 8 electrons. This shell determines the chemical, thermal, optical and electrical properties of the atom. The maximum number of electrons in a shell is $2n^2$, where n = the number of the shell, starting with K as 1.

Copper, for example, has a proton number of 29. There are 2 electrons in the K shell, 8 in the L shell, 18 in the M shell and 1 in the N shell. This single valence electron easily leaves the atom and acts as a free electron. Hence copper is a good conductor of heat and electricity.

All matter is made up of chemical substances of two kinds:

- Elements – chemical substances that cannot be broken down into simpler chemical forms.
- Compounds – the result of two or more elements linking together chemically.

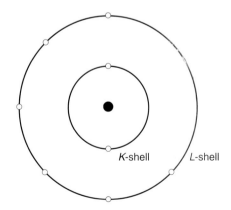

Figure 7.2 Example of an atom of oxygen.

An element is the simplest form in which matter exists. Examples include oxygen, nitrogen and tungsten. Each element only contains atoms of each particular chemical; in other words, the element oxygen only contains the specific atoms for this chemical. Most elements are unable to exist in a single form so they combine with other elements and become compounds. Examples of compounds include water, which comprises two atoms of hydrogen combined with one atom of oxygen. This is chemically expressed as H_2O.

ISOTOPES

The number of neutrons in a nucleus can vary, either occurring naturally or artificially. For example, a nucleus of carbon (proton number 6) may have a nucleon number of 11, 12, 13 or 14, with 5, 6, 7 or 8 neutrons. Each is called an *isotope* of carbon. Carbon-14 is used to date historical artefacts (e.g. the Turin shroud), whilst carbon-12 is used as a reference tool to determine the atomic mass of all other elements. Some isotopes are stable and some are radioactive, depending on the ratio of protons to neutrons.

CHEMICAL SYMBOLS

An element can be represented by its chemical symbol (Fig. 7.3) with its proton number as a subscript and its nucleon number as a superscript to the left hand side of the symbol. An element identified in this way is known as a nuclide. Expressing the nuclide in this way gives the practitioner all the information required to illustrate the number of protons and neutrons (nucleons in the nucleus) and the number of orbiting electrons. For example, carbon-14, which has a proton number of 6 but a nucleon number of 14 (i.e. it has 8 neutrons) can be represented as ^{14}C.

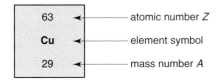

Figure 7.3 Chemical symbol for copper.

The proton number could appear as a subscript, but as carbon, by definition, has six protons, that is not strictly needed.

PARTICLE CHARGE AND BINDING ENERGY

The fundamental particles of an atom may have a small charge (1.602×10^{-19} coulomb) associated with them. Protons are positively charged (+1) and electrons are negatively charged (−1). An electrically balanced atom has the same number of protons and orbiting electrons. This charge creates a force (binding energy) which holds the electrons in orbit around the nucleus, and the atom is stable. If an electron is removed from the atom, the positive protons will outnumber the remaining negative electrons, leaving the atom with a net positive charge. This is the process of ionisation of the atom and leaves what is known as a positive ion. When an electron is removed from a shell (e.g. X-ray production), a certain amount of energy is used to overcome the attractive force of the protons in the nucleus: this is called the binding energy. The more protons in the nucleus, the higher the binding energy required to remove an electron. The closer the shell to the nucleus, the higher the binding energy. Atoms may also be ionised by X-ray photons: the energy of the X-ray is used to overcome the binding energy of one of the electrons. If atoms making up important structures in the body, such as DNA, are ionised, chemical changes occur which may cause permanent damage. This is why X-rays can be dangerous and this is why the practitioner needs to be aware of the potential damage from ionising radiation.

ELECTROMAGNETIC RADIATION

The electromagnetic radiation (EMR) spectrum encompasses a wide range of radiation types, such as X-rays, gamma rays, light, microwaves and radio waves. Figure 7.4 depicts the EMR spectrum and, as the term suggests, EMR consists of both electric and magnetic fields. These fields are at right angles to each other and travel through a vacuum at the same velocity as light (3×10^8 m s^{-1}). Outside a vacuum environment,

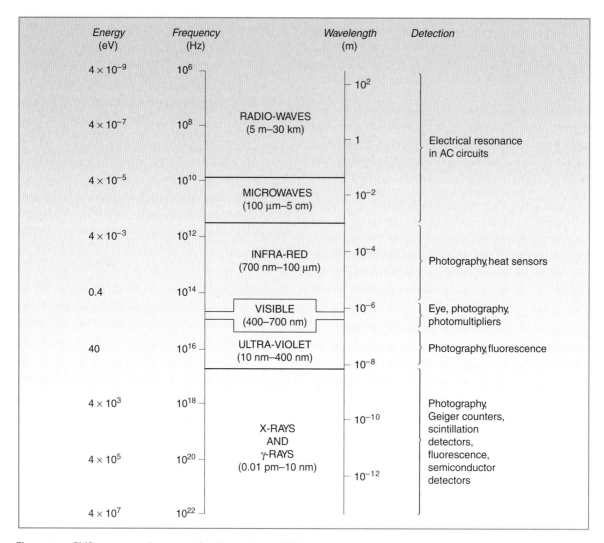

Figure 7.4 EMR spectrum demonstrating the various attributes.

EMR interacts with matter, which may absorb part of this energy and affect it.

As illustrated in Figure 7.4, the EMR has a range of frequencies and wavelengths. All EMR exhibit the same set of properties. EMR may be illustrated by plotting the energy against distance, giving a sine wave.

- Waves are composed of transverse vibrations of electric and magnetic fields (sine wave).

- The vibrations have a wide range of wavelengths (10^{-12} m to 100 m).
- The vibrations have a wide range of frequencies (10^{21} Hz to 10^8 Hz).
- All EMR travels through a vacuum at the same velocity.
- All EMR travels in straight lines.
- All EMR is unaffected by electromagnetic fields.
- All EMR may be considered as photons containing quanta of energy or waveform (duality principle).

Table 7.2   Aspects of electromagnetic radiation (EMR) within the clinical imaging department

Aspect of EMR	Clinical use
X-rays	Obtaining diagnostic images
Gamma rays	Nuclear medicine
Ultra-violet light	Conventional film–screen combinations
Visible light	Viewing radiographs
Radio waves	Radiofrequency pulses in MRI
Infra-red light	Heat transfer from the anode of a rotating anode X-ray tube

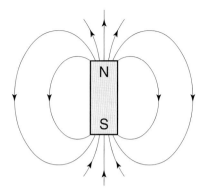

Figure 7.5 An illustration of the lines of force around a bar magnet.

In terms of diagnostic imaging, all aspects of the EMR spectrum are relevant to some area of clinical practice (Table 7.2).

MAGNETISM

Most practitioners are aware of the concept of a magnet – a piece of metal that aligns itself with magnetic north (compass). This can be used with a map to find your way when out walking. This is a permanent magnet and has a north and a south pole. It is made of iron, which has been magnetised to fulfil this function and is constructed of a series of mini bar magnets all aligned in the same direction. A piece of wire will also exhibit magnetism when an electric current is passed through it. If the wire is coiled it is known as a solenoid and will exhibit the same properties as a bar magnet providing the current is switched on. Bar magnets have no useful function in an imaging department; however, magnetism has several functions of which the practitioner needs to be aware in order to understand how the equipment functions.

Practitioners must also be aware that there are forces which exist between magnets. 'Like' poles repel each other and 'unlike' poles attract. Thus, if a north pole of a magnet approaches another north pole they will repel each other and you will be unable to get the magnets to touch. However, if one magnet is rotated they will become firmly attached at the poles. It is normal practice in physics to consider the north pole as positive and the south pole as negative. A magnet also exhibits

magnetic fields, which exert a force around it, and this can be demonstrated by using iron filings, which adhere to the lines of force (Fig. 7.5).

MAGNETIC FLUX

The number of lines of force that pass through the magnet is defined as the magnetic flux and, if we consider a unit area of the magnet, this then becomes the flux density. The SI unit of magnetic flux density is the tesla (T) and this defines the field strength in magnetic resonance imaging (MRI).

ELECTROMAGNETISM

Magnetism is associated with the alignment and movement of electrons and therefore the atom. As all atoms have moving electrons around their nucleus there are always weak magnetic forces associated with atoms. Therefore, when a current passes through a wire there are millions of electrons moving along the wire and it is this process which cause the wire to become magnetised. The wire also exhibits a magnetic field around it and this effect is known as electromagnetism. Single strands of wire exhibit a magnetic effect; however, to enable us to use the phenomenon effectively we need to coil the wire to make a solenoid. If a soft iron bar is place within the solenoid this increases the magnetic flux considerably because of the induced magnetism within the iron. The combination of a solenoid with an iron core is known as an electromagnet.

Electromagnets are used in equipment as locks for the X-ray tube mounting.

MAGNETIC MATERIALS

Some materials are easily magnetised and produce strong magnets whilst other are ineffective at producing magnets. There are three basic types of magnetic substance:

1. Diamagnetism
2. Paramagnetism
3. Ferromagnetism.

Both diamagnetism and paramagnetism are extremely weak processes and have no application in radiography.

Ferromagnetic substances can be used practically in X-ray equipment and are used in transformers, relays and MRI equipment. These materials have magnetic domains within them and all the atoms are lined up in the same direction. This can be achieved by an externally applied magnetic field; for example by stroking a piece of iron with a magnet or from an electric current.

Metals such as iron and nickel are ferromagnetic and the force required to line up all the magnetic domains is less than in other metals. This process is sensitive to temperature changes and will disappear at extreme temperatures.

ELECTROMAGNETIC INDUCTION

This is the production of an electric current by changing the magnetic field and is the opposite effect of electromagnetism, which was described earlier. It is an important concept in radiography and is the process by which transformers convert the mains voltage to the high current required to produce X-ray exposures. Transformers also isolate the X-ray circuit from the mains electricity by using an autotransformer.

ELECTRICITY

Electricity is simply moving electric charges; that is, electrons moving within a wire. Metals are good electrical conductors. The electrons in their outer shell (conduction band) are easily dislodged and these free electrons can then flow around a piece of wire, creating an electrical circuit. Insulators are materials such as plastic and rubber which have firmly bound electrons in their outer shell and are thus unable to pass an electric current.

ELECTRIC CURRENT

An electric current flowing through a material is simply a measure of the number of electrons passing from the cathode to the anode. The measure of that current is the rate of flow of the electrons. For the electrons to flow there must be a force (potential difference) to drive the electrons and a complete circuit to pass around.

The SI unit of electric current is the ampere and for a current of 1 ampere to flow a charge of 1 coulomb must pass a point in the circuit every second (i.e. 1 ampere = 1 coulomb per second).

This is a considerable number of electrons and amounts to 6×10^{18} electrons per second. The potential difference across the circuit is measured in kilovolts and determines the rate at which the electrons move. High potential differences are used in the X-ray circuit and vary between 40 and 150 kV_P (see p. 108).

TUBE CURRENT

For an X-ray tube to produce X-rays a current must pass from the anode to the cathode and this tube current is measured in milliamperes (mA). Thus the mA is the rate of flow of electrons across the X-ray tube. The total number of electrons flowing for each exposure is the product of the mA and the duration of the exposure (mA s).

RESISTANCE

Resistance is the force which tries to impede the flow of electrons. It is measured in ohms (Ω) and the resistance in any material depends upon its shape, the type of substance and the temperature of the material. Metals have low resistance to the passage of electrons whereas insulators have much higher values of resistance. The optimum shape of a conductor to reduce the resistance is one of large cross-sectional area and, of course, the longer the conductor the greater the resistance.

ELECTRICAL POWER

The SI unit of power is the watt (W) where 1 watt is equal to 1 joule per second. The power of an X-ray circuit is usually expressed in kilowatts (10^3 W). Modern X-ray rooms have a power rating of 50 kW.

INVERSE SQUARE LAW

The inverse square law is a fundamental aspect of everyday practice within diagnostic imaging and is a principle which every practitioner should understand. As previously mentioned, EMR is composed of quanta, each of which has energy. As the distance between the X-ray source (e.g. X-ray tube) and imaging receptor increases the intensity of the radiation emitted will decrease.

The intensity (I) of a diverging beam (e.g. an X-ray beam) when passing through air adheres to an inverse square law with distance (d) from the source via the following mathematical formula:

$$I \propto \frac{I}{d^2}$$

Where:
    I = Intensity of the X-ray beam
    $\propto$ = Proportional
    d = Distance

The intensity of the X-ray beam decreases with an increase in distance. This happens due to the diverging nature of the X-ray beam rather than to the interaction of X-ray photons with matter. The energy of the X-ray beam is spread over an increasing area as the distance from the source

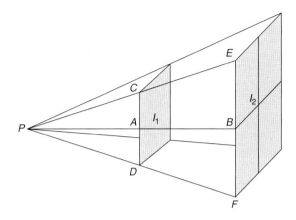

Figure 7.6 Inverse square law.

increases. By doubling the distance, the intensity is reduced to a quarter of its original value. This is demonstrated in the Figure 7.6, where the result of increasing the distance from d_1 to d_2 results in a reduction of the intensity of the X-ray beam to a quarter of that of d_1.

THE INVERSE SQUARE LAW IN PRACTICE

In practice, the inverse square law needs to be taken into consideration when undertaking examinations, which may require a large distance. For example, examinations involving the inclusion of a full-length tibia and fibula view may require the practitioner to increase the SID to accommodate this part of the anatomy. Such an increase in distance is outside the normal working distance of 100 cm SID and will require an adjustment to the exposure factors in order to provide an image with the same density and contrast as an image produced at the standard SID.

Example of inverse square law

Question: The reading from a dose area product (DAP) meter was 1041 mGy cm^2 (see Table 7.1 for SI units) for a phantom pelvis examination performed at 100 cm SID. What is the approximate DAP meter reading for the same examination (using the exact same exposure factors) at 200 cm SID?

Figure 7.7 **A** SID 100 cm. **B** SID 200 cm.

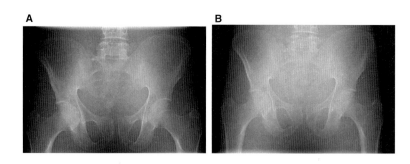

Answer: Substituting into the equation given above, we can see that $1/d^2$ increases from $1/100^2$ to $1/200^2$ when the distance doubles. So if $I \propto 1/10\ 000$ and has a value of 1041 mGy cm^2, then $I \propto 1/40\ 000$ must have a value of $1041 \times \frac{1}{4}$, which means the absorbed DAP is reduced to approximately 260 mGy $\times$ cm^2. The resultant image would, however, appear with less contrast and not as dense in comparison to the image taken at 100 cm, as only the higher energy portion of the X-ray beam would reach the image receptor. The lower energy X-ray photons would either be absorbed or scatter, potentially failing to reach the image receptor. This is demonstrated in the images in Figure 7.7.

However, with the advent of digital imaging systems, certain image algorithms may be applied to raw data and compensation for the effects of distance may be visualised by the practitioner. The practitioner should be consciously aware of the post manipulation features of modern digital imaging systems.

Recommended reading

Ball J, Moore AD. Essential physics for radiographers, 3rd edn. London: Blackwell; 1997.

A clear and straightforward introduction to physics for radiographers.

Farr RF, Allisy-Roberts PJ. Physics for medical imaging. London: Saunders; 1997.

This text provides information on medical physics, assuming you have a good base of physics knowledge.

Graham DT, Cloke P. Principles of radiological physics, 4th edn. London: Churchill Livingstone; 2003.

This book provides an in-depth introduction to the physics of diagnostic radiography. The presentation is clear and easy to understand with examples applying the theory to practice.

Website

Periodic table:
Available: *http://www.webelements.com* 6 February 2008.

Chapter **8**

The X-ray tube

Nick Oldnall

CHAPTER CONTENTS

KEY POINTS

- X-rays are produced by the rapid deceleration of fast moving electrons in a tungsten based target.
- The electrons are produced by a heated tungsten filament, the cathode.
- X-ray tube enclosures are generally constructed from glass but may be metal and/or ceramic.
- The X-ray tube contains a vacuum in order to accelerate the electrons with maximum efficiency.
- The electrons are accelerated across a potential difference ranging from 40 to 120 kV in a diagnostic X-ray tube.
- X-rays are produced as bremsstrahlung and characteristic radiation at the anode with an efficiency of around 1%.
- The anode rotates in order to spread the heat loading over a large area to prevent overheating.
- The anode is rotated by an induction motor with coils outside the glass envelope and a copper rotor inside attached to the anode.
- X-rays are produced at the focal spot on the anode, the smaller the focal spot the smaller the penumbra of the X-ray beam.
- X-rays are emitted in all directions from the tube but are constrained to a small area by a 'window' or port in the tube housing.

INTRODUCTION

Since the discovery of X-rays in 1895 by Roentgen and the heated cathode X-ray tube by Coolidge, X-ray tubes have developed into complex pieces of electromechanical engineering. They comprise around 350 parts, taking 150 assembly operations. The cost (at date of publication) can be as much as £20 000.

The production of X-rays for diagnostic imaging requires fast moving electrons to be rapidly decelerated; the design and function of the major components to facilitate this will be discussed.

The key components of a modern rotating anode X-ray tube (Fig. 8.1) are:

- Tube housing
- Vacuum envelope
- Filament assembly
- Anode
- Stator assembly
- X-ray port and collimator.

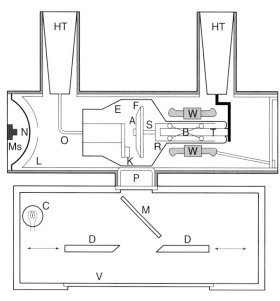

Figure 8.1 Rotating anode X-ray tube. A Anode disk, B Ball bearings, C Collimator lamp, D Collimator diaphragm, E Glass envelope, F Focal track, HT High-tension cable socket, K Cathode assembly, L Lead lining, M Mirror, Ms Microswitch, N Expansion diaphragm, O Oil, P Tube port, R Rotor assembly, S Anode stem, T Rotor support, V Plastic window, W Stator windings.

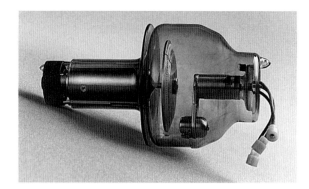

Figure 8.2 The X-ray tube.

TUBE HOUSING

The tube housing protects the delicate insert from damage during use (Fig. 8.2). It is made of steel or aluminium with an external protective coat of paint to allow easy cleaning and an internal lining of lead to reduce radiation leakage to below the required maximum. The cover has special mounting rings, trunions for attachment to the tube suspension equipment, and sealed terminals and sockets for the high-tension cables and other associated control equipment connections. On the external surface the tube is marked to indicate the position of the focus point of the anode and a plate indicates the electrical characteristics and date of manufacture.

The cover is lined with lead to reduce radiation leakage, except for the X-ray port, which is made of plastic or beryllium. Beryllium is used as it has low X-ray absorption due to its proton number of 4.

Legislation varies in different countries; however, a typical figure for the maximum radiation leakage from an X-ray tube housing at 1 meter distance from the tube, with collimators closed, is 1 mGy per hour when the tube is operating at its maximum factors.

The tube housing is earthed to provide shock proofing and contains mineral oil surrounding the insert to electrically insulate it and aid cooling. Expansion bellows within the tube housing allows expansion of the oil when the X-ray tube heats up during use.

VACUUM ENVELOPE

In order for the X-ray tube to operate, the anode and cathode need to be contained in a vacuum;

this vacuum is contained within the tube envelope. The envelope needs to be strong enough to support the anode and cathode assemblies, provide electrical insulation between the two and maintain the vacuum. The tube vacuum envelope is generally made of glass although some high-power tube envelopes are made of metal or ceramic.

Glass tube envelopes are made of borosilicate glass, which provides the required strength, low coefficient of thermal expansion and electrical insulation. Metal and combined metal with ceramic insulation are alternative methods of construction with the advantages of greater strength and mechanical stability compared to previous tubes made of glass; heat dissipation is also improved.

The X-ray window is a portion of the tube envelope which is thinner than the rest of the structure to allow X-ray output from the tube, minimising radiation absorption.

The wire penetrating the glass seals at the end of the tube is known as Dumet wire, a copper-coated alloy of nickel and iron that has the same coefficient of expansion as the glass.

FILAMENT ASSEMBLY

The filament is the source of electrons used in the production of X-rays. Electron production occurs when the filament is heated to around 2000 °C, this is achieved by passing a current through the filament. The temperature of the filament determines the number of electrons produced and is controlled by the milliamperes (mA) selected by the operator. The filament assembly is constructed as an electromagnetic lens so that it focusses the accelerated electrons to a small area of the anode – the focal spot.

There are usually two filaments: a small one with low output for better geometric resolution and a larger filament for higher output capacity, with wire diameters of 0.22 mm and 0.3 mm diameter, respectively. The filament is constructed as a spiral, with dimensions calculated to maximise the even density of the electrons produced. An alternative electron source is the flat emitter filament instead of a helix. This is used for some modern mammography tubes and

allows a better X-ray intensity distribution than with the helix, thus improving image quality.

The filament is generally made of tungsten as it is:

- dense
- hard
- relatively easy to work
- a good thermionic emitter

and has:

- low vapour pressure
- a high melting temperature (3410 °C).

Tungsten's low coefficient of linear thermal expansion ensures the dimensions change little when it is heated, and the low vapour pressure ensures little tungsten is vaporised. This is important because, when deposited on the inside of the glass tube, tungsten reduces output and increases the possibility of arcing, causing severe damage to the tube. The addition of between 1% and 2% thorium to the tungsten improves thermionic emission.

FILAMENT WIRE ARRANGEMENTS

The filaments are mounted in a focussing cup, the purpose of which is to focus the electrons produced by the filament onto the focal spot of the anode. This is achieved using electrostatic focussing.

The arrangement of the two helixes depends on the tube type and different manufacturers' tubes vary as well in the form of their focussing cup. There are general differences, which are sometimes expressed in the tube names. Siemens, for example, have Pantix tubes where both filaments are mounted parallel, or there is just one single filament; Biangulix, where both filaments are in-line; and finally a specialist tube, Megalix, with either two parallel helixes or with three – two in-line and the third parallel. In tubes with two parallel filaments both electron beams are focussed on the same area of the anode; where the filaments are in-line they are focussed on different areas of the anode.

THE FOCUSSING CUP

The filament is set centrally in a slot machined into a metal focussing cup: the cathode cup.

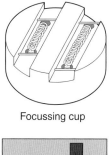

Focussing cup

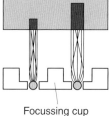

Focussing cup

Figure 8.3 Function of a focussing cup.

The shape of the cup, along with the electrostatic forces, prevents the electron beam fanning out, concentrating it on the focal spot of the anode (Fig. 8.3).

This design is called an electronic lens system with a resulting focal spot width that depends upon:

- the diameter of the filament helix
- the length of the filament helix
- the width of the cathode cup slot
- the depth of the filament in the cathode cup slot.

Cathode cups are typically manufactured from molybdenum, nickel or an iron alloy to ensure dimensional stability during use when the assembly becomes hot.

A separate filament transformer in the high-tension tank separates the primary low voltage side from the secondary high tension (HT) side of the transformer. The HT is connected to a common lead for both filaments and the focussing cup. Both filaments and focussing cup make-up the cathode and have negative polarity.

When the X-ray set is turned on the filament is supplied with a lower than operating current to heat the filament and prepare it for the higher current needed during exposure. This produces a cloud of electrons around the filament.

The electrostatic field limits the number of electrons produced at the filament, thereby limiting the maximum tube current possible; this is called the 'space charge effect'. As the tube voltage increases, the tube current increases up to a point when all the electrons in the space charge have been used up and the tube is then said to have reached saturation current.

GRID-CONTROLLED X-RAY TUBES

Specialised X-ray tubes used in capacitor discharge mobiles, cine radiography and some angiography units, where there is a need to provide rapid switching, utilise grid control of the exposure.

Normally, the focussing cup is kept at the same negative potential as the filament. In a grid-controlled tube the focussing cup may be negatively charged in comparison to the filament and so the voltage is large enough to prevent the flow of electrons from the filament to the anode. The voltage applied between the focussing cup and filament acts as a switch to turn the tube current on and off. This is known as secondary switching, as opposed to the primary switching.

THE ANODE

Original X-ray tubes were designed with a tungsten anode set in a block of copper. The tungsten produces the X-rays and the copper carries the heat away from the tungsten. This design limits the X-ray output as the rise in temperature would eventually lead to melting of the tungsten. Stationary anode designs are still used in low-output applications, such as dental radiography, as they are simpler to construct, robust and cheaper.

In 1929 Bouwers at Phillips produced the first commercial rotating anode tube, known as the Rotalix. Here the anode was a rotating disc where the area bombarded by the filament electrons – the focal spot – became a focal track with a much larger surface area and volume and with a correspondingly larger heat capacity.

The anode is the positive terminal of the X-ray tube; it serves to conduct the tube current, provide support of the target and provides a means of dissipating the heat away from the target. X-rays are produced by the rapid deceleration of fast moving electrons and tungsten is used as the material of choice for the combination of its properties.

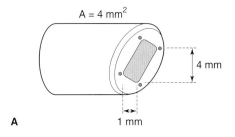

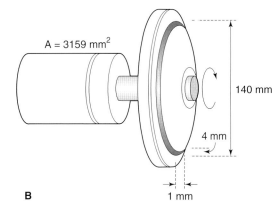

Figure 8.4 Stationary anode.

Properties of tungsten

- Proton (atomic) number 74 – the higher the proton number of the target the greater the amount of radiation that will be produced for a given tube voltage and current.
- High melting point – tungsten's melting point of around 3400 °C means it can withstand the high temperatures involved without melting and with little distortion.
- Electrical conductivity – the anode is required to conduct the tube current.
- Thermal conductivity – the target needs to dissipate the large amounts of heat produced.

These stationary anodes are found in basic X-ray tubes with low power requirements such as those in dental equipment, mobile C-arm units for fluoroscopy and low-load radiography. The low power requirements of these applications results in much lower heat generation and these requirements can be met using a stationary anode tube.

STATIONARY ANODE

The stationary anode tube has a compound anode, which consists of a tungsten target set in a block of copper, the X-rays are produced in the tungsten and the copper conducts the heat away from the target (Fig. 8.4A).

The anode block consists of a solid copper rod expanded at one end with an inclined target face end, the angle of inclination determines the focal spot size.

In a stationary anode the X-rays are produced in a small area of the anode (approx. 4 mm^2) (Fig. 8.4B), which causes the temperature to rise rapidly; this limits the loading available before damage occurs.

ROTATING ANODE

The rotating anode X-ray tube is a design improvement to allow greater tube loading (Fig. 8.5). The anode is formed as a disc mounted on a rotating stem with the rotational power provided by an induction motor system.

The anode disc is between 55 mm and 100 mm in diameter and 7 mm thick, machined to high tolerance to prevent imbalance and wobble. The disc will experience rotational speeds up to 10 000 rpm and temperatures of 2000 °C. The disc has a tungsten–rhenium target area. The addition of a small quantity (5–10%) of rhenium prevents crazing of the anode surface.

In a rotating anode the target is formed as a track near the perimeter of a rotating disc. With a typical anode disc diameter of 9 cm, the target track area is approximately 1200 mm^2. If the exposure time is long enough and the speed of rotation of the anode disc fast enough, the heating effect is spread over a much larger area and with a corresponding lower increase in temperature. Disc rotation speeds vary between 3000 rpm up to 10 000 rpm.

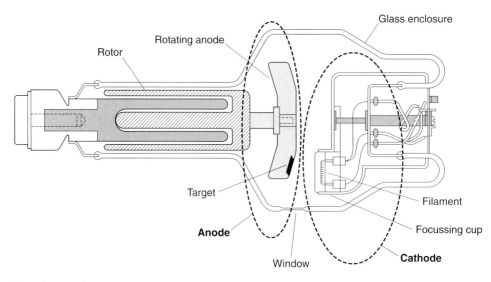

Figure 8.5 Rotating anode.

TYPES OF ANODE DISC

A basic anode disc is constructed of a tungsten disc mounted on a rotating stem; however, there are modifications of this basic arrangement designed to increase the heat capacity of the anode. In order to increase this heat capacity there are a variety of compound anode designs available; for example the tungsten track may be sintered onto a molybdenum disc (as molybdenum has a higher heat capacity), which in turn may be backed by a graphite layer providing an increase in heat capacity and a lowering of weight.

Stress relieved anodes have a series of radiating slits cut in the anode to reduce the effects of thermal expansion, permitting higher loading.

THE LINE FOCUS PRINCIPLE

In order to obtain an X-ray image with the least penumbra the X-rays must be seen to be emanating from as small a point as possible; in theory a point source will provide an image with no penumbra (Fig. 8.6).

However, the area of the anode from which the X-rays emanate is of definite size, determined by the filament size and the electronic lens system. In both stationary and rotating anode X-ray tubes the face of the anode is not parallel to the filament but at an angle. This ensures maximum efficiency from the tube and reduces penumbra further.

When visualised from a point at the centre of the X-ray beam, the area from which the X-rays emanate (the apparent focal spot size) appears smaller than it actually is (real focal spot size).

MEASURING THE FOCAL SPOT SIZE

This international standard (BS EN 60336:2005)[1] applies to focal spots in medical diagnostic X-ray tube assemblies. Methods for evaluating focal spot characteristics operating at X-ray tube voltages up to and including 200 kV are provided in this document.

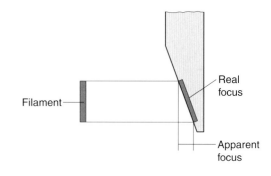

Figure 8.6 Line focus principle.

THE ANODE HEEL EFFECT

The X-ray beam is not uniform over its field – there is a gradual decrease in radiation towards the anode end of the tube. As X-radiation is emitted from the target area in a conical shape, measurements have determined that the intensity in the direction of the anode is lower (over and above the difference caused by the inverse square law) than the intensity in the direction of the cathode. The fact that the intensities vary in such a manner causes visible differences in the density produced on the radiographs. This phenomenon is called the 'heel effect' (Fig. 8.7).

The decreased intensity results from emission, which is nearly parallel to the angled target where there is increasing absorption of the X-ray photons by the target itself. This phenomenon is readily apparent in rotating anode tubes because they utilize steeply angled anodes of generally 17 degrees

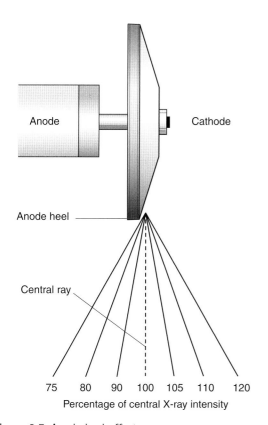

Figure 8.7 Anode heel effect.

or less. Generally, the steeper the anode, the more severe or noticeable the heel effect becomes.

THE STATOR ASSEMBLY

The anode disc needs to rotate at high speed and this is achieved by attaching the anode via a stem to a large copper rotor, which forms the armature of a motor. The target disc, or rotor, is mounted on a shaft, the stem extending from a rotor body which can spin on internal bearings on the rotor shaft. This rotor shaft extends through the end of the insert to the outside of the insert vacuum for connection to the anode wire, and also is the mounting point for the insert inside the housing.

The rotor consists of a copper cylinder and rests in ball bearings for smooth movement. The bearings cannot be lubricated with ordinary grease because it would affect the vacuum and the high-tension characteristics of the tube. Soft metals such as lead and silver are applied to separate the ball bearings and the running surfaces, in order to prevent the possibility of 'jamming' in the vacuum. This form of lubrication limits the lifetime of the bearings in the X-ray tube to about 1000 hours.

The exposure switch controls the rotation. The anode only rotates when radiation is required and is braked immediately afterwards. The high inertia of the heavy metal disc leads to some delay in the rotor reaching operational speed. The delay is up to 2.5 seconds, depending on the type of starting device and the anode. An interlock ensures exposure can only take place after the anode has reached its final speed.

The heat of the anode should be prevented from reaching the stator arrangement. The stem is designed to limit the transfer of heat to the rotor assembly; molybdenum is used as it has lower thermal conductivity than tungsten and is made as thin as possible to reduce heat conduction towards the bearings (Fig. 8.8).

THE STATOR

The stator consists of several windings, which are equally spread out around the neck of the tube. When connected to the appropriate electrical

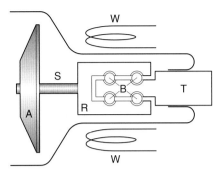

Figure 8.8 Stator assembly. A Anode disk, B Ball bearings, R Rotor assembly, S Anode stem, T Rotor support, W Stator windings.

circuit they induce a rotating electromagnetic field, which interacts with the rotor, causing it to rotate synchronously.

THE X-RAY PORT AND COLLIMATOR

X-ray tube assemblies are designed to produce radiation and confine its exit from the assembly via a well-defined portal in the lead lining.

The glass in this area of the tube envelope is ground as thin as practically possible to minimise absorption and this area of the envelope is sited close to the exit portal of the tube housing, separated from it by the cooling oil. At this point there is a window in the housing made of a low beryllium or similar low X-ray absorptive material, which is sealed to the housing to prevent loss of the oil and ingress of air. Beryllium is used due to its low mass absorption coefficient.

BEAM FILTRATION

- Inherent filtration – the aluminium equivalence in millimetres of the amount of filtration inherent within the X-ray tube assembly.
- Total filtration – the aluminium equivalence of the tube, housing and collimator and associated filters.

The total filtration of an X-ray tube assembly (without any additional added filtration) should be not less than 2.5 mm aluminium equivalent.[2] On a number of systems, a facility for introducing additional added filtration into the beam (spectral filtering) is provided within the collimator assembly. The additional added filtration may be aluminium, copper or tantalum and may be introduced manually or automatically.

Further added filtration can be particularly useful in reducing patient dose during high dose procedures, such as interventional examinations.

TUBE RATING

The major cause of tube failure can be related to the production of heat and the ability of the tube and housing to remove the heat. Tube rating charts are provided by the manufacturer to indicate safe operating conditions for the tube. The rating charts indicate the maximum exposure times possible at set kV and mA values, these charts need to be used in conjunction with anode cooling charts, which indicate the cooling time required by the anode after an exposure or series of exposures.

ANODE COOLING

The amount of heat stored in the anode at the time of exposure is measured in 'heat units' (HU) and this is calculated as a product of exposure (in kV) multiplied by the tube current and time (mA s).

As an example, a typical chest exposure of 90 kV at 2 mA s produces 180 HU, which requires only a short cooling time; however, fluoroscopy at 90 kV for 3 min at 2 mA (360 mA s) produces 32 400 HU and requires a cooling time of over 5 min. Cooling time is exponential with time and depends upon the temperature of the surrounding materials and requires a correction factor for different voltage waveforms. Tube housings also have cooling charts and these are used in a similar manner to the anode cooling charts.

HEAT PATHWAYS IN A TYPICAL ROTATING ANODE X-RAY TUBE ASSEMBLY

In an X-ray tube the point of maximum heat production is at the focal track or focal spot on the anode. The heat produced in this region has to pass from the tube to the surrounding air in order for the tube not to overheat. The heat produced at the focal spot is carried away by radiation to the glass or metal tube envelope and conduction to the body of the anode where radiation to the metal tube envelope occurs. Conduction away from the anode body is minimised by the stem construction and material to prevent damage to the motor bearings.

From the glass envelope heat is dispersed by conduction to the surrounding oil to the tube casing and thereby to the surrounding air by conduction.

The oil in some heavy-duty applications is cooled by a pumped circulation system with a forced air-cooling arrangement; some tube housings are cooled by a forced air fan arrangement to carry the hot air away more quickly.

Most tube housings include a bellows arrangement to allow for the expansion of the oil as its temperature rises in order to prevent damage to the insert or housing. This bellows arrangement includes a micro-switch interlock to prevent further exposures after the oil has expanded by a preset amount, indicating the temperature has risen to a level which could damage the tube.

References

1. British Standards Institute. X-ray tube assemblies for medical diagnosis. Characteristics of focal spots. BS EN 60336:1995.
2. Health and Safety Executive. Guidance on Equipment used for medical exposure. HSG 226. London: HMSO; 2002.

Recommended reading

Bushong S. Radiologic science for technologists: physics, biology and protection, 8th edn. Elsevier: Mosby; 2004.

A modern and up-to-date text from America; good clear descriptions, illustrated well and in good detail.

Forster E. Equipment for diagnostic radiography. Lancaster, UK: Kluwer Academic; 1985.

A very readable text covering the basis of most syllabi.

Meredith J, Massey J. Fundamental physics of radiology. Oxford: Butterworth-Heinemann; 1984.

A 'classic' text still popular after 30 years explores diagnostic and therapy physics.

Stockley S. A Manual of Radiographic Equipment. Edinburgh: Churchill Livingstone; 1986.

A popular text with students, clear diagrams outlining basic ideas.

Wilks R. Principles of radiological physics. Edinburgh: Churchill Livingstone; 1987.

A detailed text with thorough explanations of complex ideas with easy to follow mathematics descriptions.

Chapter **9**

Production of X-rays

Patti Ward

KEY POINTS

- X-rays are produced when high-speed projectile electrons collide with the X-ray tube target.
- The kinetic energy of projectile electrons transfers to target atoms. Approximately 99% of the energy converts into heat and only about 1% converts into X-rays.
- The production of X-rays comes from two interactions: bremsstrahlung and characteristic.
- A bremsstrahlung interaction involves projectile electrons that emit radiation as they slow down when passing close to the nucleus of target atoms.
- Most diagnostic X-rays are the product of bremsstrahlung interactions.
- A characteristic interaction involves the emission of radiation following a collision between projectile electrons and the orbital electrons of target atoms.
- X-ray beam quality and quantity are affected by the target material, beam filtration, distance, and prime exposure factors (kV_p, mA, and exposure time).
- The target material affects both the quality and quantity of the X-ray beam. Tungsten is the standard target material due to its high proton number.
- Beam filtration affects the beam's quality and quantity by removing low energy X-rays.
- The inverse square law governs the relationship between X-ray quantity and distance.
- The quality of radiation in an X-ray beam is the penetrating ability of the beam.

- The quantity of radiation in an X-ray beam is the number of photons in the beam.
- Peak kilovoltage (kV_p) controls the quality of the beam. As kV_p increases, X-rays are more penetrating and as kV_p decreases, X-rays become less penetrating.
- kV_p affects the quantity of X-rays produced. An increase in kV_p rapidly increases the number of X-ray photons and a decrease in kV_p rapidly decreases the number of X-rays. The amount of radiation produced is proportional to the square of the ratio of the kV_p.
- 15% rule: a 15% increase in kV_p doubles radiographic density; a 15% decrease in kV_p halves radiographic density.
- mAs (product of mA and exposure time) controls the quantity of X-rays produced.
- The relationship between the quantity of X-rays and mAs is directly proportional.
- Reciprocity law: any combinations of mA and time that give the same mAs will result in the same quantity of X-ray photons.

INTRODUCTION

Diagnostic X-rays are produced in the target of the anode when high-energy projectile electrons are rapidly decelerated. Diagnostic X-ray imaging equipment provides the means for practitioners to control the quality and quantity of the X-ray beam. Consequently, it is important to understand the process of X-ray production and the factors that influence the characteristics of the beam. Practitioners familiar with the concepts and factors that influence quality and quantity are better able to control exposure factors to produce optimal radiographic images while minimizing patient dose.

ELECTRON PRODUCTION

Four conditions are necessary for the production of diagnostic X-rays:

1. A source of free electrons.
2. A means to provide the electrons with high kinetic (motion) energy.
3. A method to concentrate the electrons into a beam.
4. A suitable material to rapidly decelerate the electrons.

In the X-ray tube, the purpose of the filament is to provide the free electrons necessary for X-ray production. As the rotor is activated the current passing through the filament heats to the point where electrons boil off. This process is referred to as thermionic emission. At this point, a space charge (cloud of electrons) forms around the filament. The focussing cup temporarily concentrates the free electrons and helps form them into a beam.

When the exposure begins, the primary circuit closes and a high voltage is applied across the anode (positively charged) and cathode (negatively charged). This causes electrons to stream towards the anode at a high rate of speed. The potential energy of each electron is one kiloelectron volt (keV) of energy for each kilovolt (kV) of voltage set for the exposure. Electrons (sometimes called projectile electrons) that travel from the cathode to anode make up the tube current.

TARGET INTERACTIONS

When the high-speed projectile electrons collide with the X-ray tube target they interact with the orbital electrons or the nuclear field of the target atoms. Kinetic energy transferred from the projectile electrons to the target atoms converts into heat or X-rays. When projectile electrons strike outer target shell electrons it puts them in an excited state and as a result, infrared (heat) radiation is emitted. Approximately 99% of the energy of projectile electrons converts into heat. Only about 1% of the energy converts into X-ray photons. Two types of interaction produce X-ray photons: bremsstrahlung interactions and characteristic interactions.

BREMSSTRAHLUNG INTERACTIONS

Bremsstrahlung in German means 'to brake radiation' or braking radiation. Bremsstrahlung target interaction occurs when projectile electrons pass

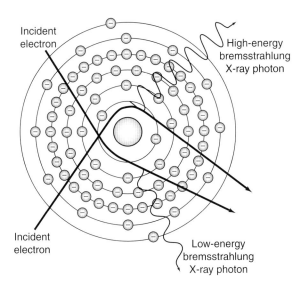

Figure 9.1 Production of bremsstrahlung radiation.

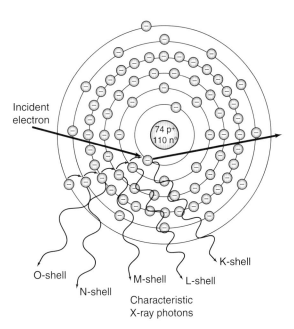

Figure 9.2 Production of characteristic radiation.

by outer shell electrons of target atoms and interact with the force field of the nucleus of the atom. Because atomic nuclei are positively charged and electrons are negatively charged, there is a mutual attraction between them. The nuclear force field causes the entering electron to slow down (or brake) and change direction. The loss of kinetic energy that occurs when a projectile electron slows down is emitted as an X-ray photon. These X-ray photons are known as bremsstrahlung photons or brems radiation (Fig. 9.1). In the diagnostic range, approximately 85% of X-ray emissions are the result of bremsstrahlung interactions.

CHARACTERISTIC INTERACTIONS

Characteristic target interaction occurs when projectile electrons interact with inner shell electrons of target atoms. Recall that orbital electrons within an atom have a specific binding energy. The binding energy, based on the size of the atom and the shell in which the electron is located, is the energy that would be required to remove the electron from the atom.

Characteristic radiation is produced when projectile electrons with sufficient kinetic energy eject an inner orbital electron (Fig. 9.2). When this

happens, the atom becomes unstable and temporarily ionised because of the missing electron. An electron from an outer shell instantly fills the void created by the missing electron and an X-ray photon is emitted. This process continues until the atom is stable. The energy of the emitted X-ray photon is equal to the difference between the binding energy of the two involved orbital electrons. Accordingly, each X-ray photon has a specific energy level. This explains why this type of emission is called characteristic radiation. The energy emitted is characteristic of the target element and the involved shells.

Higher energy X-ray photons result with target materials of a higher proton number and interactions that involve the ejection of inner shell electrons. Each target element emits characteristic radiation of a given energy. For example, the K shell binding energy for tungsten is 69.5 keV. Only projectile electrons with energies greater than the K shell binding energy are able to eject K shell electrons. Accordingly, K shell characteristic X-rays are only produced when the applied voltage exceeds $69.5 \, kV_p$. In comparison, the characteristic radiation of a molybdenum target (often used for mammography) is very different. The K shell binding energy for molybdenum is 20 keV, so K shell characteristic X-rays are produced when the applied voltage exceeds $20\,kV_p$.

With a tungsten target, only K shell interactions result in X-rays of sufficient energy to be beneficial in diagnostic radiography. All other characteristic radiation has very low energy and falls outside the useful diagnostic range. Approximately 15% of X-ray emissions are the result of characteristic interactions.

EMISSION SPECTRUM

The emission spectrum is a graphic representation of the number of X-rays plotted against the energy of the radiation, which is measured in kiloelectron volts (keV) (Fig. 9.3). The emission spectrum for bremsstrahlung radiation is continuous because bremsstrahlung X-rays include a range of energies. The emission spectrum for characteristic radiation is discrete because characteristic X-rays consist of predictable energies that are specific to the target element.

CONTINUOUS X-RAY SPECTRUM

Bremsstrahlung radiation is graphically illustrated as a continuous spectrum. The energy of a bremsstrahlung photon is the difference between the entering and exiting kinetic energy of the projectile electron. As a result, there is a continuous range of X-ray energies from zero to the maximum established by the potential difference across the X-ray tube. Maximum energy is realised if all the kinetic energy of an electron is converted into a single

X-ray photon. The maximum photon energy, determined by the maximum voltage, is the kilovolt peak (kV_p). For example, if the potential difference across the X-ray tube were $90\,kV_p$, an electron accelerated across the tube would attain a kinetic energy of 90 keV as it interacted with the target. If the electron transferred all of its energy, the energy of the X-ray photon would be 90 keV. The maximum photon energy is dependent on the potential difference across the tube (kV_p), regardless of the target material.

The size and shape of the emission spectrum reflects the quality and quantity of the X-ray beam. While the relative shape of the emission spectrum remains the same, its location along the horizontal axis can vary. Ranges located more towards the right represent X-ray beams of higher energy or quality. Graphically, the area under the curve represents the total number of X-rays emitted. A larger area represents X-ray beams with higher intensity or quantity. The greatest number of X-rays have approximately one-third to one-half of the maximum energy.[1]

DISCRETE X-RAY SPECTRUM

Characteristic radiation is graphically illustrated in the form of a line spectrum. Remember that the energy of a characteristic photon depends on the differences between the electron binding energies of a particular target material. As a result, the spectrum produced by characteristic X-rays is referred to as discrete or distinct. For example, there are only 15 specific energy levels of characteristic X-rays from tungsten: five from interactions at the K shell, four from interactions at the L shell, and the remainder from interactions at lower energy outer shells. In tungsten, only characteristic X-rays produced from the five K shell interactions are of sufficient energy to be of diagnostic value. The number of photons produced at each characteristic energy level is different because the likelihood for filling a K shell void varies from shell to shell. Often, the five energy levels are represented on the emission spectrum as a single line. As illustrated in Figure 9.3, the vertical line at 69 keV represents the characteristic K X-rays of tungsten.

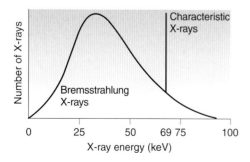

Figure 9.3 X-ray emission spectrum.

X-RAY QUALITY AND QUANTITY

The quality of radiation in an X-ray beam is the penetrating ability of the beam. The quantity of radiation in an X-ray beam is the number of photons in the beam. The terms exposure and intensity may also be used to describe quantity.

> Basic factors influencing the quality and quantity of the X-ray beam:
>
> - Target material
> - Beam filtration
> - Distance
> - Prime exposure factors

While practitioners have little control over the selection of the target material and limited options for the use of added beam filtration, it is valuable to understand how the target material and beam filtration affect the quality and quantity of the X-ray beam. Practitioners are able to control distance and prime exposure factors. Consequently, it is essential to understand how these factors influence the quality and quantity of the X-ray beam (Table 9.1).

TARGET MATERIAL

The proton number of the target material affects both the quality and quantity of the X-ray beam.

Table 9.1 Summary of factors affecting X-ray quality and quantity

Factors affecting X-ray quality	Factors affecting X-ray quantity
Target material	Target material
Beam filtration	Beam filtration
kV_p	Distance
	kV_p
	mA s

kV_p, kilovolt (peak); mA s, milliamp-second

As mentioned previously, tungsten is the chief target material used in diagnostic radiography due to its high proton number (Z) of 74. A target material with a higher proton number results in increased production of bremsstrahlung radiation. Bremsstrahlung production is also more efficient because more high energy X-rays are produced relative to low energy X-rays. A target material with a higher proton number also results in the production of characteristic radiation of higher energy. In contrast, the molybdenum ($Z = 42$) and rhodium ($Z = 45$) targets used for mammography have much lower proton numbers. These targets produce the lower energy radiation necessary for this imaging application.

BEAM FILTRATION

Filtration of the X-ray beam affects both the quality and quantity. Beam filtration changes the characteristics of the beam by removing ineffective low energy X-rays. Inherent and added filtration reduces the quantity and increases the average energy of the X-ray beam. The result is reduced patient skin dose.

DISTANCE

The distance of the anode from the image receptor (source–image distance, SID) affects the quantity of X-rays photons (see p. 91). The inverse square law governs the relationship between the quantity of X-ray photons and the distance from the target to the image receptor. The quantity of X-ray photons at the image receptor is inversely proportional to the square of the distance from the source (see p. 91). For example, if the SID is reduced by one-half, the number of X-ray photons quadruples.

PRIME EXPOSURE FACTORS

The prime exposure factors include kV_p, mA, and exposure time. The kV_p affects both the quality and quantity, while mA and exposure time affect the quantity of the X-ray beam.

Kilovoltage (kV$_p$)

The kilovoltage peak (kV$_p$) set by the practitioner determines the voltage or potential difference applied across the cathode and anode during the exposure. This setting affects both the quality and quantity of the X-ray beam. As mentioned earlier, the kV$_p$ setting controls the speed of the electrons travelling from the cathode to the anode. An increase in kV$_p$ causes greater repulsion of electrons from the cathode and greater attraction of electrons towards the anode. This increased speed means projectile electrons possess greater potential energy.

Changes in kV$_p$ affect the production of bremsstrahlung radiation, which influences both the quality and quantity of photons in the X-ray beam. An increase in kV$_p$ results in higher quality X-ray photons with a higher average energy and more penetrating ability. Keep in mind that the maximum energy of an X-ray beam remains equal to the kV$_p$ setting. With an increase in kV$_p$ there is also an increase in the quantity of X-ray photons at all energy levels. However, the increase is relatively greater for high energy X-rays than for low energy X-rays. The emission spectrum in Figure 9.4 illustrates how the area under the curve increases and shifts to the right as kV$_p$ is increased.

Changes in kV$_p$ also affect the production of characteristic radiation, which influences the quantity but not the quality of photons in the X-ray beam. Recall that no characteristic radiation is produced if the kV$_p$ is less than the binding energy of the K shell electrons. For example, no characteristic radiation is produced when the applied voltage is less than 69.5 kV$_p$ for a tungsten target because

the binding energy of the K shell is 69.5 keV. However, the quantity of characteristic radiation increases when the kV$_p$ exceeds the K shell binding energy. The increase is typically proportional to the difference between the kV$_p$ and the binding energy.

Milliamperage (mA) and exposure time

The milliamperage (mA) set by the practitioner determines the quantity of electrons in the tube current. The relationship between mA and the quantity of X-ray photons produced is directly proportional. As mA is increased, the quantity of electrons in the tube current and the number of X-ray photons increases proportionally. As mA is decreased, the quantity of electrons in the tube current and the number of X-ray photons decreases proportionally.

The exposure time set by the practitioner controls the length of time electrons are permitted to travel from the cathode to the anode. The relationship between exposure time and the quantity of X-ray photons produced is directly proportional. As exposure time is increased, the quantity of electrons and the number of X-ray photons increases proportionally. As exposure time is decreased, the quantity of electrons and the number of X-ray photons decreases proportionally.

In sum, the quantity of electrons that travel from the cathode to the anode and the quantity of X-ray photons produced are directly proportional to the mA and exposure time. The milliampere-second (mA s) is the product of mA and exposure time. The mA s affects only the quantity of photons in the X-ray beam; it does not affect the quality or energy of the X-ray photons.

Figure 9.4 Changes in the emission spectrum due to increased kV$_p$.

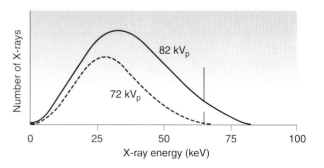

EXPOSURE MANIPULATION

Exposure manipulation includes those variables that practitioners most often employ to manage the quality and quantity of the X-ray beam. Distance, kV_p, and mAs are the primary factors considered here.

DISTANCE

As stated previously, the inverse square law governs the relationship between X-ray quantity and distance. The formula for the inverse square law is effective when the intensity of the exposure in sieverts is known. A practical alternative is to manipulate mAs to compensate for changes in distance. The square law (a derivative of the inverse square law) calls for a change in mAs by the factor of SID^2.

To maintain the same quantity of X-ray photons when the SID is altered:

$$New\ mAs = Old\ mAs \times \frac{New\ SID^2}{Old\ SID^2}$$

PEAK KILOVOLTAGE (kV_p)

The kV_p controls the energy or quality of the X-rays produced at the anode and as such determines the penetrating ability of the X-rays produced. As kV_p increases, X-rays are more penetrating and as kV_p decreases, X-rays become less penetrating. The penetrating ability of X-rays also has some bearing on the number of X-rays exiting the patient. If the penetrating ability of X-ray photons is insufficient, the quantity of photons is irrelevant. In other words, increased mAs cannot compensate for inadequate kV_p.

kV_p also affects the quantity of radiation. As kV_p increases, the number of X-ray photons rapidly increases, and as kV_p decreases, the number of X-ray photons rapidly decreases. Unlike with mAs the relationship is not directly proportional. The amount of radiation produced is proportional to the square of the ratio of the kV_p. For example, if kV_p is doubled, the number of X-ray photons quadruples.

In practice, using kV_p to manage the quantity of X-ray photons is unrealistic. Again, because kV_p affects the penetrating ability of the X-ray beam, it is important to select the optimal kV_p for a given part. However, when it is necessary to vary kV_p the 15% rule is helpful. The 15% rule states that a 15% increase in kV_p will double radiographic density, whereas a 15% decrease in kV_p will halve radiographic density.

MILLIAMPERE–SECOND (mAs)

Milliampere-seconds controls the number of electrons passing from the cathode to the anode and as such controls the quantity of X-ray photons produced at the anode. There is a directly proportional relationship between the quantity of X-ray photons produced and the mAs. In other words, as mAs is increased, the number of X-ray photons increases by the same proportion and as mAs is decreased, the number of X-ray photons decreases proportionally. The law of reciprocity states that any combinations of mA and time that give the same mAs will produce the same number of X-ray photons.

References

1. Graham DT, Cloke P. Principles of radiological physics, 4th edn. Edinburgh: Churchill Livingstone; 2003:273–287.

Recommended reading

Bushong S. Radiologic science for technologists: physics, biology, and protection, 8th edn. Mosby: St Louis; 2004: 147–160.

This provides clear descriptions on the production of X-rays, with good diagrams.

Fauber TL. Radiographic imaging and exposure, 2nd edn. St Louis: Mosby; 2004:19–32.

This text gives clear descriptions with practical tips on the effects of exposure on a radiographic image, with images to support the written content.

Chapter **10**

Effects of radiation

Sally Perry

KEY POINTS

- A beam of X-ray photons is gradually attenuated as it passes through matter by being absorbed and scattered.
- The most important interactions that result in attenuation are photoelectric absorption and Compton scatter.
- Photoelectric absorption is more likely to occur in dense materials with atoms of high proton number.
- Photoelectric absorption is responsible for differential absorption in the body's tissues that results in a radiographic image.
- Compton scatter occurs alongside photoelectric absorption and is the dominant process above a setting of 75 kV.
- Compton-scattered X-ray photons may reach the image receptor to result in image degradation.
- Attenuation in the body's tissues with the transfer of energy and subsequent ionisation may result in deterministic or stochastic biological effects.
- Radiation protection regulations aim to reduce the risk of stochastic effects and avoid deterministic effects.
- Absorbed dose is the amount of energy deposited in the body and is measured in units of gray (Gy).
- Effective dose measured in sieverts (Sv) takes into account different types of radiation and their damaging potential on different tissues and organs in the body.

- X-ray photons produce fluorescence in phosphors, a property utilised in some image recording systems.

INTRODUCTION

The beam of X-ray photons produced from the X-ray tube will lose its energy by interacting with atoms as it passes through various materials. These include the wall of the X-ray tube and its surrounding oil, the added filter, the collimators, the air, the exposed part of the patient, the couch, the image receptor and the floor. X-ray photons travel through air at virtually the velocity of light $(3 \times 10^8 \, \text{m s}^{-1})$ so they interact with these materials and transfer their energy almost instantaneously. Some of this energy will be absorbed in the various materials but some will also be scattered in different directions from the primary beam and will lose energy by interacting with other adjacent structures, such as parts of the patient not in the primary beam, the walls of the room and the lead-glass screen.

ATTENUATION

As each X-ray photon can be considered as a tiny packet of energy, the beam of X-ray photons carries energy from the X-ray target into the matter through which it passes. On penetrating matter, X-ray photons transfer energy by interacting with its atoms; this transfer of energy is called *attenuation*. The beam of X-ray photons is attenuated differently in various materials: in general, the denser the matter, the greater the attenuation. Denser materials include metals (particularly lead) and bone.

Attenuation is partly due to some X-ray photons being totally *absorbed* and partly to the energy of some X-ray photons being partially absorbed while the remainder is *scattered* in various directions (Fig. 10.1). Some X-ray photons are *transmitted* through the material unchanged, without interacting with any atoms.

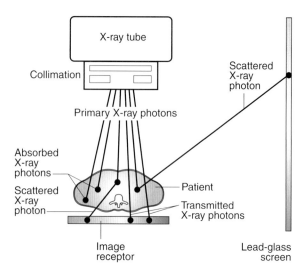

Figure 10.1 Attenuation of X-ray photons.

Attenuation = Absorption + Scatter

When a beam of X-ray photons passes through the body, the difference between parts through which X-ray photons are transmitted and those where they are absorbed results in an image.

ATTENUATION AND THICKNESS OF MATERIAL

The number of X-ray photons transmitted compared to the number attenuated in any particular type of material depends on the thickness of that material. In general, the thicker the material, the greater the attenuation. However, it is not a linear relationship where the same numbers of X-ray photons are attenuated in an equal thickness of material, but an equal percentage is attenuated in equal thickness. For example, 20% of photons may be attenuated in the first centimetre of material, then 20% of what is left in the second centimetre, and 20% of the remainder in the third centimetre, etc. This is called an exponential relationship and the percentage attenuated in each thickness is known as the linear attenuation coefficient (LAC or µ) for the specific material. This relationship is used in practice during quality control checks on X-ray equipment to measure the half value thickness/layer (HVT or HVL) of an X-ray unit. The measurement gives the thickness of aluminium that will attenuate 50% of the X-ray photons at a specific kV setting. This gives an indication of the penetrating power of the beam: the thicker the aluminium required to attenuate half of the beam, the more penetrating it is and it can be related (using published tables) to the total filtration present in the beam (see pp. 100, 107).

INTERACTION PROCESSES RESULTING IN ATTENUATION

In radiographic imaging there are two important interaction processes in matter that occur alongside each other:

- photoelectric absorption
- Compton scatter.

PHOTOELECTRIC ABSORPTION

Photoelectric (PE) absorption occurs when an X-ray photon interacts with a bound electron, usually in the inner shell of an atom, when its energy exceeds the binding energy of the electron (Fig. 10.2). The atom may be in the patient (an atom of calcium in bone, for example) or it might be an atom of carbon in the carbon-fibre tabletop; or an atom of lead in the lead-glass screen.

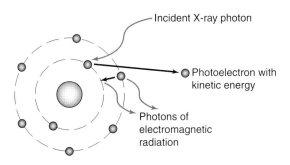

Figure 10.2 Photoelectric absorption within an atom.

The X-ray photon disappears, by transferring all its energy to the bound electron. This energy overcomes the binding energy of the electron, which then escapes the atom as a photoelectron, carrying any extra energy as kinetic energy.

As a result, the atom is *ionised* but will quickly regain stability as electrons rearrange within the atom to restore the original electron configuration, resulting in small bursts of electromagnetic radiation being released. This process is similar to that in the X-ray target following ionisation of target atoms by high-speed electrons to release characteristic radiation. In tissue, where elements have low proton numbers and correspondingly low binding energies, the characteristic radiation energies are extremely low and are usually absorbed within the atom with negligible effect.

FACTORS AFFECTING PHOTOELECTRIC ABSORPTION

An X-ray photon is more likely to undergo photoelectric absorption in dense matter containing atoms of higher proton number. It is also more likely to occur with a bound electron whose binding energy is just below the X-ray photon's energy: this means PE absorption is much more likely to occur in tissue with lower energy X-ray photons of less than 25 keV.

THE IMPLICATIONS OF PHOTOELECTRIC ABSORPTION IN PRACTICE:

The main implications to consider are:

- the radiographic image
- X-ray tube filtration
- use of contrast media
- shielding
- absorption edges
- radiation dose.

The radiographic image

Human tissue can be divided into two basic types: bone and soft tissue. There is also air within the body; for example in the lungs, and there may be pockets of air in the stomach and bowel.

Bone has a fairly high density and contains atoms of calcium and phosphorus, giving an effective proton number (Z_{eff}) of approximately 12. Soft tissues, such as muscle and fat, are lower in density and contain atoms of lower proton number (particularly carbon, hydrogen and oxygen), giving an effective proton number of approximately 7. Air is primarily nitrogen and oxygen, giving a similar effective proton number to soft tissue, but has very low density (Table 10.1).

All of these elements found in tissue have low binding energies, so typical mean X-ray photon energies of 25 keV used in radiographic imaging (corresponding to a setting of 75 kV; see p. 113) are likely to undergo PE absorption. If all these elements attenuated X-ray photons equally, we would not be able to tell the difference between bone and muscle or bone and air on an X-ray image. But the bone tissue with higher proton number and higher density will experience relatively more PE absorptions – at least eight times more than soft tissue – and air will barely experience any attenuation due to its very low density, leading to what is called *differential absorption*.

On an X-ray image, this is why bones appear white (many PE absorptions), soft tissues appear grey (some PE absorptions) and air appears black (very few PE absorptions).

X-ray tube filtration

In atoms such as aluminium ($Z = 13$), with low K shell binding energies, low X-ray photon energies are preferentially absorbed. The quality of the X-ray beam produced from an X-ray tube is increased by attenuating the low energy X-ray photons in a filter made of aluminium (see p. 100).

Table 10.1   The principal constituents of human tissue[1]

Material	Density (kg m^{-3})	Effective proton number
Bone	1700	12.3
Soft tissue (muscle)	1000	7.6
Soft tissue (fat)	900	6.5
Air	1	7.8

Use of contrast media

When it is necessary to image the walls and movements of soft tissue structures such as the gastrointestinal tract, a high density/high atomic number contrast medium is introduced. When using iodine or barium-based contrast media ($Z = 53$ and 56, respectively) K shell binding energies are much higher compared to the body's tissues, so higher energy X-ray photons are absorbed. This is why higher kV settings are used for contrast examinations.

Shielding

Lead has a very high proton number (82) and is very dense so virtually all X-ray photons are likely to undergo PE absorption in lead. However, a proportion of higher energy photons from the primary X-ray beam will penetrate lead, depending on its thickness. Photons scattered from the primary beam (that have undergone a Compton scatter interaction) will always have lower energy, so lead-glass screens and lead-rubber protective items are designed to prevent the passage of scattered photons.

Absorption edges

Photoelectric absorption is more likely to occur with a bound electron whose binding energy is just below the X-ray photon's energy, so there will be situations where some bound electrons have binding energies higher than those of the interacting X-ray photons. These electrons cannot contribute to the attenuation of the beam by PE absorption. For example, in lead the binding energy of the K shell electrons is 88 keV and of the L shell 15 keV, so a beam produced at 80 kV will not contain any X-ray photons of sufficient energy to interact with the K shell electrons, only those of the L shell and beyond. If the kV is increased to 90, the beam will contain photons of 90 keV able to interact with K shell electrons. This leads to a large increase in photoelectric absorption of the X-ray photons with energy greater than 88 keV and is known as an *absorption edge*. Photons with slightly lower energies than 88 keV are much less likely to be attenuated and therefore more likely to be transmitted. This means shielding materials using lead may be slightly less efficient at attenuating photons of this energy. Some manufacturers promote the use of protective aprons made of a composite of materials to give increased attenuation below the 88 keV absorption edge for lead.

Absorption edges also have significance in materials used for filtration. If lead or another material with a high K shell binding energy was used, in addition to attenuating the low photon energies as required, an undesirable proportion of high photon energies at the absorption edge would be attenuated.

Radiation dose

Photoelectric absorption is greater for lower energy X-ray photons and results in total absorption of the photon energy, increasing the radiation dose to the patient. In general, higher kV settings will result in less photoelectric absorption, reducing patient dose, but should not be so high that differential absorption is decreased to the extent of not producing a diagnostic image.

In mammography, where differential absorption in the breast tissue must be maximized, low kV settings are used to increase PE absorption and the contrast between adjacent structures.

COMPTON SCATTER

Compton scatter is the alternative interaction process that occurs alongside PE absorption: the two cannot be separated or prevented. In an X-ray beam of mean energy 25 keV (i.e. a setting in the region of 75 kV), approximately half of the interactions occurring will be PE absorptions and the other half Compton scatters. Compton scatter may occur when an X-ray photon interacts with a bound electron in an atom whose binding energy is negligible in comparison with the X-ray photon's energy.

Compton-type interactions may occur equally with any electron in any atom within the body – in atoms found in soft tissue and in bone as well as with electrons in higher atomic number atoms such as lead.

The X-ray photon transfers some of its energy to the electron and retains the remainder: the photon may retain virtually all of its initial energy and be very slightly deviated or scattered from its track. This is called forward scatter and occurs more frequently with photons of higher energy. Alternatively, lower energy X-ray photons may be scattered out to the side retaining less energy (side scatter) or backwards retaining least energy (backscatter). Scattered X-ray photons always have less energy than the original photon (Fig. 10.3). In all cases, an electron escapes from the atom as a Compton electron, carrying the transferred energy as kinetic energy. Electrons will rearrange in the shells with the emission of electromagnetic radiation as before.

A 25 keV X-ray photon has approximately a 50% probability of undergoing a Compton scatter, irrespective of atomic number. At higher photon energies, there is increased transmission and PE absorption is less likely, so Compton scatter dominates.

FACTORS AFFECTING COMPTON SCATTER

Compton scatter is more likely to occur where the X-ray photon energy is much higher than the binding energy of the electron with which it interacts. It dominates for X-ray photon energies greater than 25 keV. As photon energy increases, the proportion of forward scatter increases whilst back and side scatter decrease. Compton scatter is also more likely to occur in

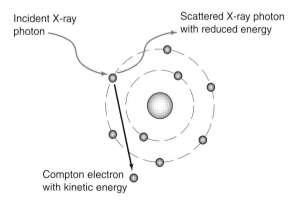

Figure 10.3 Compton scatter.

materials containing a higher proportion of hydrogen, such as water, a major component of the body's soft tissues.

THE IMPLICATIONS OF COMPTON SCATTER

The two main implications to consider are:

- image degradation
- radiation dose.

Image degradation

A forward scattered X-ray photon may leave the body and reach the image receptor. As it has not travelled in a straight line from the X-ray tube, it may be travelling in a direction as if it had penetrated bone. A large amount of scatter like this reaching the image receptor will cause what should be 'white' areas on the image to become grey, or light grey to become darker. This loss of contrast reduces the differences due to PE absorption and degrades the image.

Compton scatter can be reduced by limiting the volume of tissue exposed to the X-ray beam, by *collimating* to the area of interest. Where a large volume must be exposed, for example when imaging the abdomen, a radiation grid can be used, such as a Bucky oscillating grid built into the couch. These grids absorb (by PE absorption) most of the X-ray photons that have been scattered at a variety of angles towards the image receptor whilst allowing the linearly transmitted photons to pass.

Radiation dose

As the majority of scattered photons are produced from interactions within the patient, some of these photons will be scattered within the patient's body and will contribute to a low radiation dose to parts of the body other than that intentionally exposed. This cannot be prevented but good collimation, as mentioned above, will minimise internal scatter.

Some scatter will be produced from X-ray photons interacting with structures in the X-ray tube and casing, such as the filter, and from the collimator blades. These scattered photons may also contribute to radiation dose to parts of the body outside that being imaged. The use of appropriate shielding will attenuate most of these photons; for example to protect the gonads during chest radiography.

Compton scattered photons may travel towards the operator: the lead-glass screen is designed to attenuate these scattered photons.

THE FATE OF THE SECONDARY ELECTRONS: PHOTOELECTRONS AND COMPTON ELECTRONS

The photoelectrons and Compton electrons that escape the atom carrying kinetic energy will interact with neighbouring atoms by ionisation and excitation until all their kinetic energy is lost. A typical secondary electron will produce several hundred ionisations within a fraction of a millimetre. This transfer of energy to the surrounding atoms is responsible for radiation dose and may result in biological effects in the individual.

BIOLOGICAL EFFECTS OF X-RAY PHOTONS

Each X-ray photon that interacts in the body by either PE absorption or Compton scatter causes ionisation of the atom and releases a photoelectron or Compton electron that causes further ionisations of surrounding atoms. The majority of these ionisations will occur in atoms that make up non-critical cell structures, such as the cytoplasm. The ionised atom will quickly return to its previous state with no detrimental effect on the cell.

However, the ionisation may occur in an important atom that is part of the DNA molecule in the nucleus of a cell, resulting in a breakage of the chemical bonds between atoms. DNA, or deoxyribonucleic acid, is the part of a cell that carries the genetic code and determines each cell's type and function. Normally, the cell's monitoring systems will detect any damage to the DNA and enable a repair.

IONISATION DAMAGE RESULTING IN CELL DEATH: DETERMINISTIC EFFECTS

Sometimes, particularly if both DNA strands are broken, the damage may not be repairable. In this case, the cell will die either immediately, or when the cell attempts division, or of old age, which may be days or even years later. The death of a single cell among millions in a particular tissue does not cause any signs or symptoms. However, higher doses of radiation that might occur following certain lengthy procedures using fluoroscopy, such as angiography/angioplasty or lithotripsy, could damage a significant number of cells and lead to an observable clinical effect.

This type of damage is known as a deterministic effect, or tissue reaction, and gives symptoms related to the tissue damaged once a certain threshold dose is reached. As the radiation dose is increased, the severity of the damage increases. For example, damage to the skin where the X-ray beam has entered the body may result in a reddening in this area (erythema) that appears within a few days of exposure; further or higher doses of ionising radiation may result in a thinning of the skin (desquamation). Damage to the lens of the eye may result in a clouding of the lens in the years following exposure; with higher doses this may progress to a cataract. These types of effect do not normally occur following diagnostic imaging procedures as radiation doses are too low.

However, embryonic tissue is very sensitive to ionising radiation damage, and doses from abdominal/pelvic computed tomography (CT) examinations or a barium enema, particularly if performed more than once during the first two weeks of gestation, could result in death of the embryo or gross malformations.

IONISATION DAMAGE RESULTING IN MISREPAIRED DAMAGE: STOCHASTIC EFFECTS

There is a possibility that following ionisation of an atom making up a DNA molecule, the damage is misrepaired, resulting in a gene mutation. In most cases, the cell will die as a result. If the cell survives, the mutation may contribute to the induction of malignancy in the cell; that is, the start of a cancer. Radiation-induced cancers are usually leukaemias or lymphomas rather than the more common types, such as cancer of the lung, breast or prostate. If the mutation occurs in a sperm or egg cell, an induced cancer could occur in a subsequent child.

There is a risk of inducing cancer with any dose of ionising radiation and the risk increases with increasing dose.

RADIATION PROTECTION

The risk of stochastic effects and the potential for deterministic effects mean the use of ionising radiation for diagnostic imaging is a compromise between maximising the diagnostic information and minimising the radiation dose to the patient. All exposures should be as low as possible to reduce the risk of stochastic effects and avoid deterministic effects.

People working with ionising radiation may also be exposed to levels higher than those received from natural background radiation.

In the UK, the Health and Safety Executive enforces regulations relating to ionising radiation (see p. 13). These are in two parts: the current Ionising Radiations Regulations 1999 apply to employers using ionising radiation, such as hospital Trusts, and requires them to protect all employees by ensuring any exposures are as low as reasonably achievable and do not exceed specified dose limits. This is achieved by ensuring equipment, shielding and working practices are safe and by monitoring effective doses received by employees during their work.

The Ionising Radiation (Medical Exposure) Regulations [IR(ME)R] 2000 apply primarily to patients undergoing investigations or treatment using ionising radiation, such as radiographic imaging. Every medical exposure must be:

- justified – to give a net benefit from the exposure compared to its risk of damage to the individual
- optimised – to ensure all doses are as low as reasonably practicable.

HOW DO WE QUANTIFY 'RADIATION DOSE'?

When we use the terms 'dose of ionising radiation' or just 'radiation dose', we mean how much energy has been deposited in the organs and tissues of the body following attenuation of a beam of ionising radiation. This is called the absorbed dose and is measured in units of gray (Gy), where 1 Gy equates to 1 joule of energy deposited per kilogram mass.

However, absorbed dose does not take into account the damaging potential of different ionising radiations, such as alpha particles, nor the sensitivity to the induction of stochastic effects of different organs and tissues in the body. The International Commission for Radiological Protection (ICRP) has calculated factors to take into account both of these variables. Radiation weighting factors for different types of ionising radiations convert absorbed dose into equivalent dose. Tissue weighting factors convert equivalent dose into effective dose, measured in sieverts (Sv) or, more usually in radiation protection, a thousandth of a sievert: the millisievert (mSv). Effective dose can then be used to compare absorbed doses from different ionising radiations and to an exposed part of the body, such as the chest, in relation to the effect of that dose on the whole body.

For example, an absorbed dose of 1 mGy of X-ray photons to the whole body would include all the sensitive structures, giving an effective dose of 1 mSv. If an absorbed dose of 1 mGy was confined to the lungs, using the ICRP's tissue weighting factors, the effective dose would be 0.12 mSv, owing to no other sensitive organs in the body receiving any of the dose. If the 1 mGy were confined to the thyroid gland, the effective dose would be 0.05 mSv. This indicates the greater sensitivity of the lungs to the risk of stochastic effects compared to the thyroid. If both of these organs are irradiated but no part of any other sensitive structure, the effective dose would be 0.17 mSv.

Effective doses for the average-sized person can be approximated for radiographic imaging of all parts of the body and can be compared to the effective dose received from natural background radiation over a period of time. The

Table 10.2 Typical effective doses for diagnostic medical exposures[2]

X-ray examination	Typical effective doses (mSv)	Equivalent period of natural background radiation
Limbs and joints (except hip)	<0.01	<1.5 days
Teeth (single bitewing)	<0.01	<1.5 days
PA chest	0.02	3 days
Skull	0.07	11 days
Cervical spine	0.08	2 weeks
Hip	0.3	7 weeks
Thoracic spine	0.7	4 months
Pelvis/abdomen	0.7	4 months
Lumbar spine	1.3	7 months
Barium swallow	1.5	8 months
IVU	2.5	14 months
Barium meal	3.0	16 months
Barium enema	7.0	3.2 years
CT head	2.0	1 year
CT chest	8.0	3.6 years
CT abdomen/pelvis	10.0	4.5 years

CT, computed tomography; PA, posteroanterior; IVU, intravenous urogram

average background dose in the UK is 2.2 mSv per year (Table 10.2).

In practice, effective dose is a complicated calculation for the individual patient, so if the X-ray set is fitted with a DAP (dose–area product) ionisation chamber (see pp. 126–127), a DAP reading can be recorded. This is the radiation dose to air multiplied by the area exposed, giving a reading in Gy cm[2]. Again, it is not easily related to effective dose, but the accumulated DAP reading can be recorded for each examination and used to compare relative exposures. If other factors such as source–image distance (SID) and kV are recorded, effective dose can be calculated retrospectively if required.

FLUORESCENCE

Some materials, called phosphors, convert X-ray photons into light photons. This means they glow when exposed to an X-ray beam. As the energy of an X-ray photon is much greater than that of a light photon, one X-ray photon may be converted into hundreds of light photons. The colour of the light emitted depends on the type of phosphor. In certain phosphors this effect is instantaneous and is known as fluorescence. Fluorescent phosphors such as gadolinium oxysulphide are utilised in the intensifying screens used in conventional film-screen imaging systems (see p. 140).

Some phosphors store the X-ray photon energy temporarily and emit the energy as light over a period of time (luminescence). Other phosphors store the X-ray photon energy for an indefinite length of time. When the atoms storing the energy are stimulated by the energy in a laser beam, the energy is converted into light and emitted. These phosphors (e.g. barium fluorohalide) are known as 'storage phosphors' and are used in computed radiography (CR) imaging plates.

References

1. Johns HE, Cunningham JR. The physics of radiology, 4th edn. Springfield, Ill: Charles C Thomas; 1983:723–724.
2. Health Protection Agency (HPA)
   www.hpa.org.uk/radiation/understand/radiation_topics/medical/ted_equivalent.htm

Recommended reading

Ball J, Moore AD. Essential physics for radiographers, 3rd edn. Oxford: Blackwell Science; 1997.

This text provides useful background physics of energy, atomic structure and electricity plus deeper insights into key areas of radiographic science. Note, however, it was published in 1997, prior to the current Ionising Radiations Regulations of 1999 and 2000, as given below.

Bushong SC. Radiologic science for technologists, 8th edn. St Louis: Mosby; 2004.

Chapters 33 to 37 give a deeper insight into the biological effects of ionising radiation, including a review of human biology, radiobiology and the early and late effects of exposure to ionising radiation.

Be aware that subsequent chapters refer to radiation protection legislation in the United States and although the principles are the same anywhere in the world, the regulations are not!

The Ionising Radiations Regulations 1999 (SI No. 3232). London: HMSO.

The Ionising Radiations (Medical Exposure) Regulations 2000 (SI No. 1059) London: HMSO.

Website

International Commission for Radiological Protection (ICRP)
www.icrp.org

Chapter **11**

Diagnostic equipment

Marc Griffiths and Ken Holmes

KEY POINTS

- General diagnostic imaging systems allow practitioners to perform the fundamental clinical examinations within the radiography department.
- The flexibility and safe use of general imaging equipment is paramount in assisting the practitioner to produce optimal quality images.
- The use of an effective image capturing device and ancillary items also aid the practitioner in ensuring the lowest possible dose is given to patients.
- Grids are used to reduce the effect of scattered radiation on the image quality.

INTRODUCTION

Within the imaging department there is a range of equipment and accessory items to assist the practitioner in obtaining optimal quality images. Technological developments have seen the introduction of digital capturing systems (digital radiography, DR) and advancements in operator ergonomics, patient throughput and comfort. Modern general X-ray rooms should be spacious, permitting the examination of a wide spectrum of patients (Fig. 11.1).

The use of relatively high proton number materials to provide radiation protection measures has generally remained unchanged in the last fifteen years. Walls of a general X-ray room may be coated

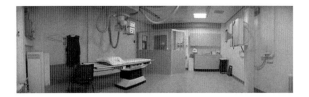

Figure 11.1 Modern general X-ray room.

with barium plaster, and lead shielding is incorporated into access routes. Consideration is also given to the ceilings and floors of any X-ray examination room if the radiology department is situated in proximity to adjoining floors within a hospital.

IMAGING TABLES

The majority of imaging tables utilised within general diagnostic departments have to meet a number of key requirements to ensure patient safety and the provision of optimal image quality. Modern imaging tables are designed to minimise unnecessary strain on practitioners during examinations and provide security and comfort for patients (Fig. 11.2). The availability of a variable height feature permits easy transfer of patients, whether they are walking, in a chair or on a stretcher. A wide range of movement is available, usually via foot control switches situated at the base of the table, and this prevents the need to move the patient around on a draw sheet and minimises injury to the practitioner. Controls positioned at either side of the imaging table also provide a universal approach to transferring and positioning patients.

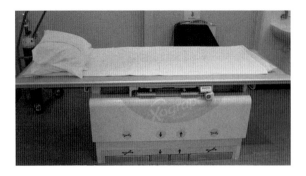

Figure 11.2 Modern imaging table of a diagnostic imaging room, courtesy of Xograph Healthcare Ltd.

Most modern imaging tables are designed using low attenuation materials, such as carbon fibre, which have the advantages of being lightweight and strong to accommodate the weight of the heavy individuals, typically up to 450 kg.[1] Using materials such as carbon fibre also absorbs less of the primary beam and reduces radiation dose when undertaking grid work. Carbon fibre is also warm to the touch and has rounded edges to prevent physical damage to patients and staff and the build up of electrostatic charge.

All modern imaging tables should encompass a good range of longitudinal and transverse travel and possess a floating top design to minimise physical strain upon the practitioner. Such designs may aid in the ability to undertake prompt and effective examinations; however, the distance between the patient and cassette unit is increased and appropriate measures need to be taken to ensure object magnification and image unsharpness does not occur. This is normally compensated by increasing the source–image distance (SID) when undertaking examinations requiring an oscillating grid mechanism. The practitioner also needs to ensure the various table and X-ray tube interlocks are observed during such examinations; all manufacturers use colour coding to indicate X-ray tube functions.

Modern imaging tables also accommodate direct capture imaging plates, which are linked to a monitor and computer unit for a near instantaneous display. The advent of digital imaging has redefined clinical practice in terms of patient positioning and appropriate use of a DR system. Traditional systems employ integrated conventional cassette units, which also act as a scatter minimisation unit. Such systems are also linked to automatic exposure devices (AED). The use of the AED has become a routine aspect of clinical work. There are normally three AED chambers integrated into the tabletop mechanism. Selection of the appropriate chamber(s) is facilitated by pre-set protocols with a manual override if the practitioner needs to change the programme to provide an optimum image, or if the patient has a metal prosthesis (e.g. hip), affecting the overall quality of the image. The density settings on the control console may be password protected to prevent changes to optimal stored values.[2]

The use of automatic cassette size sensing (ACSS) techniques ensures the collimation from the light beam diaphragm matches the size of the cassette within the Bucky mechanism. This reduces the area irradiated and produces less scattered radiation, improving image quality as well as limiting radiation dose to the patient and staff. Closer collimation can again be performed, as the diaphragms are not fixed in the position sensed by the ACSS.

TUBE SUPPORTS

Modern general X-ray tubes are supported via a ceiling track mechanism which is able to withstand the rigour and demands of a typical department workload (Fig. 11.3). Most clinical departments utilise ceiling suspended units and employ a 'cross track' mechanism to allow the unit to move swiftly over a large floor space. The tube support facilitates movement around the longitudinal, transverse and vertical axes. The telescopic column provides a flexible range of vertical movement and is supported by electromechanical locks. The ceiling in imaging rooms containing a ceiling mounted unit needs to be of a reasonable height, thus permitting the required SID for a range of examinations.

The practitioner is normally provided with colour coded functions on the X-ray tube control unit, which are associated with the same coloured indicators on the ceiling and telescopic support. Some imaging rooms which undertake basic procedures (e.g. chest room) may employ a floor mounted X-ray unit, which is cost effective but

---

Health and safety requirements for an X-ray tube

- Support the weight of the X-ray tube and associated support structures and cables.
- The utilisation of modern electromechanical interlocks and counterweight balances in order to provide a stable and safe imaging system. (Such features will lock the X-ray tube and support in position in the event of an electrical failure.)
- Encompass automated movement functions, reducing physical strain on the practitioner.
- Accurate indication of the relationship between the ceiling support, X-ray tube, imaging receptors and tables (this is crucial). Features such as inbuilt distance and angulation indicators permit accurate positioning.
- Flexible and unrestricting movement of the X-ray tube and the supporting column. This is essential for the production of quality radiographs. (Features such as angle indicators at the base of the X-ray tube support offer additional guidance when performing horizontal beam examinations.)

---

not as flexible as a ceiling mounted system. Such units are limited in their range of movement and the practitioner should take this into consideration when undertaking more complex examinations or with non-ambulant patients. Floor mounted systems are positioned on a track unit which is recessed into the floor and secured to a ceiling track for added stability. This design limits the available floor space and may present health and safety challenges.

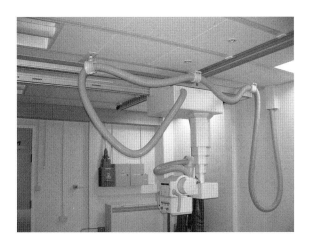

Figure 11.3 Tube support mechanism.

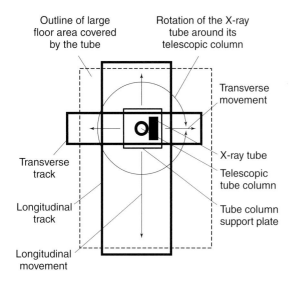

Figure 11.4 Example of wide floor coverage.

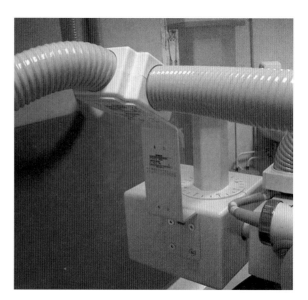

Figure 11.5 Flexible piping and high-tension support mechanism.

The major advantages of a ceiling suspended unit include:

- Flexibility and wide floor coverage, enabling the practitioner to work around immobile patients who may present in wheelchairs or on trolleys (Fig. 11.4).
- Range of examination heights to cover all examinations (e.g. standing feet and lateral cervical spines).
- Safer working environment, with all cables encased in appropriate piping and clear floor space.
- Ability to adapt radiographic technique around the type of examination.

High-tension cables are securely encased in protective flexible piping, which is supported by additional ceiling sockets (Fig. 11.5). This enables the practitioner to safely manoeuvre the X-ray unit without the risk of placing unnecessary stress upon the high-tension cables. The supports for the cables must run freely along the track to prevent any mechanical strain when the X-ray tube is rotated.

CASSETTES AND FILM HOLDERS

Modern imaging departments utilise some form of digital capturing devices (image receptor), such as computed radiography (CR) or DR. This will have some impact upon the working logistics within a general imaging room. However, some departments may still also utilise conventional film screen cassettes to capture a latent image.

Typically, if a department is employing either conventional cassettes or CR technology, there will be a range of image receptor sizes to accommodate various radiographic techniques. All image receptor devices should be stored away from primary and scattered radiation, ideally in an appropriately designed storage holder. Routine quality control assessments of the image capturing devices should also be performed, in particular the routine secondary erasure of unused CR cassettes. Direct capture units (Fig. 11.6) may either be mobile devices or fixed units (e.g. chest imaging unit). Such units are expensive and require proper storage facilities when not employed.

To undertake a range of diagnostic techniques, the modern imaging environment should include various ancillary items. These include cassette holders, foam pads, stationary grid units, sandbags and radiation protection devices (e.g. lead rubber coats). The practitioner is required to utilise a range of skills and knowledge in order to produce optimal quality images. The use of a

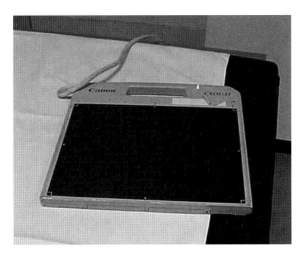

Figure 11.6 Direct capture image receptor device, courtesy of Canon Europe.

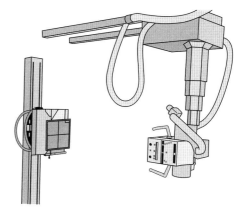

Figure 11.8 Upright Bucky unit with cassette holder unit.

cassette holder to acquire images may minimise radiation dose to staff or carers.

Cassette holders may take the form of a basic device, such as the example shown in Figure 11.7, and are generally employed for techniques such as lateral horizontal beam hip examinations. However, a modern upright Bucky mechanism with an integrated cassette holder is also a crucial feature in a general imaging room.

Figure 11.8 demonstrates the advantages of a ceiling mounted X-ray unit and upright Bucky unit. The provision of standard interlocks also ensures set geometry for chest examinations, which need to be at a standardised distance of approximately 180 cm SID. This aids in the

minimisation of geometric unsharpness for certain examinations.

A variable height facility supported by either manual or electromechanical locks enables the assembly to be moved up and down to examine a range of procedures, from lateral cervical spines to erect standing knees. The cassette support mechanism may then be removed to facilitate AED or Bucky work. The system can also be rotated 90° into a horizontal position if required for adapted techniques, such as a lateral elbow in plaster or wrists on patients who may be immobile. Modern upright DR units (Fig. 11.9), which possess an integrated image capturing

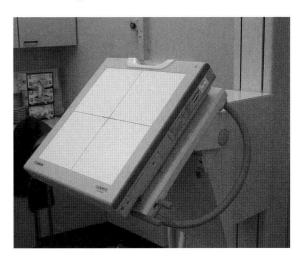

Figure 11.9 Digital radiography upright imaging unit, courtesy of Canon Europe.

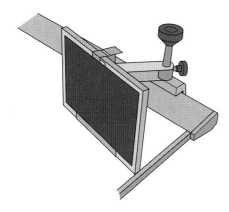

Figure 11.7 Lateral cassette holder.

device, may also be used for a wide range of examinations and allow flexible rotation. All upright units should possess patient positioning aids, such as handles and chin rests. Also the provision of electromechanical interlocks will prevent any compromise of patient safety in the event of an electrical failure.

OPERATOR CONSOLE AND DOSE RECORDING FEATURES

General X-ray units are supported with space saving control consoles (Fig. 11.10), which encompass touch screen facilities. This is coupled with the small space required for a high frequency generator to supply power to the X-ray unit. The use of solid state electronics provides accurate exposure times for examinations and improves image quality at lower patient doses by producing a nearly constant potential voltage waveform which is not possible with a single or three phase power supply.[3] The creation of a near constant potential waveform helps to reduce the possibility of movement unsharpness during radiographic procedures. This is especially true for paediatric examinations, where very short exposure times may be required.

Most operator consoles have preset anatomically programmed (APR) exposure values, which are stored on a microprocessor. The pre-set radiographic exposures provide prompt access to a digital bank of typical values used in clinical practice. However, practitioners still require the knowledge and skills to adjust these pre-set values in order to provide optimal image quality at the lowest possible dose.[4]

Typical power ratings for a high voltage generator for general radiography procedures are in the region of 30–55 kW. This is generally lower than for units such as interventional systems, which require greater power supplies due to the demands placed on them.[5]

Practitioners have a duty to ensure minimal exposure values are used in order to produce optimal diagnostic radiographs.[6] The development of radiological equipment has assisted in the promotion of minimal exposures, optimal image production and the provision of a safe working environment. Rooms are designed to ensure the operator console is at a safe distance from the examination table and erect Bucky unit. Unlike in mobile equipment, the exposure button is attached to the console, thus preventing an exposure unless the practitioner is safely behind the protective lead glass screen.

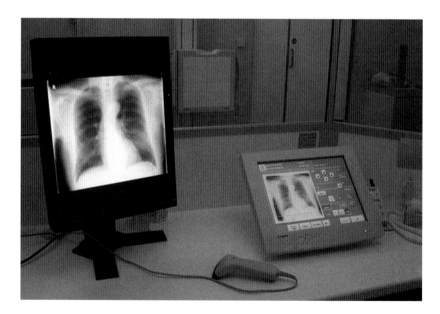

Figure 11.10 Operator console and image review workstation, courtesy of Canon Europe.

It is a legal requirement to record radiation doses to patients, and whilst an integrated dose area product (DAP) meter does not reduce radiation dose, it does facilitate easy recording of the entrance dose to the patient being examined in that room. This allows the practitioner to measure the dose and ensure it is within the diagnostic reference level (DRL) required by the Ionising Radiation (Medical Exposure) Regulations 2000.[6] The meter can easily demonstrate the effect of close collimation and this can encourage good working practices by the practitioner. DAP units display the dose given to the patient in milligrays (mGy) or centigrays (cGy) and this must be recorded for each study undertaken.

The provision of features such as exposure hold, which prevents an exposure-taking place for a number of reasons, minimises a potentially unsafe examination from taking place.[7] Reasons may include the door to the radiology department being opened during the examination, the X-ray tube not being correctly centred to the Bucky tray, no cassette in the Bucky tray or a cassette in both the upright and table Bucky systems.

MOBILE EQUIPMENT

Radiography may be performed outside the realm of the X-ray department, encompassing a range of examinations, environments and patients. Although the practitioner when performing mobile examinations may employ various adaptations upon radiographic techniques, the fundamental principles of radiation protection, image quality and patient care remain pinnacle to this service.

Mobile radiography may be performed in a wide range of environments within a hospital, including an accident and emergency department, intensive therapy unit (ITU), coronary care unit (CCU), special care baby unit (SCBU) and theatre. Working in ITU, SCBU or general ward environments requires some examinations to be performed in often small, difficult and busy environments. The practitioner is primarily responsible for obtaining a diagnostic image whilst maintaining the radiation protection of staff and patients.

Mobile X-ray units are rechargeable (capacitor discharge) in design, being generally safer than mains units, which draw power for exposures from wall sockets. This reduces the necessity for the provision of dedicated electrical sockets on wards such as ITU and CCU, where interruptions to the local power supplies are generally not recommended. However, a mains powered unit is lighter in design and has a smaller footprint, which aids with manoeuvrability of the system.[3]

Most mobile units are APR in design and encompass the majority of features located on static units (e.g. DAP meters) and have similar power outputs to general imaging rooms. Generators incorporated within mobile units work up to 40 kW peak power, allowing exposures from 40–110 kV and 0.2–360 mA s. This adds to the flexibility of mobile units, allowing them to perform a wide variety of different procedures that require a range of exposure factors, including very short exposure times (1 ms), which is a crucial consideration for various scenarios, such as trauma, CCU and ITU where involuntary patient movement (i.e. respiratory) may be an issue.

Features of a typical mobile X-ray unit are demonstrated in Figure 11.11. Mobile units may vary in design, with some units possessing extendible tube supports or adjustable-height mobile units. Extendable tube supports or adjustable-height

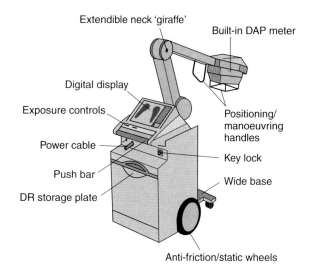

Figure 11.11 Typical design features of a mobile X-ray unit.

mobile units should aim to provide a good range of movements, including a generous source–image distance (SID) and subtle adjustments for minor angle corrections.

Modern systems should be easy to use, flexible and provide high quality images. Typically, most modern mobile units are compact in design to enable movement in confined spaces, such as in isolation rooms. Most mobile X-ray units are designed to enable the provision of an optimal imaging service and are supplied with similar X-ray tubes to those in general X-ray rooms, with typical anode angles of 15°, and provide 8500 revolutions per minute during an exposure.[6] The mobile X-ray tube and its housing are customised for its role, needing to provide the same level or radiation protection as those in the department but at a minimal weight. Modern mobile units use a single focal spot size of 0.8 mm, giving a compromise between acceptable geometric unsharpness and tube life.

The practice of mobile radiography places a great demand upon mobile X-ray units to move easily within small spaces, such as between beds and in cubicles and also over great distances between wards. Some modern machines have integrated a 'tilt-up footstep' to allow smooth transfer over thresholds and, with polyurethane tyres, are designed to glide across most floor surfaces that would be encountered throughout the hospital. Mobile machines also have built-in braking systems, usually activated by releasing the drive handle. This avoids the demand on practitioners to physically bring the machines to a halt themselves, which may otherwise have considerable manual handling consequences.

Additional features aiding manoeuvrability include a lightweight construction of the base unit and a design that enhances the operator's visibility when travelling. This is a crucial issue during transportation, where mobile units may be in close proximity with members of the public within the hospital. A small electrical motor can be used to provide a motorised drive within the unit to help promote the ease of movement.[5] Radiography is a profession that is particularly conscious of the potential manual handling risks that can be incurred while undertaking such a physical occupation on a day-to-day basis.[2]

Modern advances are aimed at improving the ergonomic design of mobiles so that examinations can be carried out easily, without any undue stress being placed upon the practitioner.

A cordless exposure device is now available, which has a proprietary infrared coding frequency and provides the operator with the ability to increase their distance up to almost 11 m.[6] The remote control provides the greatest radiation protection possible to the operator, especially when working in restricted environments, as it has the ability to function around corners. In common with conventional exposure hand switches, the remote control allows the operator to check the collimation at a distance before exposing.

The development of mobile DR units (Fig. 11.12) with amorphous silicon has enabled the instantaneous viewing of images (typical 'exposure-to-view' time = 5 s), whilst being remote from the X-ray department. The advent of DR imaging has also removed the necessity for traditional chemical processors and enhanced the storage/transportation of images. Fundamental image viewing and manipulation may be achieved using a touch screen encompassed within the mobile unit.

With the near instant availability of digital images and the ability to post-manipulate at the site of exposure, additional pressures are being placed upon practitioners to provide information in order to ensure effective patient management. It is imperative that practitioners ensure the focus

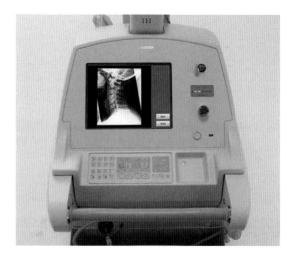

Figure 11.12 Digital radiography mobile unit.

primarily relates to the welfare of the patient during portable examinations, whilst appreciating technology advancements.

FLUOROSCOPY EQUIPMENT

The practitioner may use fluoroscopy equipment within the imaging department or in a theatre environment. Traditionally, the fundamentals of obtaining images within a fluoroscopy environment have involved the use of an image intensification unit to convert transmitted incident X-ray photons, which have emerged from the patient, into an electrical output signal. Fluoroscopy examinations result in an instantaneous 'real time' image being produced and include examinations that may employ the use of barium or iodine contrast agents, such as enemas and meals.

The process of converting an incident X-ray photon into an electrical signal involves a number of stages within a conventional image intensification unit. This process is depicted in Figure 11.13 and is performed in fluoroscopy and mobile units, which employ a 'drum' type structure aligned to an X-ray tube.

The practitioner may encounter two different types of fluoroscopy unit within the imaging department. These are under- or overcouch units (Fig. 11.14). Undercouch fluoroscopy units are designed with the X-ray tube unit underneath the imaging table and are the most popular within imaging departments. With undercouch units, the image intensification unit incorporates a handheld movement unit, allowing the practitioner to move the unit over the patient. A lead rubber protective skirt minimises the amount of primary and scattered radiation reaching the operator. Overcouch units only permit limited movement, owing to the X-ray tube being positioned over the patient,

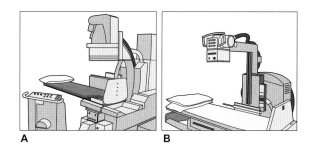

Figure 11.14 A Undercouch fluoroscopy unit. **B** Overcouch fluoroscopy unit.

but are useful for examinations with certain patient groups, such as paediatrics.

The basic purpose of an image intensification unit is to convert a weak input signal into a strong output signal within a glass vacuum environment. This conversion process begins at the input phosphor screen within the image intensification unit, which converts the incident X-ray photons into light signals. Traditionally, caesium iodide (in the form of rod shaped crystals) has been used for this purpose, as it possesses high absorption properties and is therefore able to 'stop' the high-energy X-ray photons. The caesium iodide crystals are supported on a glass plate and the emitted light is absorbed by a photocathode device and subsequently converted into a weak electrical signal. The number of emitted photoelectrons is proportional to the initial brightness of the input screen.[8]

The weak electrical signal is attracted to the output end of the image intensification unit (anode) by applying a potential difference across the input and output ends of the unit. This is similar to an X-ray tube, but the potential difference is much smaller in an image intensification unit (Fig. 11.15). The initial weak electrical signal is increased by the use of focussing electrodes, which are negatively charged and repel the electrons

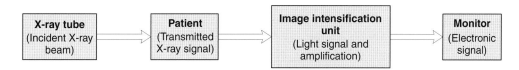

Figure 11.13 Basic process of traditional fluoroscopy image creation.

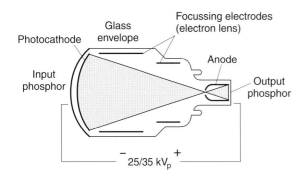

Figure 11.15 Typical design of a traditional image intensification unit.

(which are also negatively charged). This has the effect of condensing the electrical signal, which eventually reaches the output phosphor.

In traditional fluoroscopy systems, the output phosphor re-converts the electrical signal into a visible light signal. This signal subsequently appears on the viewing monitor, or may be recorded using an appropriate image-capturing device (e.g. SVHS). Modern fluoroscopy devices employ analogue to digital converter (ADC) electronics to store captured images and permit the operator to either save data onto a local or centralised system or print selected images. Advantages of digital images include the ability to manipulate and enhance the original data and potentially improve overall image quality.

Fluoroscopy equipment utilises a number of additional safety features not normally located on standard radiographic equipment. Such features include:

- a couch that has the ability to tilt and that may be operated by remote controls situated either behind a lead glass screen or as a mobile free-standing unit (Fig. 11.16)
- a lead rubber skirt, which surrounds the image intensification unit, offering some radiation protection for the operator
- mobile and static lead glass screens, which are generally thicker than those encountered within general imaging rooms
- access to appropriate radiation protection equipment, such as thyroid shield and lead rubber coats. (The lead rubber coats are normally heavier than those encountered in

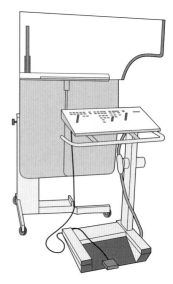

Figure 11.16 Freestanding mobile operator console with integrated lead glass screen.

general imaging rooms, owing to the higher X-ray photon energies being generated)
- a range of accessory items such as handles, straps, shoulder supports and adjustable steps in order to minimise the risk of injury to the patient during examinations
- pressure sensors to prevent patients and operators from injuring themselves and to ensure moving equipment (e.g. table tops) is not accidentally damaged by other items (e.g. wheelchairs), which may have been left in the room
- plastic trims to prevent patients from catching their hands/feet in the mechanics of a fluoroscopic unit
- integrated timers to warn the practitioner/ radiologist when a certain exposure time has been breached
- mechanical locks to ensure that fluoroscopic units cannot be driven into dangerous positions
- ceiling mounted monitors to reduce the risk of looping and being caught up in other equipment, the operator or the patient.

The fixed relationship between the X-ray tube and image intensification unit requires the patient to be positioned for certain projections. However, with the advent of modern C-arm design fluoroscopy units and the use of ultra-thin carbon fibre tabletops, the imaging unit may be positioned around the patient and can also be used for special projections, such as lateral decubitus images. The C-arm fluoroscopy design has been utilised in the theatre environment for many years and mobile image intensification units provide an essential service for various examinations, such as orthopaedic operations and surgical procedures. Advancements in technological design have provided operators with 'flat panel' image intensification units (Fig. 11.17) to replace those in the traditional 'drum' style. These incorporate amorphous silicon and so are similar to technology encountered in direct capture general radiography units. Such units are true digital systems, converting the incident X-ray photons into an electrical signal.

All modern mobile image intensification units employ a high frequency generator power supply and provide the operator with a wide range of exposure manipulation features, which may be rapidly adapted to suit the radiological procedure. The nominal output ranges vary according to manufacturer but typical values range from 3 to 8 kW.[1] Such values are lower than traditional fluoroscopy units; however, image quality is not compromised on modern digital units. Most modern systems also employ dual focal spot sizes (typically 0.6 and 1.4 mm), which are automatically adjusted according to the type of examination being performed. A broad filament is employed when high demands are placed upon the unit to provide greater amounts of X-rays. Although a number of design features have been developed on mobile image intensification units, the majority of fundamental systems still appear to house stationary anodes.

Depending upon the range of examinations being performed, different field sizes (typically 23 cm and 30 cm) are available. Larger field of view intensification units may be required for cardiac (i.e. pacing examinations) examinations. A zoom factor is normally also available for magnification purposes. A range of colour coded interlocks, measurement scales, multiple glide rails, angle indicators and laser positioning all aid the practitioner in the ensuring optimal image quality and minimal doses to patients and staff.

The operating of large electrical equipment in an environment such as a theatre introduces high risks to staff. There are many areas to consider, including the use of electricity around many compressed and combustible gases and possibly in the presence of large volumes of free fluid. The electrical supply to the unit's generator is of a high demand and therefore can only be taken from a stable circuit that can withstand it. The positioning of sockets needs to be carefully considered as they need to be placed high, but this can make them difficult to access by shorter members of staff. Conversely, if too low, they become susceptible to fluid on the floor and become hazardous to theatre staff, resulting in the plugs being kicked and cables being damaged.

Manual handling issues are becoming of great importance, with many studies demonstrating the risk incurred to their musculoskeletal system by healthcare professionals when undertaking their daily working practices.[6] Hospital trusts nationwide are now incorporating mandatory manual handling training to promote safe working practices in an attempt to protect their staff.

The majority of modern image intensification systems encompass a wide range of image manipulation features, which commonly include virtual

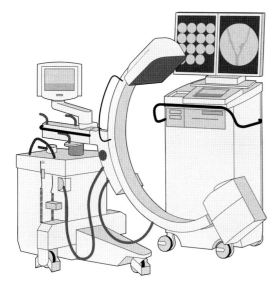

Figure 11.17 Modern 'flat panel' design mobile image intensification unit.

collimation (which permits the operator to collimate the last obtained frame in preparation for the next exposure), image rotation (virtual), zoom, flip, edge enhancement, image subtraction and a wide range of contrast and brightness tools. Advanced tools such as measurement scales, fluoroscopy reply (i.e. dynamic imaging), road mapping, noise reduction and image reversal features are also common on most systems.

With regards to radiation protection, all fluoroscopy equipment contains a number of devices similar to those found on general X-ray units, such as DAP meters. Some fluoroscopy procedures may be lengthy (e.g. tibial nailing) and consequently possibly require long screening times. It is therefore imperative that dose saving features are an essential feature on any modern image intensification unit and encompass a number of ergonomic features to enable the production of high quality images.[1] The use of a 'pulsed' stream of electrons across the X-ray tube generates a non-continuous stream of photons, which are subsequently incident upon the patient. Pulsing technology is available on all modern image intensification equipment and should be employed whenever the operator is positioning the patient or obtaining a check image (e.g. k-wire examination in theatre). Continuous beam transmission gives higher quality images at a higher dose whereas pulse imaging gives a lower dose, but as a consequence, image quality is compromised. In some situations the images gained are of high enough quality as to negate the need for postoperative films, thus reducing dose to the patients. Some degradation to image quality may occur as a result of pulsing techniques; however modern systems provide some form of compensatory factor in an attempt to preserve image quality.

CARE OF EQUIPMENT

It is the professional responsibility of the practitioner to ensure the equipment utilised in the production of quality images is safe and regularly checked. Incorrect handling may result in excessive wear and tear, such as damage to interlocks or brakes and the tube housing. Staff working within general imaging departments should undertake routine equipment checks, which may encompass:

- routine daily checks for wear and tear, damage and the inspection of interlocks and safety devices
- recording of mechanical faults on general and mobile X-ray equipment in a faults book, which is regularly inspected by the departmental quality assurance practitioner
- physical inspection and screening of ancillary and radiation protection items (e.g. lead rubber coats) on a regular basis and in line with departmental polices
- involvement in the regular performance of quality control tests, such as kV_p consistency, light beam diaphragm and beam alignment and output tests.

SECONDARY RADIATION GRIDS

Grids are a highly effective way of reducing the amount of scattered radiation reaching the image receptor (Fig. 11.18). Grids are made of strips of lead (or other attenuating material) interspaced with a radiolucent material, such as aluminium or carbon plastic fibres. The attenuating material will intercept the scattered radiation before it reaches the film, increasing the quality of the image. Up to 97% of scattered radiation can be removed through the use of a grid.

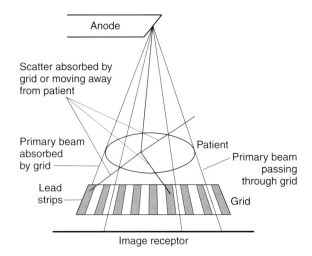

Figure 11.18 Function of a grid absorbing scattered radiation whilst allowing the useful transmitted beam to pass through.

Grids fall into a number of different categories describing their construction.

Parallel grid

This type of grid has parallel lead lines and is usually used in fluoroscopy units. It will absorb the transmitted beam towards the outer edges.

Focussed grid

A focussed grid has lead strips that match the divergence of the primary beam. This allows the transmitted beam to reach the image receptor with minimal absorption. This type of grid must be used in the correct orientation and distance to prevent detrimental effects on the image quality.

Crossed grid

A crossed grid is constructed of two parallel grids at 90 ° to each other. This improves the removal of scatter by removing the photons, which are in the same plane as the lead strips. In a single parallel grid the scatter radiation in the same plane as the lead strips will not be absorbed. Correct alignment is essential, as cut-off will occur with minimal variation from the perpendicular.

Moving grid

Grids are found in the Bucky device under the X-ray table. During exposure these grids move rapidly, blurring out the grid lines and improving image quality. This is linked to the exposure mechanism so movement starts just before an exposure is made, terminating at the end of the exposure.

TERMS USED WITH GRIDS

Grid ratio

The grid ratio describes the ratio of the grid height to the width of the interspace material (Fig. 11.19). Grid ratios range from 4:1 to 16:1. High-ratio grids remove more scattered radiation, increasing the radiographic contrast, and are ideal for high kV examinations. Low ratio grids are used for mammography examinations where a typical ratio value is 5:1.

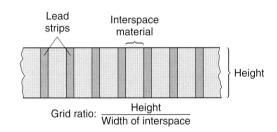

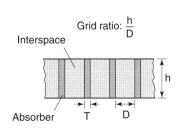

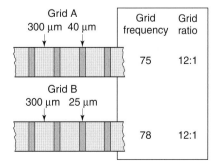

Figure 11.19 Grid ratio.

Grid factor

The grid factor describes the increase in exposure need when using a grid. The grid will decrease the intensity of the radiation reaching the image receptor. This cannot be avoided and to counteract the effect the exposure factors used will need to be increased by the grid factor. This is provided with the grid and is usually between two and six.

Grid cut-off

If certain types of grid are used at the wrong focus-to-grid distance or are not in the correct orientation to the primary beam then the beam will be 'cut-off'. This will be seen on the resultant image with a small area of the image appearing normal but the surrounding area being under exposed, with either visible lines or completely white where the attenuating material has absorbed the useful beam. This can be avoided by using grids at the correct distance and orientation. The correct orientation and distance will be marked on the grid.

References

1. Siemens Medical Solutions. Technical product information. On-line. Available *http://www.medical.siemens.com* then select UK and search for Multix swing technical info. 8 February 2008.
2. Kings Centre for the Assessment of Radiological Equipment – SafeSpecs. 2004. On-line. Available *http://www.kcare.co.uk/safespecs.htm* 23 January 2008
3. Bushong SC. Radiologic science for technologists: physics, biology and protection, 7th edn. London: Mosby; 2001.
4. College of Radiographers. Statements for professional conduct. London: College of Radiographers; 2002.
5. Siemens Medical Solutions. Product information – Multix Compact K system. Germany: Siemens Medical Solutions; 2002.
6. Department of Health. The Ionising Radiation (Medical Exposure) Regulations 2000. London, Department of Health; 1999.
7. General Electrics. Radiography – Proteus XR/a information. 2004. On-line. Available *http://www.gemedicalsystemseurope.com/euen/rad/xr/radio/products/msxpro_eou.html* 23 January 2008
8. Munkert A. The first fully digital C-Arm – 21st century mobile X-ray imaging. Medical Imaging in Bavaria, 2003:1–7.

Recommended reading

Carter P, Paterson P, Thornton M, Hyatt AP, Milne A, Pirrie JR. Chesney's equipment for student radiographers, 4th edn. Oxford: Blackwell Science; 1994.

This provides a well laid out and concise introduction to radiographic equipment. It contains excellent diagrams with clear text.

Chapter **12**

Films, cassettes, intensifying screens and processing

Brian Channon

KEY POINTS

- Radiographic film is composed of a film base with an active emulsion layer adhered using a subbing layer, with a protective super-coat.
- A cassette must be robust and light-tight.
- Intensifying screens convert the X-rays received into light, which forms the image on the film. This reduces the exposure needed to provide a diagnostic image.
- The latent image is converted into a permanent visible image through the use of developer and fixer.
- The chemicals used in processing should be replenished and replaced on a regular basis.
- Maintenance and quality assurance are essential to maintain high quality diagnostic images.

INTRODUCTION

Within the imaging department the use of automatic wet film processors to produce a visible image on a conventional film, which is exposed to light originating from intensifying screens held within a cassette, is declining. However, films exposed to a combination of light and X-radiation, using screen film, or directly to X-radiation alone using direct-exposure film, may still be encountered.

FILMS

The production of an X-ray image depends upon the existence of materials that are unstable and, when exposed to light or electromagnetic radiation, change their nature. Halogens such as bromine or iodine are combined with silver to produce silver bromide or silver idobromide.

FILM MANUFACTURE AND SENSITIVITY

Production of emulsion layer

It is essential that film manufacture is stringent and that films of the same type produced in different batches are identical. There are several stages in the formation of emulsion during which the grain size distribution and therefore the contrast and speed characteristics of film are determined. Initially silver nitrate and potassium bromide are added to a gelatin solution. Impurities are then added to create imperfections, known as electron traps or sensitivity centres, within the silver halide crystal lattice. In the latter stages of the process sensitisers that increase responses to specific colours of light or radiation and other agents, such as hardeners, bactericides, fungicides anti-foggants and wetting agents, are added.

Finally, as a result of these processes the emulsion layer, a precipitate of silver bromide within gelatine, is produced.

Spectral sensitivity

The spectral sensitivity of a specific emulsion is the range of wavelengths of the electromagnetic spectrum to which it will respond. Silver bromide crystals are inherently sensitive to the electromagnetic spectrum up to and including blue light, with other colours having a minimal impact.

During the manufacturing process the inherent sensitivity of the emulsion can be extended to other wavelengths by adding a suitable dye, usually to the surface of the crystal. The spectral sensitivity of the film emulsion can be arranged to fall into one of three categories: monochromatic, orthochromatic and panchromatic.

- Monochromatic emulsions – are blue sensitive (480 nm).
- Orthochromatic emulsions – have an extended sensitivity to include the green aspect of visible spectrum to approximately 620 nm.
- Panchromatic emulsions – have an extended sensitivity to cover all of the visible spectrum (675 nm) and thus must be handled in complete darkness. They are of limited use in diagnostic imaging.

It is essential that the colour of spectral sensitivity of the emulsion and the colour of spectral emission of the intensifying screen be matched in order to obtain maximum film blackening for the minimum exposure.

FILM CONSTRUCTION

Duplitised emulsion

The majority of screen-type film is 'duplitised'. This type of film has two sensitive emulsion layers – one on each side of base (Fig. 12.1). It is used for most general applications. However duplitised emulsions are also used for intra-oral dental film, although in this instance the film is exposed directly to X-radiation alone.

Film base

This is a thin layer of polyester (polyethylene teraphthalate), which transmits light and provides a support for the other layers.

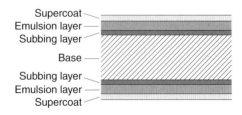

Figure 12.1 Cross-sectional diagram of duplitised emulsion.

It is essential that the base should be:

- Thin (0.08–0.18 mm depending on nature of film) – this assists in the reduction of image unsharpness caused by the parallax effect.
- Strong and flexible – to withstand stresses it will receive in film loaders and automatic processors.
- Chemically inert – so it does not affect either processing solution or sensitive emulsion.
- Impermeable to water – to aid in the reduction of processing time (and remains firm to facilitate transportation through automatic processors).
- Uniform thickness – to ensure maximal light transmission.
- Safety-base (non-flammable).

If colour tone is added it should be consistent between batches and not change tone with age. If either were to occur then density and contrast would change.

Substratum or subbing layer

This is a thin, strong adhesive layer that binds the base to emulsion. It plays a vital role in ensuring that these do not separate whilst processing, as the emulsion layer absorbs warm chemicals and swells. This layer is usually a mixture of the film base solvent and gelatin. A coloured dye may be included within this layer to reduce the amount of light transmitted from one emulsion layer to the other, reducing the crossover effect.

Emulsion layer

This is a suspension of light/radiation-sensitive silver halides suspended within a gelatin binder. The use of tabular (flat-shaped) silver halide crystals with a larger surface area–volume ratio, provides significant advantages including:

- increased speed and sensitivity of film due to a larger surface for interaction with light.
- grains lie in closer proximity, reducing the crossover effect.

Supercoat/anti–abrasive layer

This is a very thin coating of hardened gelatin. It protects the sensitive emulsion layer against

mechanical damage that can arise from handling and transport within manual and automatic film loaders and processors. However, two issues arise:

1. It must not be overly smooth as a specific amount of grip or roughness is required for the film to be transported through automatic processors.
2. If overly hard, processing fluid would be unable to penetrate it.

Single–sided emulsion

Single emulsion

Single-sided film, with one emulsion layer, may be used when a single intensifying screen is used; for example in mammography where high resolution is imperative and in instances when an image of a light source (laser source, photofluoro-graphic) is required. All films consist of a number of discrete layers.

This is similar in construction to duplitised film; however, the second emulsion layer is replaced with an anti-curl/halo backing (Fig. 12.2). Curl may occur during processing as the emulsion layer absorbs processing chemicals and water and expands to a certain degree. To avoid this a layer of gelatin of identical thickness to the emulsion layer is applied to the non-emulsion aspect of the film. During processing this will expand to the same degree as the emulsion, ensuring that the dry film will lie flat. In single-sided emulsions light can be reflected at the base–air interface, back towards the sensitive emulsion layer, thus creating a halo effect (Fig. 12.3).

To minimise the halo effect a coloured dye is incorporated within the gelatin of the anti-curl backing. This acts as a colour filter and absorbs light of specific wavelengths, increasing the

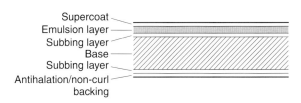

Figure 12.2 Cross-sectional diagram of single-sided emulsion.

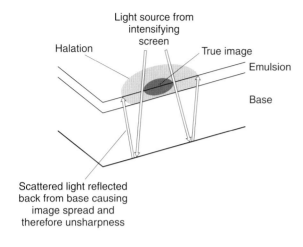

Scattered light reflected back from base causing image spread and therefore unsharpness

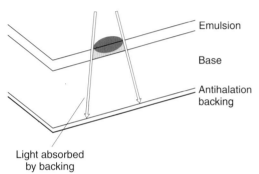

Light absorbed by backing

Figure 12.3 Halation.

resolution of the image. The dye colour utilised is always the opposite colour to the exposing light source; for example yellow dye to absorb blue light. The anti-halation dye is bleached out in the fixer during the processing cycle. Processors that process large numbers of single-sided films require a higher fixer replenishment rate than those that primarily process duplitised films, as the removal of anti-halation dye utilises more fixer energy.

Advantages of using duplitised emulsions

The use of 'duplitised' emulsions results in increased film speed and blackening for a given exposure because the amount of emulsion available for exposure enhances sensitivity. This effect is enhanced further when the film is sandwiched

between a pair of intensifying screens and provides several potential benefits in that:

- the radiation dose to the patient and the amount of scattered radiation produced is reduced – and reduction in scatter produces a safer working environment for staff
- owing to the decreased exposure, shorter exposure times can be used – providing a possible reduction in patient movement
- reduced exposures facilitate the use of a smaller focal spot size, reducing geometric unsharpness.

Image resolution and use of films

No radiographic image is truly sharp and all images are to some extent blurred as a result of imperfections within the imaging system itself.

Irradiation

This is the sideways scattering of light within the emulsion layer as a consequence of light striking the silver halide crystals (Fig. 12.4). This is a cause of image unsharpness, as the scattered light does not contribute to the primary image.

Halation

Halation occurs when an image is formed by light and some of this incident energy passes through the emulsion to the base. On reaching the base–air interface this light either passes out of the film or is reflected back towards the emulsion layer

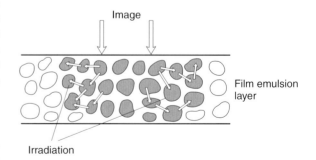

Light is scattered within the emulsion layer exposing crystals outside the image boundary thus increasing image unsharpness

Figure 12.4 Irradiation.

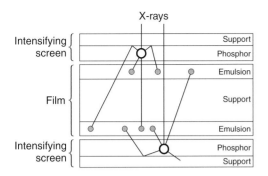

Figure 12.5 Crossover in an intensifying screen–film system.

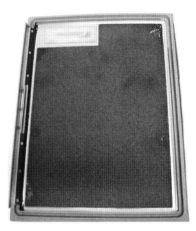

Figure 12.6 Cassette.

where it creates unsharpness by interacting with silver halide crystals.

Crossover

Crossover creates an increase in image unsharpness because light that is not completely absorbed in the emulsion layer nearest to source of light passes through the film base and subsequently interacts with silver halide crystals in the opposite emulsion layer, creating a wider and thus less sharp image (Fig. 12.5).

Parallax

Parallax is unsharpness caused by the separation of the two images recorded on duplitised film. There is an element of spatial separation between these images, and when subsequently viewed this separation creates a small degree of blur. In reality, the distance involved in image separation is very small, thus the blurring effect is negligible.

CASSETTES

In radiographic terms a cassette normally houses and provides a physically safe and light-tight environment for both the film and the intensifying screens in which the processes associated with fluorescence and the formation of the latent image can occur (Fig. 12.6). Cassettes are available in various sizes and with detailed differences between specific manufactures.

CONSTRUCTION

- The frame is either synthetic or metal to provide structural strength and support to internal features.
- Internal aspects are blackened to reduce risk of internal light reflections.
- The front recessed plate is made of carbon fibre, plastic or even aluminium to form the cassette well. Attenuation of the X-ray beam should be minimal and even across the plate; thus it is essential that the material used is of even density and thickness.
- The plate is firmly attached to the frame, providing support for the front intensifying screen.
- It may contain a small lead block, which prevents exposure reaching the film in the area designated for patient identification.
- The back is hinged to one side of the frame. This supports the back intensifying screen, which is often mounted on a foam or plastic pressure pad.
- A layer of thin lead foil may be located behind the pressure pad to help reduce backscatter.
- If the cassette can be used with a specific patient identification camera then it will include a recessed and sliding area, which should only open when within the camera device.

- Clips need to be strong and are thus frequently made of metal.
- The hinges are either plastic or metal.

The criteria for an effective cassette include:

- Light in weight, yet robust and durable.
- Rounded corners.
- Provides intimate contact between film and intensifying screen. The use of pressure pads, strong clips and hinges combined with other specific aspects used by individual manufacturers, such as a curved design or magnetic contact, help to achieve this.
- Must be individually identifiable.
- Must clearly indicate the type of intensifying screen contained within it.

CARE OF CASSETTES

Cassettes should be stored upright and away from heat. They should be cleaned and inspected on a regular basis. The outsides should be cleaned, following departmental protocols, after direct patient contact to prevent cross-infection.

INTENSIFYING SCREENS

Intensifying screens operate by converting X-ray energy into light photons. This occurs within the phosphor layer of the intensifying screen where the X-ray photons are absorbed by the phosphor crystals. This causes the crystals to become excited and luminescence occurs. Luminescence is the ability of a material to absorb short wavelength energy (X-radiation) and emit longer wavelength radiation (light). This process facilitates a gain within the imaging procedure as each X-ray photon that is absorbed releases many light photons, thus allowing the radiation dose to the patient to be reduced. In reality, approximately 95% of film blackening is created by light emitted from the phosphor layer and 5% by the direct effect of X-radiation.

Luminescence constitutes two effects:

- Fluorescence – occurs when the light emission commences (when exciting radiation starts) and terminates when exciting radiation stops.
- Phosphorescence (afterglow) – occurs when the light emission continues for more than 10^{-8} s after the exciting source has been withdrawn.

CONSTRUCTION OF INTENSIFYING SCREENS

The detailed construction of an intensifying screen can vary widely; it is, however, closely related to its planned use in clinical practice and comprises a number of discrete layers (Fig. 12.7).

Supercoat

A thin, transparent waterproof layer of cellulose acetobiturate extends around the sides (as an edge seal) and the back of the screen, encasing it completely. It forms an effective seal against a variety of fluids, any of which could seriously damage the screens. It also provides a limited degree of physical protection to the delicate phosphor layer. Light from the phosphor layer is able pass through this thin transparent layer easily, with minimal distortion, thus helping to minimise unsharpness. It is easy to clean and a poor generator of static electricity.

Phosphor layer

This layer consists of the phosphor crystals; suspended in a transparent binding material such as polyurethane. The nature of the phosphor crystals will vary depending upon the planned spectral emission of the intensifying screen. The speed of

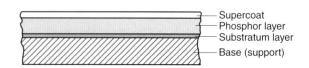

Figure 12.7 Construction of an intensifying screen.

the intensifying screen will depend upon both the type of phosphor crystal used and the density to which they are packed. Within high definition intensifying screens the use of coloured pigment or carbon granules in the binder material tends to absorb laterally scattered light within the phosphor layer. This minimises photographic unsharpness but requires an increase in radiation exposure to the patient.

Substratum

This forms the bonding layer between the base and the phosphor layer. It will vary depending on the intended use for the screens in that it may be absorptive, reflective or just transparent in nature.

When absorptive in nature a coloured dye is added to the substratum, which tends to prevent light that is travelling away from the film emulsion layer from being reflected at the base–phosphor interface back onto the film. This aids in the reduction of photographic unsharpness and is found in some high-definition type (slow) intensifying screens.

The reflective function is used in some high speed (faster) intensifying screens. Titanium dioxide or a similar white pigment is incorporated into the substratum. This acts to reflect light that is travelling away from the film emulsion layer back towards the film emulsion, reducing the radiation dose received by the patient but increasing photographic unsharpness.

Base

Frequently made of polyester, the base acts as a smooth and strong, yet flexible, support for the phosphor layer. It must be uniformly radioparent, chemically inert, moisture resistant (enhanced by coating) and ideally not discolour with age.

PHOSPHOR TYPES

It is essential that the materials used as phosphors are very efficient at absorbing X-ray photons and have high quantum detection efficiency. The phosphors should also be efficient at converting X-ray photons into light and exhibit minimal afterglow.

Modern rare earth phosphors, such as gadolinium oxysulphide, lanthanum oxybromide, yttrium oxysulphide and others, generally have both a higher detection and conversion efficiency than the older mostly blue/violet-light emitting materials such as calcium tungstate or barium lead sulphate. Rare earth phosphors are normally used in conjunction with a small amount of an activator, the combination of which determines both the spectral emission, colour of the emitted light, and its intensity of luminescence. For example a combination of gadolinium oxysulphide with terbium as an activator emits green light whilst lanthanum oxybromide with thulium emits blue light. Rare earth phosphors tend to emit the majority of light produced at discrete wavelengths and are referred to as 'line emitters', whilst older type materials, such as calcium tungstate, emit light continuously between specific wavelengths and hence are 'broad spectrum emitters' (Fig. 12.8).

MATCHING FILM SPECTRAL SENSITIVITY AND SPECTRAL EMISSION

It is essential that the film's sensitivity is matched directly to the spectral emission of the intensifying screens in order to achieve maximum film

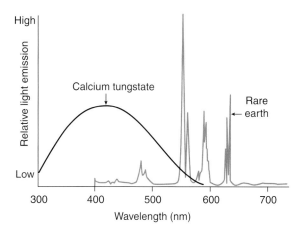

Figure 12.8 Light emissions for a broad spectrum emitter (calcium tungstate screens) and a line emitter (rare earth screens).

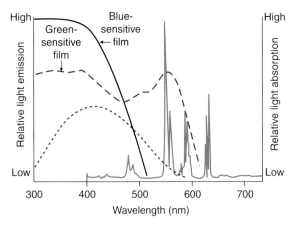

Figure 12.9 Diagram to show emission and absorption spectrums for rare earth and calcium tungstate intensifying screens, demonstrating the need to match light emission colour with film sensitivity.

blackening from a given radiation exposure to the patient (Fig. 12.9). When an orthochromatic-type film is used with intensifying screens emitting green light it can be seen that the majority of the light emitted by the intensifying screens lies within the spectral sensitivity curve of the film. This ensures optimal performance of the system. However, if a monochromatic-type film is used with the same intensifying screens, the majority of the light emitted by the screens lies outside the film's spectral sensitivity curve. Therefore, most of the emitted light will have minimal impact on the silver halide crystals within the film's emulsion.

TYPES OF INTENSIFYING SCREEN

Variations in the construction of the intensifying screen will produce screens with different characteristics for specific use.

- High-speed screens are used to image large or dense body areas or in circumstances where there is a risk of voluntary or involuntary patient movement. Increased speed is achieved by increasing the thickness, within limits, of the phosphor layer, by including a reflective layer and by increasing the size of the phosphor crystals. Therefore,

for a given exposure greater film blackening occurs but image resolution is reduced.
- High definition or detail screens are most commonly utilised for extremity imaging when a high tube loading is not necessary and fine detail is a prerequisite.

Enhanced image resolution may be achieved by the use of absorptive material within the substratum and inclusion of coloured dyes within the binding material of the phosphor layer. Except in special circumstances, intensifying screens are paired facilitating the use of duplitised film emulsions (see p. 136). In such circumstances the back intensifying screen will receive slightly fewer X-ray photons than the front screen due to absorption within both the front screen and the film itself. Thus the two images may be of a slightly different density. Manufacturers may either choose to ignore this and produce a pair of screens of identical speed. Alternatively they may opt to increase the speed of the back screen by the use of a reflective layer or greater coating weight or use a pigment to reduce the speed of the front screen.

RADIOGRAPHY WITH A SINGLE INTENSIFYING SCREEN

Mammography is the exception to the general norm that screens are always used in pairs. In this case a single-sided film emulsion is used in conjunction with a single intensifying screen with the prime aim being to reduce photographic unsharpness. The normal arrangement is for the intensifying screen to be positioned behind the film. This helps to reduce photographic unsharpness, because the light emission from the phosphor crystals has a shorter distance to travel prior to interacting with the silver halides within the film emulsion.

INTENSIFYING SCREENS AND IMAGE RESOLUTION

The use of screens plays a significant role in reducing the radiation dose received by patients. The following features of their construction make a significant contribution to the final image resolution:

- Presence of a reflective layer as part of the substratum degrades resolution.
- Presence of an absorptive layer as part of the substratum enhances resolution.
- Presence of carbon granules or coloured dye within the binder enhances resolution.
- Crossover effect. When light arising from one intensifying screen interacts with silver halides in an emulsion layer remote from it there is enhanced potential for spread due to the longer track taken.
- Size of crystals (larger crystals produce more light).
- Thickness of the phosphor layer. The potential spread of light can be greater when there is an increased distance between the phosphor and emulsion layers. (Obviously there is an overall limit to the thickness of emulsion.)

As the speed of the system increases then in general terms resolution is reduced. However, as with many aspects of imaging, a balance has to be struck between the competing considerations and the need to produce an image that is of a diagnostic quality.

QUANTUM MOTTLE

This arises when a very fast imaging system is utilised and a relatively small radiographic exposure is required. It occurs when a relatively small number of X-ray photons in the beam transmitted by the object are available to interact with the phosphor crystals. Thus the number of light photons available to interact with silver halides declines and the resultant image may be grainy, mottled or even unrecognisable.

CARE OF INTENSIFYING SCREENS

Intensifying screens are relatively delicate and as such must be handled with care. Most opening/closing occurs within film loaders, reducing the opportunity for damage to screens. If a need to open a cassette arises then this should occur in areas away from dust or liquid, which may cause contamination.

Internal cleaning is necessary to remove small artefacts that often appear as small white spots on the subsequent image and have a detrimental effect on image quality. The manufacturer's instructions relating to the procedure and cleaning agent should be followed. It is essential that the cassette is not reloaded and closed until both screens are completely dry. If a screen becomes damaged then it is irreparable and both screens within the cassette will need to be replaced, which is time consuming and expensive.

PROCESSING

The final stage in the production of a hardcopy X-ray image is processing. Automatic processing is often linked to a daylight handling system for the loading and unloading of cassettes.

Whilst passing through the automatic processor the film is subjected to a number of processes during which the latent image is changed into a visible format.

DEVELOPMENT

Development is the initial stage in the processing cycle which converts the latent image into a visible form. This involves a process of electron donation by which the exposed silver halide crystals are reduced to metallic silver whilst the unexposed silver halides remain unchanged. An exposed silver halide crystal possesses a weakness in its negatively charged ion barrier caused by a collection of silver atoms at the crystal's sensitivity centre. Electrons from the developing agent are able to penetrate the exposed silver halide and convert it into silver. Unfortunately, the developer is not entirely effective at differentiating between exposed and unexposed silver halide grains. The development of unexposed crystals contributes to the overall image density whilst reducing the contrast of the film.

The developer solution has various constituents including:

- Developing agent, which supplies electrons for the process of reduction. It is normally a combination of two specific developing agents – phenidone and hydroquinone – producing a PQ developer. They are used in precise proportions in order to utilise the specific features of each.
- Accelerator provides an alkaline environment, pH range 9.8–11.4, to allow the developer to function effectively. This is achieved by the use of potassium carbonate or potassium hydroxide. The pH of the developer, along with solution temperature, plays a major role in controlling the activity of the developing agent. The activity of developer is greater at higher pH levels.
- Restrainer (anti-fogging), usually benzotriazole, acts to aid the selectivity of the developing agent, helping to prevent conversion of unexposed silver halides. This is achieved by strengthening the negatively charged barrier that surrounds the silver halide. Potassium bromide, an effective restrainer, is produced as a by-product of the development process.
- Water is used as a solvent as it is clean and free from chemical deposits and is the medium in which the other developer constituents are mixed.
- The use of potassium sulphite as a preservative acts to reduce the rate of aerial oxidation of the developing agent and to facilitate the regeneration of phenidone by hydroquinone.
- Bactericides and fungicides act to restrain growth of organisms within the solution.
- Hardeners reduce the chances of damage to the emulsion layer during transportation or of the film becoming stuck in the processor. The hardening agents are usually aldehydes or sulphates. In addition, films are pre-hardened during manufacture.

Undesirable changes to the pH level of developer solution may occur as a result of both aerial oxidation and the acid by-products of the development process. Within modern developers the use of carbonates as accelerators and sulphides as preservatives counteracts the potential effects that could arise from changes in the pH of the solution.

Factors influencing development rate include:

- pH of the solution
- solution temperature – developing agent is more active at higher temperatures
- nature of the developing agent (controlled by the manufacturer)
- development time.

FIXATION

Major functions of fixation include:

- continuing the process of film hardening
- terminating further development
- converting undeveloped silver halides into a soluble silver complex
- making the image permanent.

Constituents of fixer

- Ammonium thiosulphate – the fixing agent is rapid acting and combines with undeveloped silver halides to form a soluble silver compound that then migrates through a process of osmosis into the fixing solution. Fixer therefore becomes rich in silver complexes.
- Acetic acid – ensures development is terminated and provides an appropriate environment, pH 4.0–4.5, in which hardener functions. If the pH of the solution is below 4.0 the fixing agent breaks down.
- Aluminium salts are commonly used as hardeners to reduce the drying time and enhance the hardening effect.
- Water as a solvent.

- Preservative reduces the rate at which the fixing agent decomposes. This is known as sulphurisation.
- Boric acid is used as an anti-sludging agent to reduce the rate at which the aluminium salts may precipitate out of solution.
- Buffers act to control the pH of the solution by neutralising the effects of the alkaline developer solution that is carried over within the film emulsion.

Factors affecting fixation rate include:

- presence of hardeners (slows process)
- high concentration of silver complexes in solution (retards process)
- variation in pH (pH should be constant)
- nature and concentration of fixing agent.

WASHING

This stage is designed to remove both residual fixer chemicals and silver salts from the film emulsion. This process is not 100% effective and residue salts can adversely affect the archival permanence of the resultant image, causing a brown stain. Therefore, the aim of washing is to reduce level of the residual salts to such an extent that they will not create staining during the expected life of the film. Washing is most effective when the film is exposed to a continuous flow or spray of uncontaminated water, as the diffusion of residual salts from the emulsion layer is more effective in clean water.

DRYING

If film completely dries it becomes brittle, so approximately 15% of the dry film is actually moisture. Air is used to evaporate excess moisture from the film. Air of low humidity (dry air) accelerates the process, as does air circulation.

AUTOMATIC PROCESSORS

The basic components within an automatic processor are very similar despite the differences that occur between manufacturers products in relation to design and film capacity (Fig. 12.10).

MAIN CONTENTS OF THE PROCESSOR

The processor is essentially a light-tight box containing:

- a series of processing tanks and a roller transport mechanism (Fig. 12.11). (Movement of film is achieved by racks of rollers. These are delicate and may be made of various materials and arranged in a variety of formations)
- an electric motor to ensure that all racks are driven at a constant speed. Plastic or stainless steel guide-plates assist movement at top and bottom of tanks where film changes direction
- crossover assemblies, located between adjacent processing tanks, utilise 'squeegee' rollers to remove much surface liquid (Fig. 12.12)
- Arrival of a film into the entry roller system can activate a number of processes,

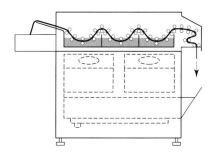

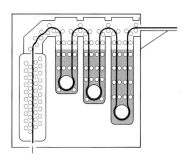

Figure 12.10 Processor types.

A

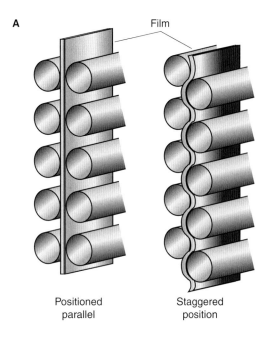

Film

Positioned parallel

Staggered position

B

Film

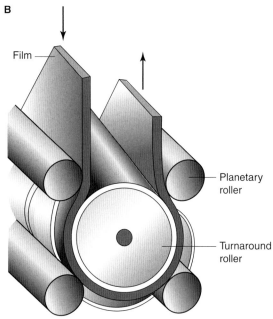

Planetary roller

Turnaround roller

Figure 12.11 A: Roller system from a processor. B: Roller from the bottom of the system to allow return of the film.

including replenishment of processing fluids, activated by either a microswitch situated above the higher entry roller or by an infra-red detector.

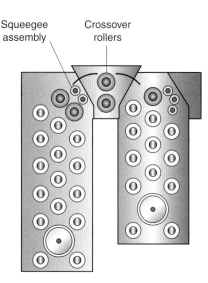

Squeegee assembly   Crossover rollers

Figure 12.12 Crossover assembly.

DEVELOPER SECTION

Temperature control

To maintain image quality temperature must be maintained within 0.5°C. An immersion heater working in conjunction with a thermostat may achieve this. Alternatively, a heat exchange unit may be used.

Drainage system

This facilitates the emptying of the tank for routine cleaning and maintenance. It is usually a length of plastic tubing which is screwed into a drain hole in the base of the tank. It may also act as an overflow pipe.

Replenishment system

This pumps fresh developer solution into the tank, maintaining the activity and quantity of developer within the tank.

Recirculatory system

This system requires inlet and outlet pipes, an electric pump and possibly a filter to ensure agitation and recirculation of the solution.

FIXER SECTION

The fixer section contains drainage, recirculatory and replenisher systems that are similar in function to those within the developer section (Fig. 12.13). The temperature control will be dependent on the design of the processor and may utilise heat exchange from the surrounding warm developer and wash tanks. In the case of cold-water wash units the temperature control is achieved by using an immersion heater thermostat device, with insulation provided in the dividing wall between the fixer and wash sections. The precise control of fixer temperature is not as critical as it is for developer solution.

WASH SECTION

This section aims to remove both residual fixer complexes and silver complexes; thus improving archival permanence of the film. Differing types are available including:

- a spray rinse that directs clean water at both surfaces of film as it transverses the tank. This is microswitch activated so it only operates when there is a film in the section
- a tank of running water with a flow rate of 7 L min^{-1}. This is not ideal as large quantities of water passing through the processor use considerable resources.

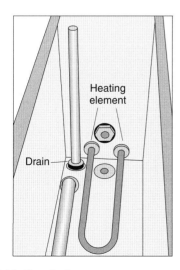

Figure 12.13 Fixer tank.

DRYING SECTION

There is danger to the film emulsion if the air used for drying is too hot. A microswitch is present to prevent film damage. There are a number of different systems available to dry films (Fig. 12.14).

- Infrared drying – this is where the heat from electrically heated elements is radiated onto the film whilst the air blown from a fan removes vapour.
- Hot air drying – this ensures heated, filtered air is directed onto the film from a series of cylindrical tubes, located between transport rollers. Some of the waste moist hot air is ducted to an external source as it can contain residual chemicals, whilst the remainder is re-heated and used again.

TRANSPORT SYSTEM

The film transport system comprises a series of rollers arranged in racks, driven by an electric motor at a constant speed (Fig. 12.15).

The arrangement of the rollers may vary and includes staggered or face-to-face. The deep or vertical rack system is the most common and is associated with high-capacity processors. During the processing cycle the film is required to change direction at the top and bottom of the tanks. In these situations plastic or stainless steel guide plates are utilised to guide the film through 90° directional changes. Rollers fit into distinct categories:

- Hard – made from PVC-type material, these guide the film.

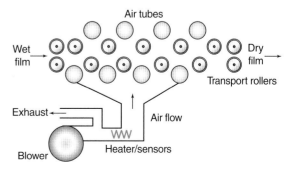

Figure 12.14 Dryer section.

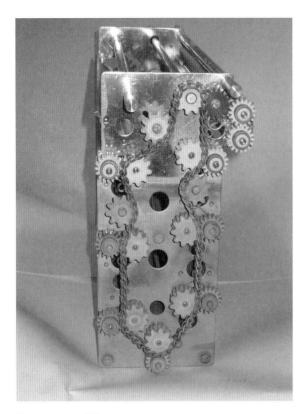

Figure 12.15 Film transport system.

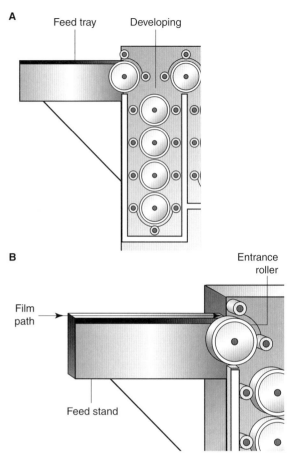

Figure 12.16 Film feed system.

- Soft – made from neoprene-type material. These include both the squeegee rollers and those needed for where extra grip is necessary to change direction of movement.

Squeegee rollers play an important part in reducing carry-over rate of chemicals. As a safety measure, a microswitch prevents roller operation if the lid of the processor is not in place.

FILM FEED SYSTEM

This system activates all the main processor functions and, in instances when manual loading of the processor occurs, gives an audible signal that it is safe to feed another film into the processor (Fig. 12.16). Different systems are utilised to achieve this, including:

- Entry roller detection – which occurs when a film activates a switch in the entry roller.

- Infrared detectors – which are placed just inside the processor behind the entry roller assembly.

REPLENISHMENT SYSTEM

As a film passes through the beam is broken. This calculates the film size and the required amount of replenishment. As films are processed then the nature of both the developer and fixer solution is subject to change. This occurs because the by-products of the process can alter the nature of the solution. Some solution is carried over on the film, reducing the amount present in the tanks and causing some contamination. Developer solution can become less active as it oxidises in the air and so constant replacement

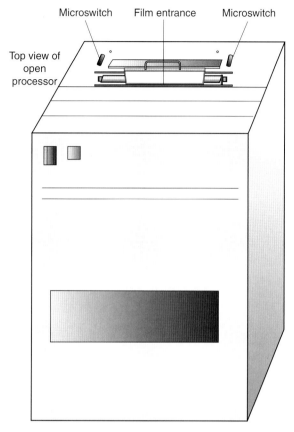

Figure 12.17 Replenishment system.

is essential. In order to maintain both solution activity and level, replenishment of solutions is essential (Fig. 12.17). Replenishment may occur whilst each film is fed into the processor when the microswitch is activated or is related to the area of film processed as calculated by infrared detector. The latter is the most accurate method.

MICROPROCESSOR CONTROL

Microprocessors can be used to monitor and display the performance of specific aspects of the unit, including temperature of solutions, dryer temperature, solution levels and transport speed.

STANDBY SYSTEM

This is designed to save energy and water, thus enhancing the efficiency of the operation of the processor by reducing the operating costs. Wear and tear on the system is also kept to a minimum. The system automatically shuts down some of the processor functions, including water supply, transport and circulation systems and dryer, if a film has not entered the processor within a prearranged time interval. The system will switch on again once a film enters the processor or after a predetermined time out of use, thus maintaining processors in a state of immediate readiness for use.

AUTOMIXERS (CHEMICAL MIXERS)

Mixers (Fig. 12.18) may differ in construction and mode of operation but all systems provide:

- mixing (replenishment tanks) of 34–40 litre capacity
- visible and audible warnings, given when the solution is low
- colour-coded replenishment chemical bottles that fit onto the top of the unit
- replenishment bottles that are pierced once they are placed in the correct position on the unit
- chemical drainage into the tank whilst water flushes out the bottle
- a pump that operates during filling to ensure mixing of the water and chemicals
- termination of the water supply when the solution level reaches the full sensor (the circulation pump continues for up to 10 min to ensure thorough mixing of the chemicals).

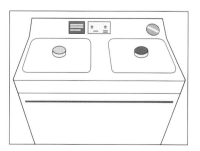

Figure 12.18 Automixer.

ADVANTAGES OF AUTOMIXERS

- Reduced chances of operator contact with chemicals and thus potential for skin/eye contamination.
- Accuracy of mixing in that the amount of solvent used is measured precisely on each mix, providing replenisher solution of the same constituency at all times.
- Time saving.
- Reduced potential for spills.

CARE AND MAINTENANCE OF THE AUTOMATIC PROCESSOR AND CHEMICAL MIXER

Routine maintenance, including regular servicing and actions taken by departmental staff, plays a vital role in the maintenance of image quality. Departmental protocols and manufacturer's instructions relating to care and maintenance may vary considerably. It is vital that these instructions are followed. It is *essential* that the unit is switched off and isolated from the mains prior to any work commencing.

Safety equipment for processor cleaning:

- Goggles (eyewash should be available)
- Aprons
- Gloves
- Suitable plasters to cover any cuts.
- Canister mask.

AUTOMATIC PROCESSOR CARE

These are guidelines; the specific care provided by manufacturers should be followed.

Daily

- Use colour coded cloths to avoid contamination.
- Clean the entry and crossover rollers and the solution level – dried chemical deposits can damage films.
- Some protocols require the water tank to be drained at the end of the working day, especially if the unit is not used for a period, or an antibacterial tablet may be added to the wash tank.

Weekly

- Daily procedure.
- Remove deep roller racks and clean under running water; do not use abrasive fluids. (Roller racks are heavy and manual-handling risks should be considered. Also it is essential to ensure that chemical contamination of processing tanks does not occur when removing or replacing racks into processing fluid.)
- Clean drained wash tank, again avoiding the use of abrasive materials.

In addition manufactures recommend the periodic drainage and cleaning of fixer and developer tanks.

PROCESSOR QUALITY CONTROL

Slight variations in operating parameters can produce a significant effect on final image quality. Many processors are capable of displaying a range of information relating to their operating parameters. It is vital that a record is kept of all checks and data obtained during processor monitoring activity. During all routine maintenance activities a general visual check should be made of all aspects, especially those relating to the drive mechanism.

Routine assessment should also be made of:

- drive time
- replenishment rates
- fluid agitation
- operating temperature.

A change to the nature of processing solutions occurs as a result of use; solution replenishment is designed to maintain the maximum function of both developer and fixer. Checks on processing chemistry include:

- assessment of pH levels – both developer and fixer solution function most effectively within a narrow pH range. pH should be tested on a regular basis
- estimation of silver content of fixer solution
- specific gravity testing – useful in determining the accuracy of dilution of neat chemicals. The expected figure is obtainable from the manufacturer.

SENSITOMETRIC TESTS

These may be used to determine the actual function of the processor. This involves the production or purchase of 21-step control strips. The process may be computerised or manual.

Computerised

In these circumstances a strip reader is utilised to determine fog level, speed and contrast when a processed 21-step sensitometric control strip is fed into the unit. The information gleaned from the strip is used to produce and evaluate a characteristic curve. The unit may also indicate whether the curve is within normal limits and, if not, the potential remedial action that should be taken.

Manual

This requires the use of a densitometer, and as the density of specific parts of the image must be recorded manually it is a somewhat lengthy and time-consuming procedure. Results are used to plot graphs that investigate trends by recording the fog levels, density and contrast (Fig. 12.19).

Parameters assessed

Fog is determined by measuring the density of a part of the film that has not been exposed during the production of the strip. This density is used to form a base line for subsequent records. The test is performed daily and on subsequent days the

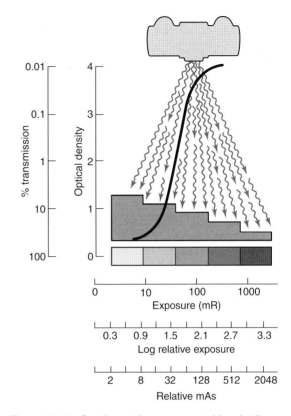

Figure 12.19 Sensitometric curve created by plotting optical density values obtained from exposure to a step-wedge tool.

density of an identical part of the film is measured and plotted on the graph.

Film speed is a sensitive indicator of variations in developer solution activity. The density of steps is determined and the step with the nearest to a density of 1.0 plus basic fog is selected. The density of this step is recorded on the graph. On subsequent days the density of the same step number is measured and recorded on the graph.

Selecting two steps and measuring the density of each can assess contrast. It is better to avoid the use of adjacent steps because density differences may be very small. The lowest density figure is then subtracted from highest, with the difference being plotted on the graph. On subsequent days the density of the same step numbers are measured and the differences recorded on the graph.

CHEMICAL MIXERS

- Should be cleaned at regular intervals, with the tanks drained by the use of circulation pumps.
- The overflow drain should be used to remove any residual chemicals.
- The removed solution is stored for further use.
- Clean tanks by using water and a brush – but avoid contamination.
- Replace overflow drain and refill.

HEALTH AND SAFETY CONSIDERATIONS

It is essential that an assessment of the health and safety risks associated with a given procedure be undertaken prior to working with processing chemicals. Staff must be adequately instructed to undertake the task and safety equipment should be provided and utilised. Information relating to the actions to be taken in the event of an accident should be clearly displayed. Regular monitoring of the working environment should occur to ensure that occupational exposure standards are being maintained.

Further reading

Ball J, Price T. Chesneys' radiographic imaging, 6th edn. Oxford: Blackwell Science; 1998.

This text provides a clear description of all aspects of processing and films.

Gunn C. Radiographic imaging: a practical approach. 3rd edn. Edinburgh: Churchill Livingstone; 2002.

Environmental Protection Act 1990. London: HMSO.

Water Act 1989. London: HMSO.

The Control of Substances Hazardous to Health Regulations 2002 (SI 2002/2677). London: HMSO.

These three documents should all be consulted, as their contents are applicable to the use and disposal of processing chemicals and water.

Chapter **13**

Digital radiography

Fiona Chamberlain

KEY POINTS

- Most hospitals within the UK are now completely film-less or in the process of replacing film with various digital systems.
- Digital images can be viewed rapidly, manipulated quickly (annotated, cropped), then sent to a computer network for reporting and viewing.
- The introduction of teleradiography means that images can be viewed and reported on around the world, thus making use of international expertise and collaboration.
- Some DDR imaging plates are fragile and susceptible to temperature variation.
- Mammography is currently one area where film is still being used quite extensively, although this is expected to change within the next few years.
- There are two types of digital imaging in use: computed radiography (CR), and digital radiography (DR).

INTRODUCTION

As with the recent developments with general photography, where digital cameras are replacing film, this technology is also being used to replace X-ray film with digital imaging. Digital imaging has already been in use for many years in computed tomography (CT), magnetic resonance imaging (MRI), nuclear medicine (NM), fluoroscopy and

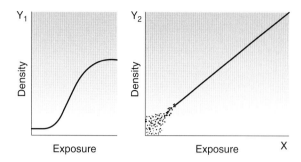

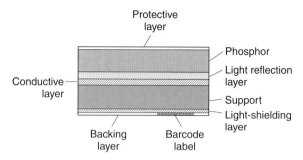

Figure 13.1 A film characteristic curve with the limited latitude for a diagnostic X-ray film (*left*) compared to that of digital imaging (*right*).

Figure 13.2 Construction of the imaging plate showing the photostimulable phosphor (PSP) layer.

ultrasound, but only recently has conventional X-ray equipment started to use digital technology.

Digital radiography has greater exposure latitude than X-ray film; therefore any over- or underexposure of an image can still be viewed. However, there is a trade off between radiation dose and image quality, as high exposures will give a very clear image but an unacceptable dose to the patient. Low exposures will result in a noisy (grainy) image and may miss diagnostically significant information. This is an advantage over the traditional film–screen combination where any exposure in the foot or shoulder areas of the characteristic curve will result in no usable image being obtained (Fig. 13.1).

COMPUTED RADIOGRAPHY

Computed radiography (CR) has been used as a direct replacement in areas where previously film was used. It uses storage phosphor cassettes in standard X-ray rooms and has allowed radiology departments to make the transition from film to digital imaging without significant equipment changes.

THE IMAGING PLATE

The imaging plate is coated with a photostimulable phosphor (PSP), which captures X-rays once they have passed through the patient or object being imaged (Fig. 13.2). The PSP material has been

'doped' with small amounts of impurities which alter the physical properties of its crystalline structure.

A PSP material has a high absorbance at the energies used for diagnostic radiology and is able to store the irradiated energy and then release it as visible light in response to the stimulation of a beam of laser light within the reader. The family of europium doped barium fluorohalides fits these criteria – BaFX, where X can be chlorine (Cl), bromine (Br) or iodine (I).

As the X-rays pass through the PSP material, they interact with the electrons in the crystalline structure, giving them energy, which enables them to enter the conduction band. Some electrons return immediately to the valence band, but others remain 'trapped' in the forbidden zone between the two bands (Fig. 13.3). This trapped signal is proportional to the amount of radiation incident on the plate; these electrons form the latent image in the PSP.

RETRIEVING THE LATENT IMAGE

To retrieve the latent image from the PSP it is placed in a CR reader, where a laser scans it (Fig. 13.4). The laser gives the electrons enough energy to return and leave the traps and to decay down to the ground or valence state. As these electrons move down in energy a blue light is emitted. This light is collected by a light guide and directed towards the photomultiplier tube. The light moves through the photomultiplier, is then amplified and then the signal is digitised using an analogue-to-digital converter, allowing the temporary storage

Photostimulable phosphor (PSP)

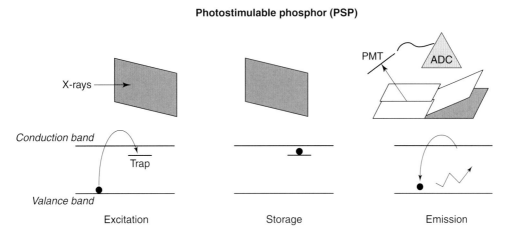

Figure 13.3 Schematic sequence of images of conduction and valence bands showing 'trapped' electrons.

of the image in digital format. This can then be sent to a monitor for viewing or to a printer.

ERASURE OF THE PLATE

Unfortunately the read out with the laser does not clear all the trapped electrons, as there are traps at many different energy levels that do not respond to the energy of the laser light beam. The remaining electrons are removed using a bright white light, which has enough energy to pass through the PSP and all the traps will respond. This removes any residual signal from any previous images. It should also be exposed to this bright light, a 'primary' erase, to prevent build-up of background signals over time.

CARE OF THE IMAGING PLATE AND CASSETTE

All manufacturers have a suggested cleaning and maintenance procedure and it is important to follow their guidance and use the recommended products in order not to invalidate any warranty or guarantee.

CR plates should be checked regularly for damage, as part of a departmental quality assurance programme, and removed from use or repaired if damage is found. The imaging plates also need regular checks because they are removed from the cassette each time they are read – edges tend to get damaged, cracks can appear and they can be vulnerable to scratches. Once again any damaged plates must be removed from service. There have been reported problems with cassette catches opening

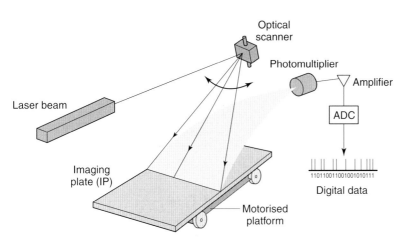

Figure 13.4 Schematic of a computed radiography (CR) plate reader.

and the plates dropping out, so these must be checked and cleaned before being returned to service. Imaging plates have an estimated life of 10 000 exposures (manufacturer dependent), so it is important to make sure cassettes are rotated and used evenly throughout a department.

With CR the detector is separate from the imaging device and incorporates extra stages to the production of an image, digital radiography removes the need for a cassette and a reader from this process.

IMAGING THE PATIENT USING CR

The patient is registered to each imaging plate used by means of an individual barcode on each plate, using the patients' hospital number. X-rays are then taken, the operator inputs into the CR reader the views that have been taken (e.g. chest X-ray (CXR), abdominal X-ray (AXR)) and the plates are then placed in the CR reader, which picks up the barcode and allocates images to the correct patient, along with the correct protocol for image processing (Fig. 13.5).

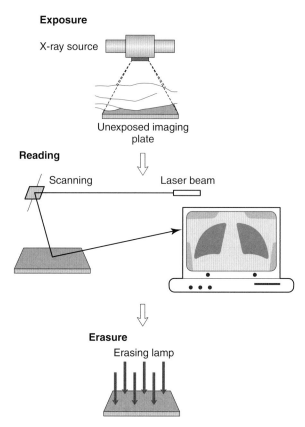

Figure 13.6 The sequence of events during a diagnostic examination using computed radiography.

The CR reader then removes the plate from the cassette and this is read out as previously described. The image is subsequently viewed on an acquisition workstation where it is cropped and markers applied (i.e. L or R, PA, AP, etc.). The image can be checked for quality and dose indicators, such as sensitivity or exposure index (manufacturer dependent). Once the radiographer is satisfied that the image is correctly identified, manipulated and annotated, it is then sent on to the network for reporting and storage for retrieval at a later date from anywhere within the network (Fig. 13.6).

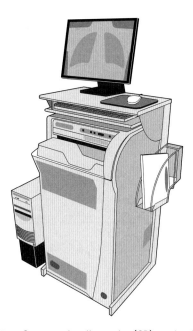

Figure 13.5 Computed radiography (CR) reader for single cassette use.

DIGITAL RADIOGRAPHY

Currently there are two types of system utilised for digital imaging:

- Indirect digital radiography – produces an analogue signal that is then converted by an analogue-to-digital converter
- Direct digital radiography – transforms the incoming X-ray photons directly into an electronic signal.

The image receptor is usually an integral part of the X-ray equipment so it is more expensive to implement than CR.

INDIRECT DIGITAL RADIOGRAPHY

Indirect digital radiography (IDR) uses a phosphor (caesium iodine, CsI), which is coated over an active matrix array (AMA) of amorphous silicon (a-Si) (Fig. 13.7).

Image production

- The X-ray photons are absorbed by the phosphor material where they are converted in to light photons.
- The amorphous silicon array converts the light into an electrical signal.
- This signal is then sent to an image processor (photo-diode) to allow image display and storage.

- The signal strength is proportional to the number of X-ray photons, which then produces the image.

Disadvantages of using IDR systems

Scatter can be a problem with this system and the amount can depend on the thickness and structure of the phosphor material; however, this will be less than with screen film. Noise on the image can also be an issue but cooling the detector can reduce this. Systems are currently restricted by size as each photo-diode represents one pixel in the image, and images are several mega- or even giga-pixel sized. Therefore spatial resolution is restricted due to the physical size of the photo-diode and the pixel.

DIRECT DIGITAL RADIOGRAPHY

Direct digital radiography (DDR) does not use a phosphor material; the X-ray photons are directly converted into an electrical charge. The detector material used is amorphous selenium (a-Se) which is coated on a thin-film-transistor (TFT) array (Fig. 13.8).

A bias voltage is applied across the detector structure and as the X-rays pass through they directly generate positive and negative charges which are in proportion to the level of X-ray exposure. The positive charge is drawn to the capacitor where it is stored and readout by the customised electronics within the array. The imaging plate is made up from millions of these detectors causing

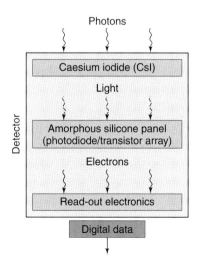

Figure 13.7 Amorphous silicon detector.

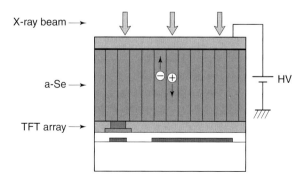

Figure 13.8 Amorphous selenium detector.

variations between them. Software is available to smooth out the differences between the detectors on the plate. This smoothing process is known as 'stitching'. As with CR, the patient images are checked, annotated and sent onto the computer network for reporting and storage.

Advantages of an amorphous selenium detector

- This detector type has better spatial resolution as there is no scatter in a phosphor layer.
- There is only one energy conversion, compared to the two needed for IDR, so it has greater efficiency.
- The design is simpler so manufacturing is slightly easier.
- Each pixel does not need a photo-diode.

Disadvantages of an amorphous selenium detector

- This type of detector is very temperature dependent and extremes of heat or cold can damage it.
- It is quite fragile so is not suited to mobile units.

COMPUTED RADIOGRAPHY VERSUS DIGITAL RADIOGRAPHY

Computed radiography is cheaper to implement than any DR system and CR is seen as a direct replacement for film. In some areas it can be seen as being cost neutral, owing to the saving made from not purchasing processing chemicals and film. There have also been health and safety gains by the removal of film processing equipment, the reduction in chemical vapours in the workplace and disposal of used chemicals.

DR necessitates the replacement of the entire X-ray unit (normally), so the process of implementation will be slower as it is probable that it will be installed as part of an overall equipment replacement plan, which could take many years. Radiology departments which are film-less tend to have a combination of CR and DR technologies. This helps with training issues, as CR is less of a step from the conventional film-screen techniques than

DR. Staff need to be able to utilise the new technology and get accustomed to softcopy viewing and reporting. This must be factored into the installation costs and timescales in order to ensure full and best use of the equipment.

Both CR and DR have the scope to reduce the radiation dose, when compared to film-screen imaging, although they have not yet shown significant dose reduction. In fact it has been reported that a phenomenon known as 'dose creep' has started to happen; operators have been increasing the exposure factors to improve image quality, and radiologists and consultants have come to expect to see good high quality images. CR and DR have fairly comparable resolution and efforts are being made to improve this with new technology and materials used.

PACS – PICTURE ARCHIVING AND COMMUNICATIONS SYSTEM

PACS is the system predominately used for the image acquisition, image display, the network and storage and retrieval of images in most hospitals and clinical environments. Implementation of PACS has become widespread and has resulted in the use of softcopy display for reporting and display (Fig. 13.9).

IMAGE DISPLAY

As with the image production, the viewing display must be seen as the final part of this process for the reporting workstations. These displays must be able to manage large data files, be able to show the full resolution and greyscale levels of the image and have a fast response to manipulation of the images. For subsequent image reviewing the high quality is not so important so standard PC monitors are acceptable.

Viewing conditions must be optimised where possible for reporting workstations: they must be in an area of low ambient light, with little or no reflection off the screen from other light sources. They should be part of a quality assurance programme to ensure viewing conditions remain satisfactory throughout the monitor's lifespan.

The reporting monitors must be checked daily using a recognised test pattern such as the

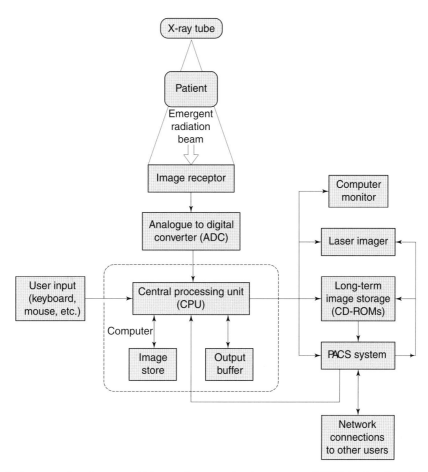

Figure 13.9 Typical set-up of a picture archiving and communications system (PACS) in the clinical environment.

SMPTE test pattern (Fig. 13.10). There should be checks for distortion and centring, by verifying that all 11 luminance patches are visible. It should be checked that the 5% and 95% patches can be seen and the visibility of the high and low contrast line pair patterns should be assessed.

DICOM – DIGITAL IMAGING AND COMMUNICATIONS IN MEDICINE

This is the industry standard for protocols between different systems. It enables modalities within a radiology department to communicate with each other and so would apply, for example, between CT and ultrasound. DICOM enables images to be displayed on the PACS system regardless of the type of image and the equipment manufacturer. It

is therefore important that during any equipment purchase phase the DICOM standard must be stipulated as an essential requirement to ensure compatibility.

EPR – ELECTRONIC PATIENT RECORD

The EPR is a programme available in many NHS hospitals and it is planned to be linked to all UK hospitals, allowing patients' records and notes to be available wherever they may be treated. PACS will become a part of this and allows the radiology images to be viewed alongside the patients' notes. The EPR has been designed to integrate the existing HIS (hospital information systems) and RIS (radiology information systems) into one single system.

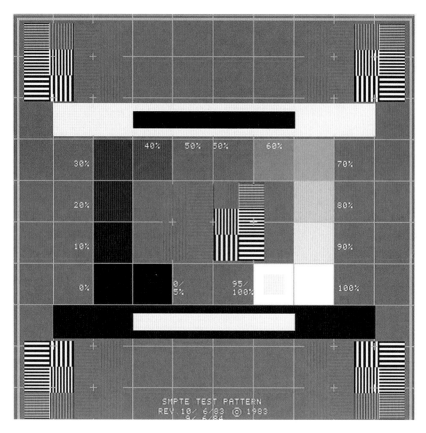

Figure 13.10 SMPTE test pattern.

Further reading and information

Bushong SC. Radiologic science for technologists. 8th edn. St Louis: Mosby; 2004.

This text provides a well-illustrated and informative chapter covering all aspects of digital imaging.

Oakley J. Digital imaging. Cambridge: Cambridge University Press; 2003.

An informative and extensive text covering everything you need to know about digital imaging in one place.

Website

www.kcare.co.uk

This website provides extensive and useful information on all aspects of equipment. Research is carried out to assist in the development of protocols and identify areas of best practice.

Chapter **14**

Image quality

Ken Holmes and Marc Griffiths

KEY POINTS

- Image quality affects the ease of extracting information from an image.
- Good image quality will ensure the maximum amount of diagnostic information is gained from the image.
- Sharpness is essential as blurring of an image will lower the image quality.
- Contrast describes the difference in density between two adjacent structures.
- Density is the degree of blackening on the film.
- Fault finding is essential to ensure that image quality is optimal.
- Understanding the cause of faults will ensure rectification of the cause and improved image quality.

INTRODUCTION

One of the fundamental roles of practitioners in radiography is to produce optimum radiographs for reporting. Image quality is difficult to define because it is subjective in its nature, but an optimum quality image enables the observer to extract information from the image and make an accurate diagnosis. Poor quality images have a poor signal-to-noise ratio and detract from the process of extracting information. However, there are characteristics of a radiograph, which may be evaluated, and enable the practitioner to distinguish the diagnostic quality of the image. These factors include:

- magnification and distortion
- sharpness
- radiographic density
- contrast
- latitude of the film or the resolution of the monitor (VDU).

These factors can be affected during the production and processing of the image (both analogue and digital processing) and once the image has been produced or displayed. It is essential that if a film is produced it is viewed under optimum viewing conditions and must not be held up to the nearest light bulb! Digital images must also be viewed on an appropriate monitor with diagnostic resolution.

SIGNAL–TO–NOISE RATIO

One concept used to define image quality is the signal-to-noise ratio. The signal is the useful information from the patient being imaged and the noise is anything that detracts from accessing the information. Useful information is derived from photoelectric interactions within the patient (absorption by body structures) and noise is derived from scattered photons, because the image receptor does not have the ability to determine their origin. In radiographic images if the signal level is high compared to the noise, structures within the body will be clearly seen, but if the signal level is similar to or less than the noise level then the structure will become obliterated.

Images produced in radiography are often a compromise between obtaining a perfect signal and reducing the noise. The production of images is constrained by a number of factors including the radiation dose level and each component of the imaging chain. For example, a faster film-screen system is utilised when imaging the abdomen than for the extremities and this enables the practitioner not only to produce a diagnostic image with minimal noise but to minimise the radiation dose to sensitive organs.

MAGNIFICATION

When producing a radiographic image all objects in the image are larger than the object being X-rayed. This magnification is due to the geometry of imaging. The ideal situation is to have the object being X-rayed as close as possible to the image receptor, parallel to the X-ray tube and the image receptor, with the radiation beam at right angles to the object. This minimises the magnification of the image but also, more importantly, the magnification of the unsharpness in the image (Figs 14.1 and 14.2).

If the object being imaged is not parallel to the image receptor it will be magnified; however, each end will be magnified differently and this will produce distortion. This may be elongation or foreshortening of the image (Fig. 14.3).

The focus to image receptor (SID; see p. 91) should be as long as possible and the distance between the patient and the image receptor (object–film distance, OFD) as short as possible. For practical reasons the SID is usually 110 cm for techniques on the X-ray table and 180 cm

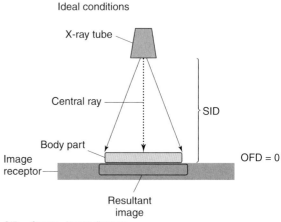

SID   Source–image distance
      This should be as long as possible
OFD   Object–film distance
      The object should be as close to the image receptor as possible. As the object moves away from the image receptor the magnification increases. This makes the object bigger but also magnifies any unsharpness in the image

Figure 14.1 Image with minimal magnification.

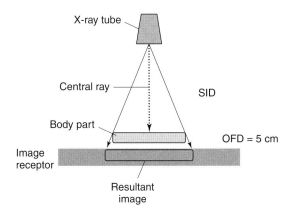

Figure 14.2 Image demonstrating magnification – if the body part is not in contact with the cassette, the result is magnification.

for chest and cervical spine erect film work. The OFD should be as close as possible and ideally the object is in contact with the image receptor. Using a Bucky assembly also causes magnification of the image but the grid is necessary to reduce scatter and improve the contrast of the image. Practically, the mechanism which moves the grid and houses the Bucky is kept as small as possible.

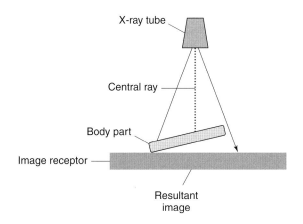

Figure 14.3 Image demonstrating distortion – if the body part is not parallel with the cassette, the result is distortion. Distortion also occurs when the X-ray beam is angled across the object being X-rayed.

SHARPNESS

In order to determine the image quality the image must be sharp. Blurring will reduce the image quality and also reduce the diagnostic quality of the image. The factors affecting sharpness are:

- movement
- the resolution of the imaging system (film-screen combination or VDU)
- the geometry of the imaging system (relationship between the focus, patient and imaging system).

MOVEMENT UNSHARPNESS

Movement unsharpness should be kept to a minimum by careful radiographic technique. Making the patients comfortable, giving them precise instructions on breath holding and planning the procedures all help reduce this. Using short exposure times also helps reduce blur in the image. Exposure times as low as 0.003 seconds for a chest radiograph enable the practitioner to ensure minimum movement, even in paediatric patients.

RESOLUTION OF THE IMAGING SYSTEM

This is covered in more detail in other chapters of the book (see pp. 141, 154). However, it should be noted that the fastest film-screen combination or exposure index compatible with diagnostic quality should be used. When determining the quality required in an image the practitioner must be aware of what structures need to be defined. An image to determine the position of bones in a plaster cast following an orthopaedic reduction needs less resolution than the original image to diagnose the fracture. Ideally the smaller of the foci of the X-ray tube should be used (fine focus) but if this does not enable a short exposure time to be used on a patient likely to move then the practitioner may need to use a broad focus. This is another example of where the practitioner needs to make a decision that is a compromise between the ideal conditions and getting a diagnostic image.

GEOMETRY OF IMAGING

The positioning of the patient (geometry) to produce an image has a direct relationship to the quality of that image. The section on magnification (p. 162) outlined the ideal conditions needed to produce radiographic images and dealt with the requirements to reduce magnification (p. 163). It also emphasised that any increase in the size of the object also increases the unsharpness of the image and this will be explored in this section.

Figure 14.4 is a diagrammatic representation of image production and shows that a penumbra (unsharpness) is formed with any image that is produced from a finite source (focal spot). The diagram uses a large distance between the object and image receptor to illustrate the principle of the penumbra. In practice the amount of geometric unsharpness (U_g) in an image is small and may be much less than 1 mm.

Measurement of the penumbra (U_g) is a straightforward calculation using similar triangles. Figure 14.5 demonstrates the diagrammatic representation of similar triangles and the calculation to determine unsharpness in an image of

- Focal spot size 0.5 mm
- SID 100 cm
- OFD 1 cm

Calculate: Ug

Formula: $Ug = \dfrac{\text{Focal spot size} \times \text{OFD}}{\text{FOD}}$

$\dfrac{0.5 \text{ mm} \times 1 \text{ cm}}{99 \text{ cm}} = 0.005 \text{ mm}$

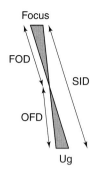

Figure 14.5 Diagram to demonstrate geometry unsharpness when taking an X-ray of a finger.

a finger due to geometric unsharpness. The values used are typical in radiography and the unsharpness is only 0.005 mm.

MEASUREMENT OF UNSHARPNESS IN AN IMAGE

The sharpness of the image can be measured using a test tool (resolution) or by viewing the image and determining whether fine structures can be visualised (definition). The resolution can be determined by measuring the ability of the imaging system to resolve the smallest object of the test tool and is expressed in line pairs per millimetre ($lp\ mm^{-1}$). This is perhaps an abstract concept to illustrate sharpness and it would be more sensible to determine the definition within the image; for example, can I see the bony trabeculae?

Again, however, definition within the image is subjective and depends on a number of factors including the viewing conditions and the experience of the practitioner viewing the image.

RADIOGRAPHIC DENSITY

Radiographic density is generally applied to hard copy images and can be defined as the amount of overall blackening on the film.

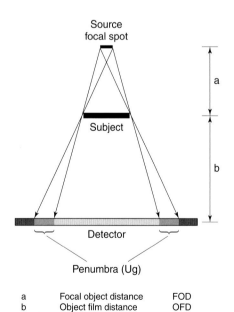

a	Focal object distance	FOD
b	Object film distance	OFD
a + b	Source–image distance	SID

Figure 14.4 Diagram to demonstrate the geometry of imaging.

It is an easy concept to understand at each extreme of density. All practitioners will be familiar with an image which has so much blackening that it is impossible to see any detail within the image, making it undiagnostic. Similarly, a film which has insufficient blackening, where the structures cannot be defined at all, has no diagnostic value. The secret to good practice is to produce an image with the 'optimum density', enabling the practitioner viewing the film to make an accurate evaluation of the patient's condition and therefore the correct diagnosis. Unfortunately in conventional film-screen radiography, once the image is processed there is little that can be done to rectify a poor quality image except use a bright light to look at images with too much blackening.

The equivalent term when viewing digital images is 'brightness' and this may be defined as the intensity of light that represents the individual pixels in the image. Brightness is controlled by the processing software and can be adjusted following image processing.

Numerous factors can affect the radiographic density, as shown in Box 14.1.

When viewing a radiograph that is suboptimal, due to the radiographic density, it can be difficult to define the reason for the problem. This will be discussed at the end of the chapter.

CONTRAST

Contrast is a more difficult concept to understand in an image and can be influenced by a number of factors (Box 14.2). There are a number of ways of defining contrast in an image. Generally when we refer to contrast we mean the radiographic contrast, but practitioners should be precise in their terminology.

Box 14.1   Factors affecting the radiographic density

Milliampere–second (mA s)	This is the product of the mA and duration of the exposure (exposure time). The mA s directly affects the density of the image. Increasing the mA s increases the intensity (number of photons) in the X-ray beam and hence the number incident on the image receptor.
Kilovoltage (kV$_p$)	Increasing the kV$_p$ increases the intensity of the X-ray beam. Unlike mA s there is no direct relationship between density and kVp. Changes in the kV$_p$ also affect the quality of the beam (the range of photons) and the radiographic contrast.
Source–image distance (SID)	The intensity of the X-ray beam changes due to the inverse square law. As the distance to the source of the radiation (focus) increases the intensity decreases as a product of the square of the distance.
Use of grids	These absorb both the primary beam but, more predominantly, the scattered radiation. Grids reduce the overall density of the image and improve the radiographic contrast.
Film–screen speed	When using a film-screen combination the relative speed of the system will affect the density. Higher film-screen speeds are more efficient and increase the density of the image.
Collimation	Increasing the area of the patient that is irradiated will produce more scattered radiation and hence reduce the density of the image. Good collimation increases the contrast of the image.
Tube filtration	This is fixed in modern tubes but altering the filtration may affect the range of photons produced and hence the density.
Processing	Both the development of film in a film processor and the operating characteristics of the digital processor can affect the density.

Box 14.2   Factors affecting radiographic contrast

Kilovoltage (kV$_p$)	Increasing the kV$_p$ increases the intensity of the X-ray beam. The predominant process above 60 kV$_p$ is Compton scatter. Generally speaking, as the kV$_p$ increases the radiographic contrast decreases and this is due to the increased scattered radiation produced.
Subject contrast	The composition of the patient varies depending on the anatomical area. Images of the chest and abdomen have very different inherent contrast.
Collimation	It is essential to collimate (restrict the size of the beam) to the area being X-rayed. Increasing the area irradiated increases the scatter produced and therefore reduces the contrast.
Film–screen combination	The type and speed of the film-screen combination determines the inherent contrast of the image.
Grids	Grids eliminate scattered radiation and increase the contrast of the image.
Air gap	Air gaps have a similar function to grids. If there is a large distance between the object and the image receptor (OFD) a number of scattered photons, as they travel forward, will miss the image receptor.
Processing	Both the development of film and the manipulation of the digital image can affect the contrast.
VDU characteristics	The contrast can be adjusted by windowing the image post acquisition. Together with brightness adjustment, windowing allows the practitioners to view a wide range of structures.
Contrast agents	These are used to enhance the contrast of the image. They generally occupy an internal structure of the body, e.g. bowel. The subject contrast is therefore altered, affecting the contrast of the image.

Radiographic contrast

Differences in optical density on a radiograph:

- A high contrast image has few differences in density and is black and white (Fig. 14.6).
- Low contrast images have a large range of densities and more shades of grey (Fig. 14.7).

The radiographic contrast of any image will affect the ability to make an accurate diagnosis: if it is not optimum important structures may be poorly defined and an incorrect diagnosis made.

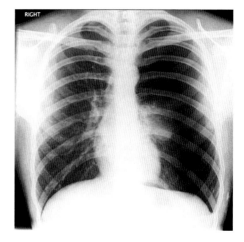

Figure 14.6 High contrast images with few shades of grey and large differences in densities.

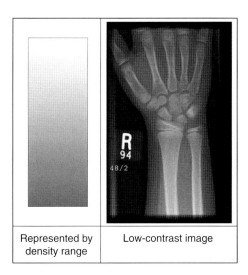

| Represented by density range | Low-contrast image |

Figure 14.7 Low contrast image with many shades of grey and small differences in densities.

1. Subject contrast (differences in densities within the patient):
   - depends on the proton number of the structures and the electron density (see p. 112)
   - varies depending on the area of the body
     - the thorax has high inherent contrast and adjacent areas have large differences in proton number (air in lungs vs. dense heart muscle)
     - the abdomen has low inherent contrast with adjacent areas having a similar proton number (muscle, fat and organs).

2. Subjective contrast (how we perceive the contrast in an image):
   - depends on a number of factors including
     - radiographic contrast
     - viewing conditions
     - experience of the practitioner viewing the image.

3. Objective contrast:
   - is where the optical density is measured using a densitometer and two areas compared to determine the contrast. The results are then generally illustrated by a characteristic curve.

Practitioners may think that resolution of an image is dependant on the contrast qualities of the image. Unfortunately, due to the subjective nature of viewing images, the concept that these two factors are dependent on each other still confuses inexperienced practitioners. High contrast images appear sharper (higher resolution) to the inexperienced practitioner. When viewing images the ability to see small structures is the true measure of definition. The resolution should always be measured in an image, which has an optimum radiographic density and contrast.

LATITUDE

The latitude of the film–screen combination is determined during manufacture. Latitude can be defined as the region of useful exposure which will produce an image in the diagnostic range of densities.

In film–screen imaging an optimum exposure will produce an image with the details required in the useful density range (Fig. 14.8). Unfortunately it is not possible to manufacture a film with both

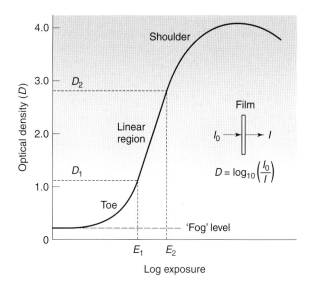

Figure 14.8 Characteristic curve for a film–screen imaging system.

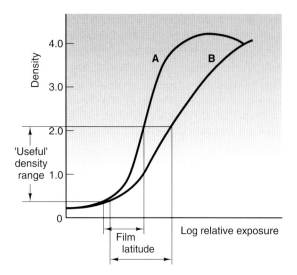

Figure 14.9 Characteristic curves for a high and low latitude film-screen imaging system.

high contrast and wide latitude. Generally speaking, the faster the film (the less exposure it needs to reach the maximum density) the higher the radiographic contrast and the narrower the latitude. A film-screen system with a speed index of 100 has the highest resolution and a wide exposure latitude. A film-screen system with a speed index of 400 requires less exposure to produce an image and has less resolution and narrow latitude. Figure 14.9 demonstrates the characteristic curves for two films – film A is a 400-speed system and film B a 100-speed.

Overexposure will produce an image with too high a radiographic density whilst underexposure will produce an image with one that is too low. In a faster speed film-screen combination, which has narrower latitude, it is easier to over- or underexpose the image as the useful density region is narrow. The contrast of the image in both of these circumstances is reduced, affecting the practitioner's ability to see detail within the image.

VIEWING A RADIOGRAPH

Having taken all the knowledge and skills of the practitioner to produce an optimum image it is essential that the image produced is viewed under optimum conditions. The equipment used and the environment used to view the image will affect the practitioner's ability to extract information from the image. It is important not only to have correct viewing conditions but also to concentrate on viewing the image without distraction from colleagues.

The viewing box is the main equipment for viewing hard copy images. It is essential that all viewing boxes are part of a Quality Assurance programme and that the colour and intensity of light output are comparable. The viewing box must have even illumination, with a northern or tropical daylight output and a colour temperature of 6500 K.

There are six specific factors associated with the viewing of images that need to be considered when viewing images. The following information is taken from EUR 16260EN:

'The proper assessment of image quality and accurate reporting on the diagnostic information in the radiographs can best be achieved when the viewing conditions meet the following requirement:

- The light intensity incident on the viewer's eye should be about 100 cd/m^2. To achieve this, the brightness of the film illuminator should be between 2000 and 4000 cd/m^2 for films in the density range 0.5 to 2.2.
  – This can be measured with a photometer.
- The colour of the illumination should be white or blue and should be matched throughout a complete set of film illuminators.
- Means should be available to restrict the illuminated area to the area of the radiograph to avoid dazzling.
  – Only one viewing box should be illuminated and small images masked using black templates.
- Means for magnifying details in the displayed radiographic image should be available. These means should magnify by a factor of 2 to 4 and contain provisions to identify small image details of sizes down to 0.1 mm.
  – This is achieved using a magnifying glass.
- For viewing exceptionally dark areas in the radiographic image an additional spotlight with iris diaphragm providing a brightness of at least 10 000 cd/m^2 should be available.
- A low level of ambient light in the viewing room is essential.'

ACCEPTABLE IMAGE GUIDELINES

Image quality is normally considered in terms of the practitioner's ability to perceive normal anatomy or detect any potential pathology. The image must have optimum contrast and density, maximum image sharpness and minimal noise. The image should demonstrate the anatomy or pathology of interest as conspicuously as possible; for example in extremity radiography this is bony trabeculae and for a chest radiograph a sharp reproduction of the vascular pattern in the whole lung, particularly the peripheral vessels, is required.

EUR 16260 EN gives details of guidelines for quality criteria for a number of radiographic examinations (chest, skull, lumbar spine and pelvis)[1] and EUR 16261EN outlines quality criteria for paediatrics.[2] Images should only be repeated if they are not of diagnostic quality (Box 14.3). If the clinical question is answered by the image but it is of poor aesthetic quality the image should not be repeated.

Box 14.3   Factors affecting acceptable image quality

Image annotation	The patient identification, the date of examination, positional markers and the name of the facility must be present and legible on the film. These annotations should not obscure the diagnostically relevant areas of the radiograph.
Patient positioning	Correct patient positioning plays a major role in determining the success of any radiographic examination. The area of interest must be included and the patient must be correctly positioned to demonstrate the relevant anatomy.
Image definition	The relevant anatomy is visualised and the area of interest sufficiently penetrated, e.g. bone trabeculae, skin surface. The structures are shown without misleading distortion.
Collimation	Image quality is improved and the radiation dose to the patient is reduced by limiting the X-ray beam to the smallest field giving the required diagnostic information. Radiosensitive organs need to be excluded whenever possible from the primary beam. On no occasion should the X-ray beam fall outside the image receptor area.
Protective shielding	For radiation protection purposes, standard protection devices should be available to shield radiosensitive tissues or organs whenever possible.
Film blackening and contrast	This has a major influence on image quality. The range of the mean optical density (D) of a clinical radiograph should normally lie between $D = 1.0$ and $D = 1.4$ and the optical densities of fog and film base should not exceed $D = 0.25$. For the diagnostically relevant parts of the film, the overall range of optical densities should lie between 0.5 and 2.2. These densities are difficult to assess subjectively; therefore the definition of one or a few critical points of the particular radiographic projections would be desirable where the optical density of a specific anatomical feature and its contrast relative to the surrounding image could be measured; e.g. bony trabeculae and skin surface.
Film processing	Optimal processing of the radiographic film has important implications both for the diagnostic quality of the image and for the radiation dose to the patient. Film processors should be maintained at their optimum operating conditions as determined by regular and frequent (i.e. daily) quality control procedures.
Radiographic exposure conditions	Knowledge and correct use of appropriate radiographic exposure factors, for example kV_p, focal spot value, tube filtration, and source–image distance (SID) is necessary because they have a considerable impact on image quality.
Artefacts	The image should be free from artefacts, especially clothing which may obscure relevant details.

COMMON FAULTS WITH REMEDY

This is a difficult concept to articulate and I would strongly advise the practitioner to perform the task of image evaluation with an experienced radiographer or clinical tutor. Often it is difficult to determine the exact cause of the fault and a systematic approach is desirable to determine what may have caused your image to be of poor quality (Table 14.1).

Table 14.1 Common faults with remedy

Fault	Possible causes and remedies
Poor contrast	Poor collimation – collimate to the area of interest Obese patients – consider compression binder or using a grid
Artefacts	Clothes, ECG leads
Unsharp image	Imaging geometry, patient movement, poor screen/film contact (only affects limited areas of the image) Increase source–object distance ● Use fine focus ● Use short exposure times ● Give clear instructions ● Make patient comfortable ● Consider immobilisation with pads/sandbags ● Good QA and identify cassette responsible and remove from practice
Increased film blackening (too dark an image)	Overexposure (this is the most obvious reason for an image with increased film blackening and the easiest one to remedy) Simply check the exposure factors on the control panel Incorrect film/screen combination Again, check the cassette for the film/screen speed. You may have used a regular (400 speed) cassette for an extremity (100 speed) Automatic Exposure Device (AED) This may occur for a number of reasons: ● Collimation within the chamber selected ● Incorrect chamber selected (the structure selected has a higher proton number or is thicker than the structure of interest) e.g. an outside chamber over the chest when undertaking a spine image Film fogging Fogging of films may occur along the edge of the film due to light leakage into the cassette or globally due to light leak or faulty safelights in the darkroom. Neither of these processes are likely in a modern department due to QA programmes Film processing There are a number of reasons for dark images due to faulty processing Overactive developer may be due to over-replenishment, too high a developer temperature or too long in the developer. These faults are unlikely to occur due to processor QA but will affect several images, not just the one the practitioner is concerned about.
Reduced film blackening (too light an image)	Underexposure This is the most obvious reason for an image with decreased film blackening and the easiest one to remedy; simply check the exposure factors on the control panel Incorrect film / screen combination

Continued

Table 14.1 Common faults with remedy—cont'd

Fault	Possible causes and remedies
	Again check the cassette for the film/screen speed. You may have used an extremity (100 speed) cassette for a shoulder (400 speed) Automatic Exposure Device This may occur for a number of reasons: • Too short an exposure time to allow the density to be achieved • The incorrect chamber selected (area selected has a lower atomic number or is thinner than the required area), e.g. an inside chamber over the chest when undertaking a spine image • Area of body does not cover the relevant chamber Film processing There are a number of reasons for light images due to faulty processing: • Underactive developer due to over-replenishment • Too low a developer temperature • Contamination of the chemistry These faults are unlikely to occur due to processor QA but will affect several images, not just the one the practitioner is concerned about.

References

1. European guidelines on quality criteria for diagnostic radiographic images. June 1996 EUR 16260
2. European guidelines on quality criteria for diagnostic radiographic images in paediatrics. July 1996 EUR 16261 EN

Further reading

Whitley AS, Sloane C, Hoadley G et al. Clarke's positioning in radiography, 12th edn. London: Hodder Arnold; 2005.

The definitive work on radiographic technique. Comprehensive information presented in a logical manner with excellent illustrations.

Gunn C. Radiographic imaging: a practical approach, 3rd revised edn. Edinburgh: Churchill Livingstone; 2002.

Covers all aspects of imaging technology, easy to use, learn from and an easy reference.

Fauber T. Radiographic imaging and exposure, 2nd edn. St Louis: Mosby; 2004.

Thorough yet practical approach to fundamental principles. This is an American text so you need to be a little cautious of terminology.

Website

http://health.gulfcoast.edu/chest2/image.htm [Accessed 28 February 2008]

Interesting definition of terms with images.

http://www.nde-ed.org/EducationResources/Community College/Radiography/cc_rad_index.htm [Accessed 28 February 2008]

Excellent website with a comprehensive range of information.

Chapter 15

Mammography

Karen Dunmall

CHAPTER CONTENTS

KEY POINTS

- A knowledge of the structure of the breast is essential to allow accurate positioning and interpretation of images during a mammography examination.
- Breast positioning follows clear protocols to ensure reproducible and diagnostic images.
- Equipment used during mammography is designed specifically for the examinations performed.

INTRODUCTION

Mammography is the general term for the imaging of the breast using X-radiation as a diagnostic tool to identify benign or malignant lesions. It can, however, be divided into two distinct categories:

1. Symptomatic – where an individual (usually a woman) presents with a breast symptom, for example:
   a) Palpable lump – rubbery and easily moveable, high probability of benign.
   b) Skin-pitting, puckering, ulceration and thickening.
   c) Veins – asymmetry and increase may indicate tumour.
   d) Nipples – discharge or inversion.
2. Screening – where the woman is invited for screening for breast cancer. This is routinely

initially between the ages of 50 and 64 and through age extension projects to 65–70. Women can 'self refer' after the age of 70.

SOFT TISSUE RADIOGRAPHY

Within general radiography the differences in density of varying parts of the subject (the subject or patient contrast) is usually visible at 45 kV. This is due to the attenuation of the X-ray beam by various tissues being dependent on the cube of the proton number of the structure (Z^3):

- Adipose tissue, $Z = 6$
- Fibrous/glandular tissue, $Z = 7$
- Calcium, $Z = 20$

Therefore bone and soft tissue structures attenuate X-rays at quite different rates and produce an image with visible contrast between 50 kV and 70 kV.

Soft tissue radiography is utilised when imaging structures where the proton numbers of the tissues are very similar to amplify the differences in density to allow the different tissues to be identified.

The relative radiolucency of breast tissue also demands an X-ray beam of penetrating ability (beam quality) of 20–35 kV_p. In mammography the lowest kV_p should be selected so as to give the highest subject contrast, as the absorption coefficient of soft tissue falls rapidly with an increasing kV at low energies. However, if the energy is too low, there will not be enough intensity to penetrate the breast to produce an image. This will just increase the radiation dose and time of the exposure. So there will be a compromise between good image quality and keeping radiation doses as low as reasonably practicable. Therefore, to optimise the image the breast must be compressed; this helps reduce the overall thickness and, consequently, the radiation dose (as there is improved beam penetration), reduce the risk of movement unsharpness, and improve the contrast resolution, by reducing scatter. The compressed breast will be closer to the image receptor, which improves the spatial resolution.

With larger compressed breast thickness there is a need to use a higher energy kV_p, which does cause a slight loss in contrast, but is acceptable due to the dose saving.

ANATOMY OF THE BREAST

The adult breasts are two hemispherical organs situated on the anterior and lateral aspects of the chest wall, on the surface of the pectoralis major muscle (Fig. 15.1). The breast extends from the second rib superiorly (and clavicle) to the sixth rib inferiorly, and laterally from the mid-axillary line to the sternal edge medially. The glandular tissue in the upper outer quadrant of the breast, which extends into the axilla, is known as 'axillary tail'. The nipple usually lies at the level of the fourth/fifth rib space; however, the breast is

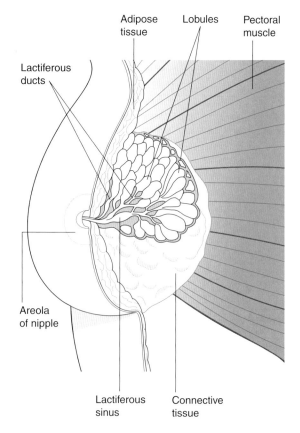

Figure 15.1 Internal structure of the breast.

a mobile structure, which varies considerably in size and shape, so this should not be seen as a reliable surface marking.

The adult breast is composed of glandular tissue and fatty tissue, which accounts for the variation in size and shape. The glandular tissue is formed from 15–20 lobes, each consisting of several small lobules. A lobule has a number of secretory alveoli, which open into lactiferous ducts. The lobule and the duct form the basic unit of histopathology as the majority of benign and malignant lesions arise in the terminal ductal lobular unit (TDLU). Each lobe of the breast is drained by one lactiferous duct, which passes upwards to form dilated sinuses (ampulla) behind the areola. The areola is the area of pigmented skin surrounding the nipple. The lactiferous sinuses exit by individual orifices onto the nipple surface. The fatty tissue lies under the skin, separating it from the irregular boundary of the anterior surface of the glandular tissue known as the superficial fascia. Fibrous strands, which extend from the skin to the superficial fascia, form the suspensory ligaments (Cooper's ligaments).

Figures 15.2 and 15.3 depict, respectively, the venous drainage and arterial supply of the breast.

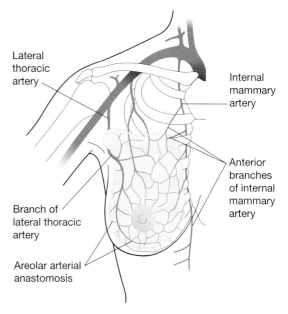

Figure 15.3 Arterial supply.

LYMPHATIC DRAINAGE

The lymph drains from the central portion of the breast, the circumareolar region and the skin surface, into a plexus of vessels on the surface of the pectoral muscle (Fig. 15.4). Approximately 75% of lymph drains into the axillary glands with only 25% passing from the medial half of the breast into the internal mammary nodes. There is also a limited amount of crossover between breasts and into the abdominal lymphatics. The relatively high occurrence of cancers in the upper outer quadrant and central areas of the breast and the fact that the majority of the lymphatic drainage passes into the axillary region have a direct importance in the selection of the mediolateral oblique as a screening position for breast cancer.[1]

HISTOLOGY OF THE BREAST AND RADIOGRAPHIC APPEARANCE

The structure of the breast, with its varying amounts of glandular, fibrous and adipose tissue, holds the key to the best age for imaging the breast using X-radiation.

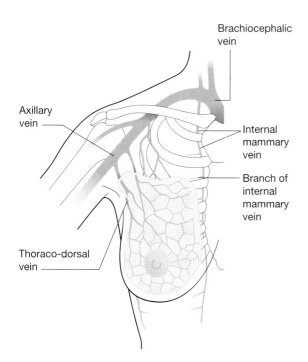

Figure 15.2 Venous drainage.

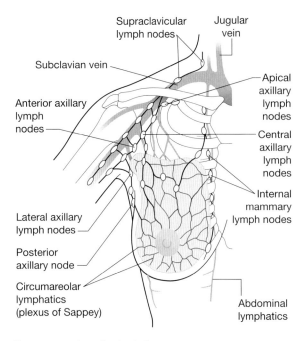

Figure 15.4 Lymphatic drainage.

There are three main types of tissue within the breast:

1) Adipose (fatty) tissue – this tends to be radiolucent as it has a proton number of 6 and results in areas of relatively higher optical density on the image.
2) Fibrous tissue – this is indistinguishable from glandular tissue on the radiographic image as it has a similar proton number (7) but does appear as an area of lesser optical density than adipose tissue.
3) Glandular tissue – as above; it is usually referred to as fibro-glandular tissue due to the similarity of radiographic appearance. Cancers arise from the epithelial lining of the TDLU and are defined dependent on the varying degrees of proliferation and abnormal growth.

BREAST DEVELOPMENT AND STRUCTURAL CHANGES

The adolescent female breast develops from rudimentary tissues that start to form during fetal development. There are varying periods of inactivity; however, the process speeds up during pre-puberty and puberty. The adolescent breast has a greater amount of developing glandular tissue but the shaping is usually caused by the accumulation of adipose tissue. The breast is a radiosensitive organ that is at greatest risk from radiation between 10 and 19 years of age, but there is also a risk between the ages of 20 and 39.

The adult breast is less dense than that of the adolescent and has a greater fat content. The exception to this occurs during pregnancy and lactation when the TDLU increase in size and the epithelial cells prepare for the secretion of milk. After lactation ceases the TDLU reduce in size and number.

During the menstrual cycle changes occur in the breast which relate to the hormonal effects on the epithelial cells in the TDLU. Although the changes do not appear on the image the discomfort experienced during the pre-menstrual period may produce difficulties in positioning and compression of the tender breast.

The density of the breast tissues on a mammogram image depends on the relative amounts of glandular, fibrous and adipose tissue present (degree of obesity of the patient). There is a gradual decrease in the glandular tissue of the breast, which is termed as involution. This can begin to occur as early as 35 years and is associated with the decline and cessation of ovarian function. In the menopausal and postmenopausal period (45–75 years) there is a more noticeable increase in fat deposition and glandular tissue reduction. Screening mammography is carried out between the ages of 50 and 64+; this correlates to the menopausal/postmenopausal phase of the breast. On a mammogram this is indicated by the majority of the dense tissue occupying the upper outer quadrant, hence the indication for the mediolateral oblique. This also becomes important in the positioning of the automatic exposure control (AEC) chamber (sometimes also referred to as an automatic exposure device, AED), as the exposure will be insufficient to penetrate the dense tissue if the AEC is under an area of adipose tissue.

MAMMOGRAPHY EQUIPMENT

Figure 15.5A shows a typical mammography unit and Figure 15.5B is of an X-ray unit showing the AEC position.

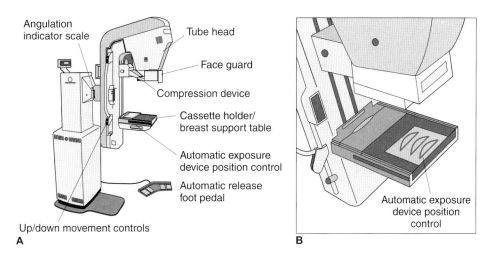

Figure 15.5 **A** A mammography unit. **B** A mammography X-ray unit showing position of automatic exposure control (AEC).

X-RAY TUBE AND HOUSING

A constant potential generator supplies the X-ray tube. The source–object distance (SID) is shorter than normal diagnostic X-ray examinations (45–60 cm) and the use of a fine focal spot of between 0.15 and 0.4 mm reduces geometric unsharpness. Image quality needs to be of an absolute high standard (i.e. micro calcifications, fine details).

With mammography equipment the tube housing is more compact than a standard X-ray tube (Fig. 15.6). The lower kV_p employed is a favourable

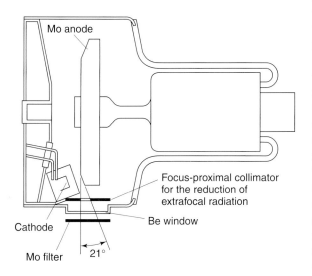

Figure 15.6 X-ray tube.

factor in permitting a smaller tube housing. Both high-tension cables enter the tube housing via the anode end to avoid patient contact. One particular type of unit has a system whereby the tube head moves out of the way during procedures such as biopsy or stereotactic localisation. As well as being able to move the X-ray tube head there is also a Perspex face guard to prevent the head from moving into the X-ray field. The tube is orientated with the anode further away from and the cathode closer to the patient, thus utilising the 'anode heel effect'. The increased output at the cathode side of the X-ray tube is directed at the thicker chest wall edge of the breast whilst the 'heel effect' is over the thinner nipple edge.

The main difference to a normal diagnostic tube is the use of molybdenum (Mb) as the target material. Traditionally, the only way to reduce the beam quality was to use a lower kV_p; however, varying the target material and filtration can improve the penetrating power whilst reducing the glandular tissue dose in dense breasts. Tungsten (W) does not have any characteristic radiation at low voltages, unlike molybdenum (Fig. 15.7). Despite the lower intensity of brehmsstrahlung from molybdenum, this reduction in intensity is offset by the characteristic X-ray emission of molybdenum. Rhodium (Rh) is now also used as a target material and filter, its characteristic radiation is slightly higher than molybdenum,

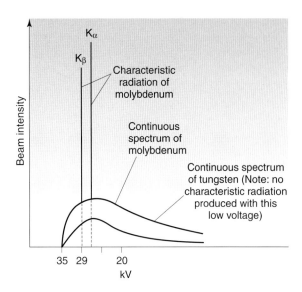

Figure 15.7 Graph to show characteristic radiation of molybdenum.

which makes it useful for patients with dense breast tissue or who have undergone radiation treatment or hormone therapy.

- Molybdenum target tube voltage: 24–30 kV$_P$ (K characteristic 20 keV)
- Rhodium target tube voltage: 26–32 kV$_P$ (K characteristic 23 keV)
- Tungsten target tube voltage: 22–26 kV$_P$ (K characteristic 69 keV)

The filtration of the beam is essential to remove the low energy photons and minimise skin dose. By utilising multiple target and filtration combinations it is possible to tailor the beam quality to the specific tissue-type requirements. The beam penetration can be improved by employing the same material as a filter and target material. The material used for the exit port is also important in 'hardening' the beam in general X-ray equipment; however, in mammography a beryllium (Be) window permits the softer radiation to pass through and enhance the subject contrast.

EQUIPMENT – FITNESS FOR PURPOSE

Overall, the equipment should be non-threatening in appearance and have a quiet operation level. This is important to reassure the woman and thus encourage the uptake rate and re-attendance. Mammography, by virtue of the technique, may be uncomfortable due to the compression of the breast; however, there are various adaptations, which should enhance the experience.

The anatomical size and shape of breast makes imaging more difficult than other parts of the body. In order to ensure reliability and reproducibility the mammographic image must demonstrate the whole of the breast. The shape of the breast tends to create variation in image density gradients, which have the potential to lead to misdiagnosis.

COMPRESSION PLATES

Compression plates ensure improvement in overall density and minimise motion unsharpness. The breast support table and compression devices must have rounded edges to aid in patient comfort and safety. The radiographer controls the compression, which is normally applied gradually and is indicated by an LED display showing the force in newtons; there is also immediate postexposure auto-release. 'Hands-free' compression is enabled by a dual control foot pedal that allows the operators' hands to be used to guide the positioning of the patient. During biopsies and stereotactic localisations the immediate release of the compression device is overridden, to keep the patient immobilised. In some units a sudden large movement of the patient during compression will trigger automatic release from compression. There are pressure sensor interlocks to prevent overcompression of breast tissue but these can be overridden by a manual control.

SUPPORT TABLE

The support table is connected to the mammography unit and directly centred to the X-ray tube. The beam is automatically collimated by means of a cone which produces a D-shaped field in order to ensure consistent accuracy, protect the patient and enhance the contrast by reducing the area irradiated and hence scatter produced.

The breast support plate must be height adjustable and rotate in different planes to accommodate the different needs of the patient. A digital display indicates the angulation of the breast support, which assists the radiographer in reproducibility of images. Within the support table there is the AEC, which corresponds to D-shaped areas on the Perspex compression plate so that its position relative to the underlying breast tissue can easily be seen. The AEC system has an array of eight solid-state measuring cells. The breast support table also houses the anti-scatter grid mechanism and the cassette tunnel (or the digital imaging system). There is an interlock to prevent double exposure of a cassette or the irradiation of a patient without a cassette in place.

TUBE COLUMN

There are handgrips on the tube column, which are aids for stability of the patient. There are also fail safe interlocks and brakes which act during power cuts to prevent sudden movement of equipment and potentially serious consequences for the patient. The movement of the X-ray tube housing and support table may be motorised to aid the radiographer and reduce strain on the upper arms. The equipment is earthed for electrical safety.

RADIATION PROTECTION FOR STAFF AND PATIENTS

A lead equivalent glass screen affords radiation protection for staff. The presence of a pre-determined collimation area, the automatic optimisation of parameters (GE units) and combinations of target material/filter all assist in minimising the exposure and hence dose to the breast and patient.

Automatic optimisation uses the first 0.015 seconds of the exposure to automatically determine and apply the optimal kV, filter and track selection according to the composition of the breast under study. This results in a potentially lower dose to the patient and a reduction in the number of exposure related repeats.

Some units utilise the digital acquisition of mammography images. This gives the ability to manipulate images (magnification and windowing) and to transfer and digitally archive. Amorphous selenium (aSe) is the next generation of detectors, offering higher digital quantum efficiency with lower dose and higher resolution.

COMPUTER AIDED DIAGNOSIS (CAD)

CAD is a sophisticated tool that identifies suspicious lesions and assists the radiologist/reader in the early detection of breast cancer. Triangular markers indicate possible microcalcification clusters and asterisk-shaped markers highlight regions suggesting masses or architectural distortion. The advantages of CAD may include the reduction in the number of individuals needed to interpret the images, together with an increase in sensitivity. However, research carried out has yet to show clear benefits from this technological advance.[2,3]

TECHNIQUE

The initial part of any radiographic procedure should be to gain consent from the patient to have the examination performed. Screening mammography is no exception, so before any woman is screened an explanation should be given as to what will happen and an indication of the discomfort which may occur. In some screening centres a questionnaire is completed by the mammographer indicating:

- whether there is a family history of breast cancer
- the existence of any known pathology or unusual symptoms; e.g. nipple discharge, pitting, etc.
- menstrual history
- pregnancy history
- any noticeable scars or skin lesions; e.g. moles, skin tags.

It may also be the policy to carry out a manual breast examination prior to mammography.

THE CRANIOCAUDAD PROJECTION

Stage 1: Woman stands in front of the X-ray equipment

1. The breast support table (Bucky) is parallel to the floor.
2. The cassette is in place if using a conventional unit.
3. The marker is in place for craniocaudad (RCC or LCC) projection on the outer lateral aspect of the support table.
4. The woman stands in front of the mammography machine with the breast support table adjusted to be at the same height as the inframammary fold, approximately nipple level.
5. The mammographer stands to the opposite side of the patient being imaged.
6. The hand on the side of the breast being imaged is guided to lie across the abdomen to help achieve a relaxed pectoral muscle.
7. The woman is asked to walk forwards towards the support table, where the mammographer raises the breast under examination by placing a hand gently underneath the breast to simulate the craniocaudad position. The woman is requested to turn her head to one side so that it is parallel to the face guard (Fig. 15.8).

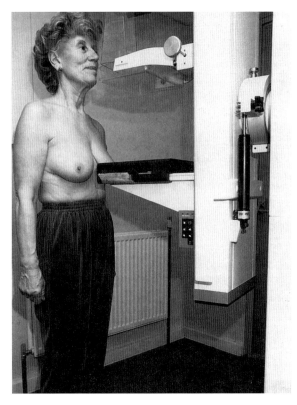

Figure 15.8 Stage 1 position. The breast support table is at the same height as the infra-mammary fold, at approximately nipple level.

Potential areas for errors in positioning at stage 1

- If the breast support table is too high, the woman may feel the need to raise herself to fit on the support but during compression may settle back into a lower position. This would pull the breast away from the unit and result in the area adjacent to the chest wall being missed. In addition, the nipple might not be in profile.
- Alternatively, the breast support may be too low, causing an area of inframammary fold to be hidden under the breast and the nipple not to be in profile.
- If a woman is turned too far medially or laterally this would result in partially missing off the medial or lateral quadrant of the breast.

Stage 2: Lifting the breast onto the support table

1. The breast should rest on the support table with the woman's anterior abdominal wall in contact with the edge of the breast support table.
2. The mammographer guides the woman towards the support table by placing her hand on the woman's back. Care must be taken not to turn the woman too far medially or laterally, which might result in the omission of breast tissue from the X-ray.
3. The breast is eased forwards so that the skin on the under surface is not folded (Fig. 15.9).
4. The breast is held in place by the mammographer's hand whilst compression is commenced, ensuring that the nipple remains in profile.

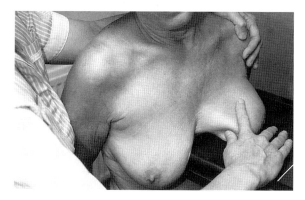

Figure 15.9 Lifting the breast onto the support table.

5. The shoulder of the side under examination is guided back so it does not clash with the compression plate.

Potential areas for errors in positioning at stage 2

- The shoulder is too far forwards and prevents commencement of compression.
- The shoulder is moved too far away from the unit and the outer sector of the breast is not in the field of image.
- The nipple is not in profile – this can be due to the support table being either too high or too low, resulting in an excessive amount of breast tissue superiorly or inferiorly and thus causing the nipple to be positioned too far along on the superior or inferior surface. In some instances it may not be possible to gain a nipple in profile due to position of the nipple on the breast. This should be noted and care take to ensure that the nipple is seen in profile on at least one projection and, possibly, a separate image taken of the nipple in profile if required (Fig. 15.10A, B).

Stage 3: Compressing the breast onto the support table

1. The mammographer applies compression by continuous pressure on the foot pedal whilst using a hand to immobilise the breast (Fig. 15.11).
2. There is a point at which the breast cannot be held – when the compression touches the chest wall edge of the breast at its thickest part. Where possible hold the breast at the nipple edge until the compression is at its maximum (preset no greater than 200 newtons).
3. Whilst the compression plate is coming down check that:
   - the nipple is in profile

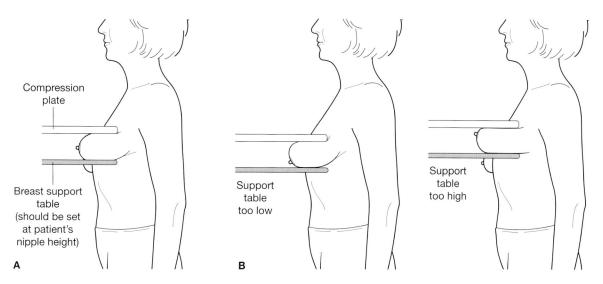

Figure 15.10 A Nipple in profile. B Breast incorrectly positioned.

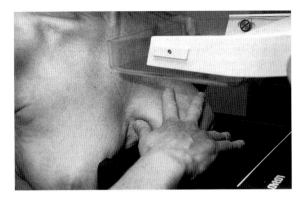

Figure 15.11 Compression of the breast.

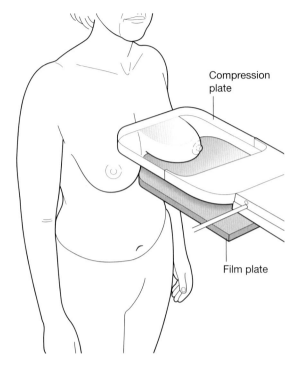

Figure 15.12 Breast in the craniocaudad position.

- there are no skin folds under or on top of the breast
- there are no omissions of the medial or lateral aspect of the breast
- the AEC position indication on the compression plate shows it is in the middle of the breast
- there is no shoulder, head or fat overlying the image.

Potential areas for errors in positioning at stage 3

- Movement of the breast when the mammographer removes her hand to prevent it being trapped under the compression plate.
- Overlying fat/axillary tissue at the lateral aspect – this can be removed by moving the patient's shoulder backwards or putting the patient's hand on her hip. Care must be taken in the latter not to pull vital breast tissue from under the compression plate.

Stage 4: Compressed breast on the support table

The breast should feel tense under the compression plate and there should be a slight blanching of the superior breast surface, accompanied by a slight reddening of the edge of the breast (Fig. 15.12).

Stage 5: Exposing and viewing the image

The breast is exposed and the compression released immediately post exposure, unless the woman is undergoing a localisation procedure.

The craniocaudad projection/image is evaluated using the following criteria (Fig. 15.13):

1. Identification
   - correct name and date
   - correct anatomical marker
   - correct projection marker.
2. Breast image to include:
   Anteriorly – nipple in profile
   Laterally/medially – skin edges and medial/lateral glandular tissue edges.
   Posteriorly (chest wall) – the pectoral muscle on image margin and retroglandular fat tissue.
3. Symmetrical images.

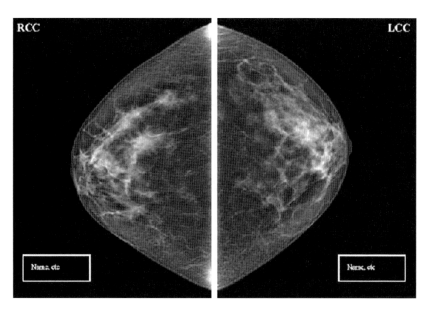

Figure 15.13 Craniocaudad radiographs of the left and right breast.

4. Adequate compression – should be able to visualise skin pores along the pectoral muscle.
5. Exposure showing adequate density to penetrate through glandular tissue and contrast existing between various structures within the breast; e.g. glandular tissue, fat, vascular structures and calcification (if present).
6. Visually sharp resolution of pectoral muscle, vessels.
7. Absence of any skin fold.
8. Absence of artefacts arising either from the breast (e.g. scarring, moles) or from anatomy interposing between X-ray tube and cassette.
9. Processing faults if using a conventional film-screen combination.

THE MEDIOLATERAL OBLIQUE PROJECTION

This is a routine mammographic projection which demonstrates all the breast tissue (including the axillary 'tail'). The preparation for the patient is the same as for the craniocaudad; cooperation is vital in mammography as a relaxed patient is somewhat easier to image than someone who has a tense pectoral muscle and stiff upper body. The angle required on the support table can be estimated using the general body shape of the woman so that there is not a lot of alteration of the equipment occurring.

PATIENT TYPES

Hypersthenic individuals

Short and stocky, with broad shoulders (Fig. 15.14), these patients benefit from an angle between the compression plate and horizontal of less than 45° and, potentially, 40°. The support table will then be at an angle, making it parallel to the middle axis of the breast tissue and thereby reducing the degree of foreshortening.

Hyposthenic and asthenic individuals

Taller, narrower shoulders benefit from an angle between the compression plate and horizontal of more than 45 °, and potentially 50–55 ° (Fig. 15.15). Asthenic individuals are very tall and slender and benefit from increased angulations of the compression plate.

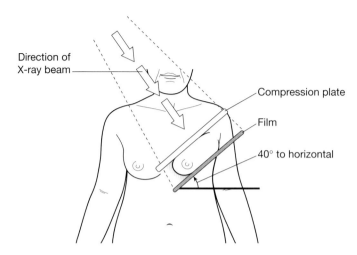

Figure 15.14 Hypersthenic individuals.

MEDIOLATERAL OBLIQUE TECHNIQUE

Stage 1: Woman stands in front of X-ray equipment

1. The breast support table (Bucky) is at the required angle to the floor (see above).
2. The cassette is in place if using a conventional unit.
3. The marker is in place for mediolateral oblique (RMLO or LMLO) projection on the outer upper aspect of support table.

4. The woman stands in front of the mammography machine (approximately 15 cm away) feet facing forward with the breast support table adjusted so that the lateral border of the chest wall is in line with the support table. When using isoscentric units there may be no need to alter the height of the support table between CC and MLO as the nipple level should remain in the centre of the film (Fig. 15.16).

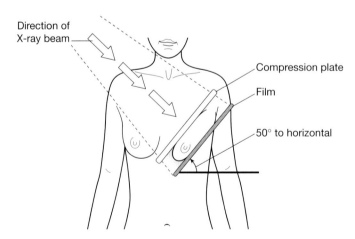

Figure 15.15 Hyposthenic individuals.

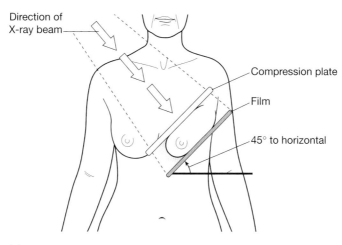

Figure 15.16 Stage 1 position.

Potential areas for errors in positioning at stage 1

- If the breast support table is too high the woman's breast will be positioned in the top half of the film and therefore miss the pectoral muscle and, possibly, the 'axillary tail'.
- Alternatively, the breast support may be too low, causing the top edge of the support table to dig into the woman's axilla, and the breast may be missed from the lower edge of the film as compression will contact the shoulder and not be able to hold the breast.

Stage 2: Lifting the breast onto the support table

1. The mammographer stands to the opposite side of the patient being imaged.
2. The hand and arm on the side of the breast being imaged are guided to lie across the top of the support table to help achieve a relaxed pectoral muscle.
3. The woman is asked to walk forwards and the mammographer guides her towards the support table by placing her hand on the woman's back. The mammographer raises the breast under examination by placing a hand gently in a cup movement to secure the lower edge of the breast between the thumb and forefingers. Care must be taken not to turn the woman too far medially or laterally, which might result in the omission of breast tissue.
4. The breast rests on the support table with the woman's anterior abdominal wall (inframammary angle) within the radiation field.
5. The mammographer's free hand should run along the mid-axillary line of the woman to ensure there are no skin folds trapped there.
6. The free hand can then move upwards to the axillary aspect and remove any axillary folds (Fig. 15.17).

Potential areas for errors in positioning at stage 2

- The nipple is not in profile. If the woman is too far in front of (or rotated towards) the support table there will be an unequal amount of breast tissue medially, causing the nipple to be too far on the lateral surface. Conversely, if the woman is too far from (or rotated away from) the support table, the nipple will appear to be on the medial aspect of the breast.

A

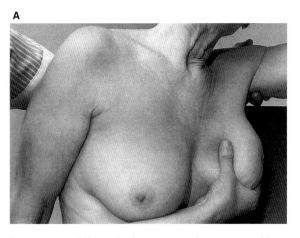

B

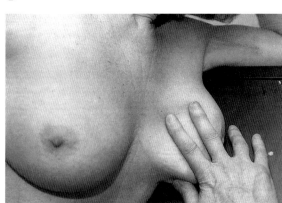

Figure 15.17 Lifting the breast onto the support table.

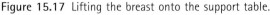

- There may be skin folds along the mid-axillary line; lifting the breast forwards or moving/rotating the woman from the hips towards or away from the support table can remedy this.
- The inframammary angle is not visualised in field of radiation – this can be due to the woman standing too far away from the support table. It can also be as a consequence of the above-mentioned positioning errors.

Stage 3: Compressing the breast onto the support table

1. The breast is held in place by the mammographer's hand whilst compression is commenced, ensuring that the nipple remains in profile.
2. The shoulder of the side under examination is guided back so it does not clash with the compression plate.
3. The mammographer applies compression by continuous pressure on the foot pedal whilst using a hand to immobilise the breast (Fig. 15.18).
4. There is a point at which the breast cannot be held, when the compression touches the chest wall edge of the breast at its thickest

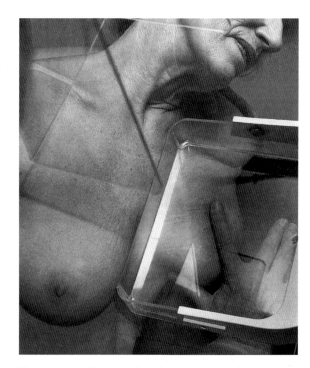

Figure 15.18 Compressing the breast onto the support table.

part. Where possible, hold the breast at the nipple edge until the compression is at its maximum (preset no greater than 200 newtons).

5. Whilst the compression plate is coming down check that:
   - the nipple is in profile
   - there are no skin folds under or on top of breast
   - there are no omissions of the axillary aspect of breast by the inclusion of the pectoral muscle; the compression plate should sit in the 90 ° angle that is formed by the chest wall and the arm of the breast under examination.
   - the AEC position indication on the compression plate shows it is in the middle of the breast.
   - the inframammary angle is in the field of radiation.

Potential areas for errors in positioning at stage 3

- The nipple is no longer in profile and/or the inframammary fold is missing – woman rotated or film too high. Re-adjust the position.
- Folds are present at the axilla – this may be due to an excess of fat in the axilla region. Try lifting the arm causing the folds or attempt to smooth skin and 'pull out' folds as compression occurs.
- Folds at inframammary angle – this may be due to an excess of abdominal wall fascia overlapping the angle. Try to push the excess flesh off the film or ask the woman to move her hips backwards.

Stage 4: Compressed breast on the support table

The breast should feel tense under the compression plate, with a slight blanching of the medial breast surface accompanied by a slight reddening of the edge of the breast (Fig. 15.19).

Potential areas for errors in positioning at stage 4

- Overlying fat/axillary tissue prevents compression of breast tissue and the breast

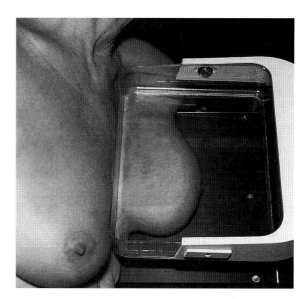

Figure 15.19 Breast in the mediolateral oblique position.

droops uncompressed. The film being too high and the head of humerus being compressed can cause this. Correct by lowering the support table or easing out axillary tissue until compression occurs at the breast. Care must be taken not to ease out breast tissue or it will not be imaged.

Stage 5: Exposing and viewing image

The breast should be exposed and the compression released immediately post exposure, unless the woman is undergoing a localisation procedure (Fig. 15.20).

The mediolateral projection or image is evaluated using the following criteria:

1. Identification
   - correct name and date
   - correct anatomical marker
   - correct projection marker.
2. Breast image to include:
   Anteriorly – nipple in profile.
   Inferiorly – skin edges and glandular tissue edges.

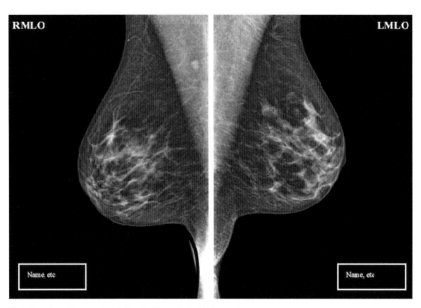

Figure 15.20 Mediolateral radiograph of the left and right breast.

Posteriorly (chest wall) – the pectoral muscle on image margin and retroglandular fat tissue.

Superiorly – axillary tail and pectoral muscle.
3. Symmetrical images.
4. Adequate compression – should be able to visualise skin pores along the pectoral muscle.
5. Exposure showing adequate density to penetrate through glandular tissue and contrast existing between various structures within the breast; e.g. glandular tissue, fat, vascular structures and calcification (if present).
6. Visually sharp resolution of pectoral muscle, vessels, etc.
7. Absence of any skin fold.
8. Absence of artefacts arising either from the breast (e.g. scarring, moles) or from anatomy interposing between the X-ray tube and cassette.
9. Processing faults if using a conventional film-screen combination.

PATHOLOGY

Breast cancer is the most common cancer detected in women in the UK. It currently accounts for 17% of annual female cancer deaths (13 000); however, this has been reduced from 15 000 per annum when the screening programme was first introduced in 1988. There is evidence from randomised-controlled trials of a significant reduction in mortality in the population with breast cancer.[4]

QUALITY ASSURANCE

The quality assurance (QA) system in place for breast screening units covers not only the quality of the X-ray equipment and images. The daily, weekly and monthly QA processes that are carried out on the mammography equipment are seen in Table 15.1. Processing QA is carried out following the standard QA programme for all processors.

Table 15.1   Routine QA tests for mammography equipment

Test tool	Purpose	Frequency	Equipment	Data recorded
4 cm Perspex	Consistency of output and optical density, (OD)	Daily + • after service • after moving mobile unit • if malfunction suspected	• 4 cm Perspex blocks • QA test cassette (18 × 24 cm), (24 × 30 cm) • + current film • Densitometer	mA s, target material, filter material, kV resultant film density, beam alignment, grid lines, artefacts (including processing marks)

Remedial values

• mA s > ± 5% of baseline
• deviation in OD >0.2 (target OD 1.5–1.9)

Suspension of service values

• mA s > ±10% of baseline
• OD > range 1.3–2.1 and not correctable by AEC density control adjustment

Test tool	Purpose	Frequency	Equipment	Data recorded
2 cm, 4 cm and 6 cm Perspex	Consistency of AEC for varying thickness	Monthly + • after service • after moving mobile unit • if malfunction suspected	• 2 cm, 4 cm and 6 cm Perspex blocks • QA test cassette (18 × 24 cm), (24 × 30 cm) • + current film • Densitometer	mA s, target material, filter material, kV, resultant film density, beam alignment, grid lines, artefacts (including processing marks)

Remedial values

Max deviation of OD from 4 cm value > 0.20
or Maximum OD − Minimum OD > 0.30 or any thickness producing OD outside range 1.3–2.1
Local protocols may cover mA s deviation values

Suspension of service values

Max deviation of OD from 4 cm value > 0.40
or Maximum OD − Minimum OD > 0.60
Local protocols may cover mA s deviation values

Continued

Table 15.1 Routine QA tests for mammography equipment — cont'd

Test tool	Purpose	Frequency	Equipment	Data recorded
Leeds TORMAS or TORMAX phantom	Image quality test	Weekly + • after service • after moving mobile unit • if malfunction suspected	• 4 cm Perspex block + Leeds TORMAS/TORMAX • QA test cassette (18 × 24 cm), (24 × 30 cm) • + current film • Densitometer • Magnifying glass or resolution	Resolution in line pairs/mm OD, artefacts Details within test tool. Record mA s [Test carried out at fixed kV and automatic mA s (28 kV, Mo target, Mo filter)].

Remedial values

High contrast resolution:
- < 12 line prs mm^{-1} for 5–6 mm detail
- > 25% decrease in contrast resolution from baseline

Threshold contrast:
- > 1.2% for 5–6 mm detail
- > 5% for 0.5 mm detail
- > 8% for 0.25 mm detail

Suspension of service values

High contrast resolution:
- < 10 line prs mm^{-1}

Threshold contrast:
- > 1.4% for 5–6 mm detail
- > 8% for 0.5 mm detail
- > 11% for 0.25 mm detail

AEC, automatic exposure control

References

1. Lundgren B, Jakobsson S. Single view mammography. Cancer 1976; 38:1124–1129.
2. Gur D, Sumkin JH, Rockette HE, et al. Changes in breast cancer detection and mammography recall rates after the introduction of a computer-aided detection system. J Natl Cancer Inst 2004; 96:185–190.
3. Khoo L, Taylor P, Given-Wilson R. A prospective study of computer aided detection in one United Kingdom National Breast Screening Programme. Radiology. In press 2008.
4. Advisory Committee on Breast Cancer Screening. Screening for breast cancer in England: past and future. NHSBSP Publication no 61. Sheffield: NHS Cancer Screening Programmes; 2006.

Further reading

Lee L, Strickland V, Wilson AR, Roebuck E. Fundamentals of mammography. Oxford: Churchill Livingstone; 2003.

Written by superintendent radiographers and consultant radiologists, this textbook provides the knowledge which is vital to an assistant practitioner and radiographer in the provision of a high quality mammography screening service. It outlines the quality assurance measures for X-ray and film processing equipment, the techniques for basic and complementary projections and the psychological considerations required when carrying out breast screening. Finally, it also contains the basis for mammography image interpretation, which is necessary in the developing role of the advanced practitioner.

NHS Breast Screening Programme (NHSBSP) On-line. Available www.cancerscreening.nhs.uk/breastscreen/index.html 13 February 2008.

The NHSBSP website has a marvellous range of information both for National Health Service personnel and the public, with easily accessible and downloadable publications covering all aspects of breast screening.

Bushong SC. Radiological science for technologists: physics, biology and protection, 8th edn. St Louis: Mosby; 2004.

Carter P. Chesneys' equipment for student radiographers, 4th edn. London: Blackwell Scientific; 1994.

Cox J. The impact of technology on working practice. Synergy 2001; (June):24–26.

Duthie S. Stereo core biopsy of the breast. Synergy 2001; (June):14–19.

MDA Evaluation Report (02103): Mammography X-ray unit, Instrumentarium Imaging Diamond; 2003.

Young KC, Oduko JM. Review of computerised radiography systems in the NHSBSP. NHS Cancer Screening Programmes, NHSBSP Equipment Report 0501; 2005.

Websites

Siemens Medical website:
http://www.siemensmedical.com

GE Medical website:
http://www.gemedicalsystemseurope.com/euen/rad/xr/mammo/index.html

Philips Medical website:
http://www.medical.philips.com/main/products/xray/products/radiography/mammography/

Xograph website:
http://www.xograph.com

Chapter **16**

Nuclear medicine

Vicki Major and Marc Griffiths

KEY POINTS

- The radiation dose from any diagnostic procedure should be as low as reasonably practicable, consistent with diagnostic results.[1]
- This is governed in nuclear medicine by the administration of strictly controlled amounts of radioactivity under a licensing arrangement and the use of optimum imaging conditions.[2]
- Any person working within the nuclear medicine environment should have an awareness of the practical radiation protection considerations.
- Nuclear medicine studies require the administration of less than a microgram of the radioactive substance under test. This has the advantage that it does not interfere with the physiological pathways but demonstrates their function.
- The radioactive substances may be given in one of two forms: in their radionuclide form or attached to a drug and known as a radiopharmaceutical.
- The radiopharmaceutical or radionuclide determines which system or organ the radioactive substance targets.
- Most radioactive substances used in diagnostic imaging emit gamma radiation, which can subsequently be detected externally to the patient, and an image is produced of the uptake in the specific area.
- Nuclear medicine studies can often detect certain disorders earlier than other diagnostic imaging procedures because they rely on functional rather than structural changes.

INTRODUCTION

Nuclear medicine is concerned with providing diagnostic information about patients following the administration of a radioactive product. The patient is imaged using a gamma camera. Images are produced of the distribution of the radioactive substance within different organs and systems. This can be compared with normal distribution to diagnose if a medical condition is present and assess its extent or severity.

A multidisciplinary healthcare team, comprising medical staff, hospital physicists, radiopharmacists, medical technologists, radiography practitioners, nurses and clerical support staff, delivers the nuclear medicine service. Nuclear medicine departments can be autonomous or part of a diagnostic imaging department.

Key terms

Radionuclide: a species of atom whose nucleus disintegrates by the emission of alpha particles, beta particles or gamma radiation.

Radiopharmaceutical: a medicinal product dependent for all or part of its action on a radioactive ingredient. It may be used for diagnostic, therapeutic or research purposes.[2]

Half-life: the time taken for the radioactivity to decay to half its original value. In the body this depends on the physical properties of the radionuclide and how quickly it is excreted from the body.

Gamma camera: the instrument used to detect the radiation and produce images.

Technetium: the most common radionuclide used in medical imaging.

RADIONUCLIDES USED IN MEDICAL IMAGING

TECHNETIUM

Technetium-99m (abbreviated to ^{99m}Tc) is the most common radionuclide used in medical imaging. ^{99m}Tc is attached to a pharmaceutical to produce a radiopharmaceutical, which is normally injected intravenously into the body. ^{99m}Tc is used because:

a) It has a half-life of 6 hours.
- If a radionuclide had a very short half-life, such as 30 minutes, it would be very difficult to transport it from its site of manufacture in time to use it. If it had a long half-life, such as 30 years, the dose to the patients would be too great because their bodies would be receiving a radiation dose for the rest of their lives. The radiation dose to the patient to achieve a diagnostic medical image should be 'as low as reasonably practicable' (ALARP). A very short half-life would mean that the physiological uptake of the radiopharmaceutical could not be observed because it can take several hours for physiological uptake to occur in some systems. It is easy to deal with articles and waste contaminated with ^{99m}Tc because it has a short half-life. After a few days of storage the radiation dose is low enough to be considered insignificant and therefore articles can be disposed of or used again in the department.

b) It is a pure gamma emitter.
- Gamma emitters are part of the electromagnetic spectrum. This means that they do not damage cells as much as alpha and beta particles, which are charged. Radioactive decay occurs when an element has an unstable arrangement of protons or neutrons and transforms into a stable element.[3] Most elements emit alpha or beta particles as well as gamma radiation. The gamma radiation emission is normally instantaneous, but with some elements the atom stays in an excited state for a prolonged period of time. These are called 'metastable radionuclides' and they emit radiation at a discrete energy level that is characteristic of the radionuclide and normally only emit gamma radiation. The 'm' in ^{99m}Tc indicates that technetium is metastable.

c) It has a 140 keV energy level.
- The energy level characteristic of ^{99m}Tc is 140 kiloelectron volts (keV). This means that the energy is high enough to go through the patient and interact with the gamma camera. If it were too low, it would be attenuated in the patient and would not be able to interact with the camera. An energy level of 140 keV

is low enough to be attenuated by the distance of a normal gamma camera room and therefore the practitioner will not be over-irradiated by the radionuclide.

d) It is cheap and easy to produce.

- ^{99m}Tc is produced in the morning, before work begins in the hospital, by passing saline over a column containing the radioactive element molybdenum in a radiopharmacy (Fig. 16.1). The molybdenum is contained in a radioactive generator. As the saline passes over the column of molybdenum the saline takes off the daughter product technetium, forming a radioactive saline. The parent molybdenum stays on the column.
- The radioactive saline is then tested to make sure it has not been contaminated by the parent because this would be dangerous to

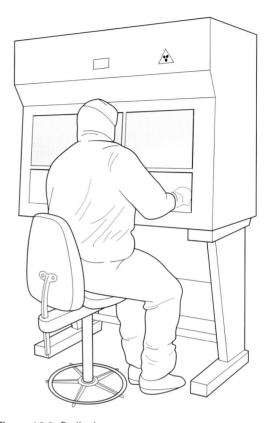

Figure 16.2 Radiopharmacy.

the patient due to the fact that molybdenum has a half-life of 67 hours and emits beta radiation. The ^{99m}Tc is produced in sterile radiopharmacy (Fig. 16.2).

e) It binds easily to pharmaceuticals.

- ^{99m}Tc in radioactive saline is added to freeze-dried pharmaceutical kits in the radiopharmacy (Fig. 16.3). The kits take about 10 minutes to bind to the radionuclide and then they are ready to sub dispense, so they can be injected into patients. Some kits have to be boiled before they bind. The radiopharmaceuticals are tested for chemical binding and sterility.

f) They are non-toxic.

- Unlike radiographic contrast media, technetium does not contain iodine and therefore reactions are very rare. Technetium radiopharmaceuticals contain microscopic amounts of pharmaceuticals and therefore allergic reactions do not normally occur.

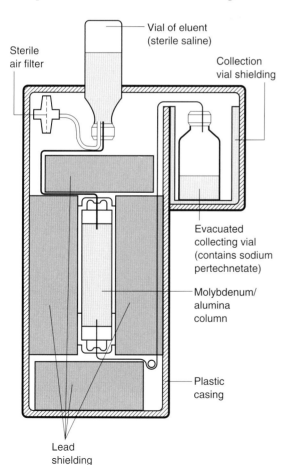

Figure 16.1 Molybdenum generator.

Sterile air filter

Vial of eluent (sterile saline)

Collection vial shielding

Evacuated collecting vial (contains sodium pertechnetate)

Molybdenum/ alumina column

Plastic casing

Lead shielding

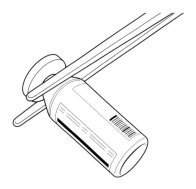

Figure 16.3 Freeze dried radiopharmaceutical kit.

OTHER RADIONUCLIDES USED IN DIAGNOSTIC IMAGING

^{81m}Krypton

Krypton is used for scanning the lungs as it can show the ventilation. It is metastable like technetium and also a pure gamma emitter. It has an energy level of 190 keV, but has a half-life of 13 seconds. This means that the radionuclide has to be produced and then administered directly to the patient. In this case the patient inhales the radionuclide. Air is passed over a column of rubidium, which results in krypton being produced.

^{201}Thallium

Thallium is used for imaging the heart muscle (myocardium). It has a half-life of 73 h and has a principal energy level of 81 keV. It is not an ideal imaging agent due to the multiple energy levels and can be toxic in large amounts.

^{111}Indium

Indium is used for scanning a patient with infections. It is attached to the patient's white blood cells. Indium has energy levels of 171 and 245 keV and a half-life of 2.8 days.[4]

EQUIPMENT

The instrument used to detect the radiation and produce images is a gamma camera. An image can be formed from the information gathered by the camera and displayed in either a static or whole body form (planar images) or dynamic mode (related to time; e.g. renal). Modern imaging systems can also create images in three dimensions (single photon emission computed tomography, SPECT), similar to those observed in computed tomography (CT) or magnetic resonance imaging (MRI).

The basic design of a gamma camera has not significantly changed for over 40 years and the use of devices such as sodium iodine crystals and photomultiplier tubes are the main reasons why nuclear medicine images have such low resolution in comparison to CT. However, technology advancements may see the development and production of solid-state gamma cameras in the future. The modern gamma camera consists of a large detector (or two detectors in dual head systems, Fig. 16.4), which is positioned as close to the patient as possible during examinations.

Other features of a modern gamma camera system include an imaging couch, which is curved for patient comfort, a gantry for the detector heads to manoeuvre and a positioning monitor. The gamma camera is linked to a computer system which reflects the relative uptake of radiopharmaceutical tracer within the patient in the form of a visual image.

Many nuclear medicine departments will utilise one gamma camera to undertake a range of

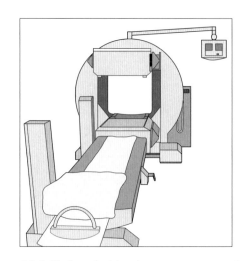

Figure 16.4 Modern dual head gamma camera system with an imaging couch and collimator cart.

examinations. Some larger departments may employ a dual and a single head gamma camera to perform clinical examinations. Dual head gamma camera systems allow the operator to perform certain examinations (e.g. whole body bone scans) quicker than single head units, which is particularly useful for patients who may be in considerable discomfort.

The detector unit comprises a number of components, which enables the visualisation of radiopharmaceutical uptake within the patient. The gamma camera is a robust piece of medical imaging equipment; however, there is a requirement to ensure the working temperature of the examination room is kept constant and extreme fluctuations in temperature are avoided as this may have an impact upon the quality of the images produced.

The basic components of a modern gamma camera detector unit are:

- collimator
- crystal
- photomultiplier tubes
- shielding and cooling devices
- remote operating monitor.

Collimator

This is employed to localise accurately the radiopharmaceutical uptake within the patient. The collimator is designed from perforated or folded lead and has a 'honeycomb' appearance. Of all the gamma photons emitted by a patient over 99% of them are wasted and not recorded by the final processing computer. The collimator is an essential component of the detector unit and a nuclear medicine department may have a range of parallel hole design collimators to suit the type of examination being performed. The term 'parallel hole' refers to the perpendicular design of the collimator's long axis holes to the detector crystal. The walls (septa) between the holes of the collimator are made of lead and subsequently absorb any gamma events that are not perpendicular to the crystal. Parallel hole collimators are the most commonly used collimator within most nuclear medicine departments. Some departments may employ a pinhole collimator for thyroid

examination. Pinhole collimators work in the same manner as traditional pinhole cameras, with the image being inverted on the monitor. Investigations involving the use of higher energy isotopes, such as indium-111 or gallium-67, require the use of collimators with thicker lead septa between the holes.

The majority of investigations performed within a nuclear medicine department involve the use of technetium-99m based radiopharmaceutical agents. Technetium-99m has a photopeak energy of 140 keV and low energy collimators are used to absorb any gamma events that are not perpendicular to the crystal. For dynamic renal examinations a 'low energy all purpose' (LEAP) collimator may be employed and the holes are of a particular design to allow more gamma events to interact with the crystal than a 'low energy high resolution' (LEHR) collimator. The collection of counts on a dynamic examination is crucial if image processing is to take place afterwards. Figure 16.5 depicts a set of collimators being exchanged on a dual head gamma camera system. This process is mainly automated and requires minimal practitioner involvement. Caution should, however, be exercised when collimators are being exchanged, as the detector crystal

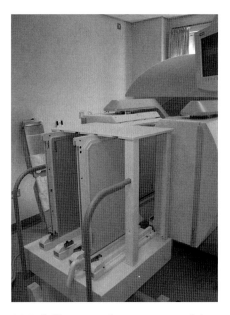

Figure 16.5 Collimator exchange cart containing a set of collimators.

is exposed and the collimators themselves are very heavy.

Crystal

Gamma events passing through the collimator holes interact with the sodium iodide crystal and this subsequently produces a pulse of fluorescent light. The brightness of the pulse is proportional to the initial intensity of the incident gamma event. The crystal within a gamma camera is extremely fragile and is protected by an aluminium container within the detector head. Standard sodium iodide crystals are sensitive to humidity, moisture, external light and extreme temperature changes. Maximum caution needs to be exercised by practitioners when the collimator has been removed from a detector unit during routine quality control tests. The aluminium container will only protect the crystal from very minor physical damage. Most modern crystals are rectangular in design and are approximately 9.5 mm thick.

Photomultiplier (PM) tubes

The fundamental purpose of a PM tube is to convert a light pulse into an electrical signal. A number of PM tubes are positioned behind the crystal and protected with black plastic covers (Fig. 16.6).

These covers protect the PM tubes from any potential external light, which may be incorrectly processed. A scintillation event within the crystal

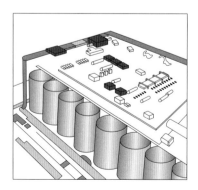

Figure 16.6 Detector head with outer casing removed demonstrating electronic circuitry and PM tube covers.

is detected by a PM tube and is converted into a weak electrical signal. This weak signal is amplified using a series of dynodes within the PM tubes. The electrical outputs from the PM tubes are converted into the spatial coordinates (X and Y) required for the image appearance on the monitor (pulse arithmetic circuitry) and a Z signal, which identifies the incident gamma photon energy value during its interaction with the crystal. The Z signal passes through a pulse height analyser (PHA), which is able to discriminate against background or scatter radiation from a particular isotope. It is normal practice in nuclear medicine to place a 10% 'window' either side of an isotope's photopeak value. For example, with technetium-99m, which has a photopeak energy value of 140 keV, the lowest 'accepted' gamma photons would be 126 keV and the highest 'accepted' gamma photons would be 154 keV.

Shielding and cooling devices

The shielding encases the detector head and accommodates the collimator. On modern gamma cameras it is lead lined to prevent any radiation interference occurring during scanning. Due to the amount of electronics on most modern gamma cameras, a number of cooling fans may also be situated near the top of the detector head. The filters surrounding these fans should be checked routinely and cleaned if necessary. Caution must be exercised during examinations involving the use of radioactive respiratory gases (e.g. technetium-99m aerosol ventilation gas), as particles may become lodged within the cooling fans and have an adverse affect on image quality.

Remote operating monitor and gantry/table controls

This small, flat panel monitor is situated on a boom from the gamma camera gantry, which permits the practitioner to commence an examination remotely rather than having to do so from the main operator's console. This is particularly useful if the practitioner is performing a dynamic examination, requiring a quick start after intravenous injection of a radiopharmaceutical.

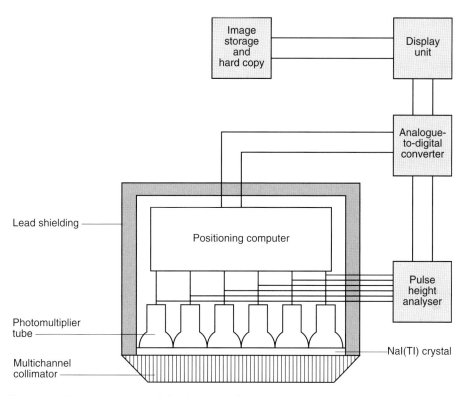

Figure 16.7 Diagrammatic representation of the features of a gamma camera.

Figure 16.7 gives a representation of a gamma camera system.

CREATION OF AN IMAGE

Gamma events leaving the patient's body may be travelling at various angles – some may be perpendicular to the detector of the gamma camera (gamma event A in Fig. 16.8). Gamma events that are perpendicular to the crystal within the detector unit have to pass through the collimator; those that are not perpendicular to the crystal are absorbed by the collimator (gamma event B in Fig. 16.8). The collimator is the first tool used to ensure the accurate representation of physiological tracer uptake within the patient and without it there would not be any recognisable image on the monitor.

The second tool is the PHA, which as previously mentioned, discriminates against scatter or background radiation. Like in most clinical examinations, the nuclear medicine practitioner will have access to a number of preset protocols, which are stored on an operator's computer console. Modern computer consoles use software driven platforms and graphical user interfaces (GUI). These permit quick access to a range of common clinical protocols and radioisotopes. The photopeak energy value per

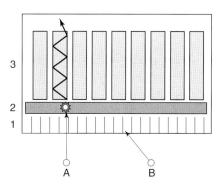

Figure 16.8 Schematic diagram demonstrating the pathway of two gamma ray events; perpendicular to the crystal (A) and not perpendicular to the crystal (B).

second of these isotopes is stored within the gamma camera's computer and, as a result, determines the energy 'window' for that particular isotope. The practitioner has the ability to adjust the energy window if circumstances require this action. Nuclear medicine images may also be presented in different colour scales. Grey scale is normally utilised for skeletal and respiratory images and colour may be used for renal and cardiac examinations. Colour intensity scales are also presented with the images to assess the degree of tracer uptake within a particular part of the area under examination (Figs 16.9 and 16.10).

ACCESSORY EQUIPMENT FEATURES

A typical nuclear medicine department will utilise a range of ancillary items to position patients and ensure the production of optimal quality images. Paediatric patients require considerable preparation for examinations within nuclear medicine and the practitioner may employ the use of

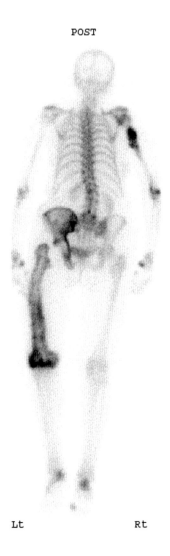

POST

Lt   Rt

Figure 16.9 Skeletal scan demonstrating Paget's disease with intense uptake in multiple areas of the left femur, pelvis and right humerus.

Figure 16.10 Cardiac scan demonstrating a patient who had experienced a myocardial infarction.

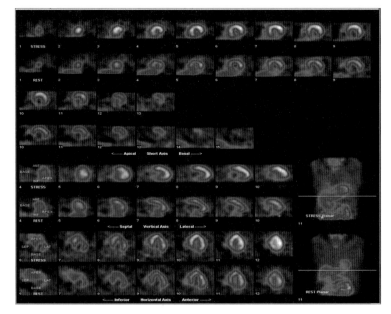

special imaging pallets, sandbags and immobilisation devices during the scan. It is crucial that patients do not move during examinations, as image unsharpness will occur. If patient movement occurs during a dynamic renal examination, this could potentially lead to an incorrect assessment of renal function. Some departments also use DVD and audio equipment to distract paediatric patients during examinations. The use of such equipment also reduces the close contact between the practitioner and patients and therefore helps to reduce the radiation dose received.

SPECIALISED EQUIPMENT

As previously mentioned, the majority of nuclear medicine departments also perform SPECT imaging. Common SPECT procedures undertaken within clinical practice include cardiac and skeletal examinations. However, some departments may also use SPECT techniques to perform neurological and oncology related procedures. SPECT imaging involves the collection of a number of views around the patient using the detector head/s. Most gamma cameras employed in clinical practice are dual head and can be configured to perform different SPECT examinations. As the detector head/s move around the patient (normally in a step fashion) each view collects a preset number of gamma photon events. Figure 16.11 demonstrates the set-up for a cardiac

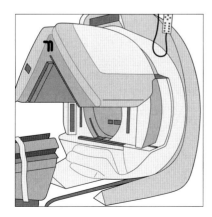

Figure 16.11 Dual head gamma camera with the detector heads prepared for a cardiac examination.

examination, with the detector heads presented in an inverted 'V' fashion. Performing SPECT examinations permits the presentation of data in three image planes: transaxial, sagittal and coronal. Powerful computers process the collected data and the practitioner may manipulate the generated data to provide the final images.

Recently the use of 'hybrid' gamma cameras has been introduced into clinical practice. Inherently, nuclear medicine images possess inferior spatial resolution compared to computed tomography. This is mainly due to the aforementioned inefficiencies of current gamma camera technology. The introduction of a low power X-ray tube and detector bank on the same gantry as the gamma camera heads is allowing practitioners to 'fuse' anatomical and functional data from the same imaging environment. Such technology is beginning to redefine the physical layout of nuclear medicine departments (given the use of an X-ray source) and is assisting in the localisation of certain physiological tracers. Figure 16.12 demonstrates an example of hybrid imaging.

HANDLING AND SAFETY

SAFETY OF THE GAMMA CAMERA

The area of camera movement should be free from any objects. If a chair or other object is left in the path of travel the camera or object could be damaged. Some centres mark the footprint of camera movement on the floor to clearly show the extent of the exclusion zone.

The gamma camera interlocks should be checked every day and every time the collimators are changed.

RADIATION SAFETY

Radiopharmaceuticals can be shielded before they are injected into the patient. Tungsten syringe shields and lead and tungsten pots can be used. Radiopharmaceuticals are unsealed sources and therefore have the potential to

Figure 16.12 Anatomical, functional and 'fused' data sets from a SPECT/CT system.

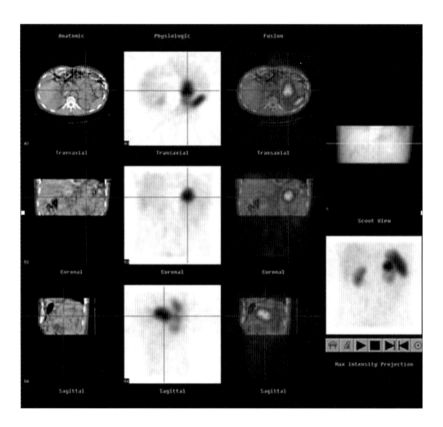

contaminate through spillage. Pots and shields may be contaminated with radioactivity and therefore should not be touched. Treat all pots and shields as if they are contaminated and wear gloves and use tongs or other devices to keep a distance from them.

Gloves should be worn for handling radioactive materials, contaminated objects and if a suspected spillage has occurred. It is important to check for contamination: hands should be monitored after contact with radioactive products and departments should be monitored regularly (Fig. 16.13). A radioactive trefoil sign indicates areas containing radioactive materials or patients.

Radioactive waste has to be disposed of in the correct manner. ^{99m}Tc waste is normally stored for at least a week. Empty syringes and needles may also be radioactive these should be disposed of in a shielded sharps box.

After the radiation has been injected into the patient then the best radiation protection is distance from the patient. The inverse square law means that if the distance is doubled then the radiation dose will be reduced by 75%.

A spill kit should be available in case some unsealed radioactivity has been spilt (Fig. 16.14). The nuclear medicine department should have a contingency plan in case of a spill.[1] If a spill has occurred, the radiation may have been spread and door handles and the bottom of shoes should be monitored as well as any area that might have been contaminated. The area of any spillage should be demarked. After donning protective clothing the spill should be wiped up, from the outside in, to avoid further spread. If the radiopharmaceutical is short lived it might be easier to close the area until decay has occurred. Records should be kept of the incident.

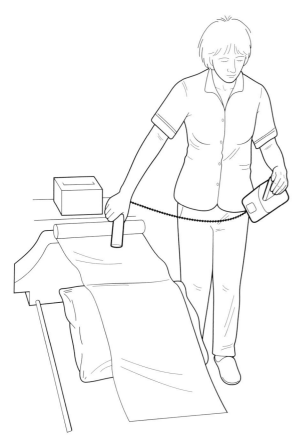

Figure 16.13 Radiographer monitoring a gamma camera room.

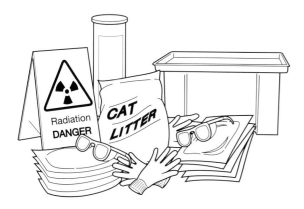

Figure 16.14 A spill kit for radioactivity.

EXAMINATION OVERVIEWS

BONE SCANS

Main indications

Metastases, Paget's disease, infection, loose prosthesis, primary bone tumours, osteomyelitis, fractures, avascular necrosis, osteomalacia and hyperparathyroidism.

For fractures, avascular necrosis, osteomyelitis and prosthesis an image can be taken at injection and at 5 minutes post injection to give an idea of the blood supply to the area, as well as an image at 3 hours. This is called a three-phase bone scan.

Radiopharmaceutical and rationale

^{99m}Tc-MDP (methylene diphosphonate) or ^{99m}Tc-HDP (hydoxydiphosphonate):

- Clearance occurs by combination of skeletal uptake and urinary excretion. There is fairly rapid blood clearance – less than 10% remaining in the blood 1 h post injection.
- Skeletal blood flow influences local uptake of the radiopharmaceutical.
- Crucial influence on uptake appears to be osteoblastic activity. Osteoblasts build new bone, osteoclasts resorb bone.
- Radiopharmaceutical accumulates on bone surface, tracer being incorporated into the bone mineral crystal hydroxyapatite.

Procedure

- The patient is injected intravenously.
- The patient is scanned 3 h post injection. (Children can be scanned from 2 h; patients with poor renal function are better scanned at 4 h post injection).
- The patient is encouraged to drink plenty of fluids and micturate frequently. This clears the radiopharmaceutical from the soft tissues.
- The patient should remove metal objects and have an empty bladder prior to the start of the scan.
- The patient lies supine.

- The scan normally includes the whole of the skeletal system (Fig. 16.15).
- Radiation protection instructions should be given to the patient prior to injection and instructions sent to the ward with inpatients.

Collimators used

- Low Energy High Resolution.

STATIC RENAL SCANS

Main indications

Scarring from urinary tract infections, ectopic kidney, horseshoe kidney, failure to visualise a kidney with other imaging modalities. Renal failure, evidence of functioning renal tissue.

Radiopharmaceutical and rationale

^{99m}Tc-DMSA (dimercaptosuccinic acid):

- Radiopharmaceutical binds to plasma proteins and accumulates in renal cortex.

Procedure

- The patient is injected intravenously.
- The patient is scanned 3 h post injection.
- The patient is encouraged to drink plenty of fluids and micturate frequently. This clears the radiopharmaceutical from the soft tissues.
- The patient should remove metal objects and have an empty bladder prior to the start of the scan.
- The patient lies supine (babies may lie prone).
- Left and right posterior obliques are acquired of the kidneys, as well as anterior and posterior images (Fig. 16.16). The relative function of each

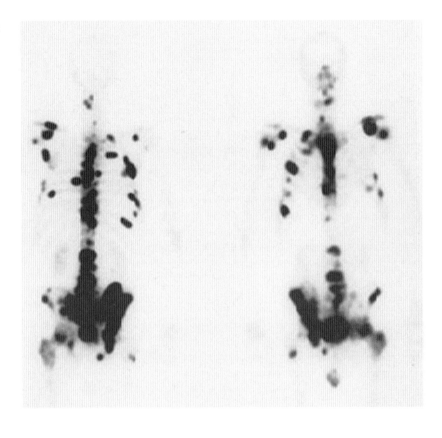

Figure 16.15 Whole body bone scan of patient with multiple metastases.

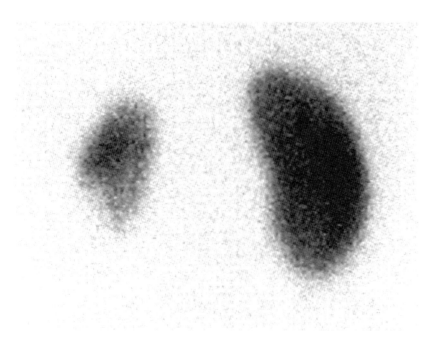

Figure 16.16 Posterior image of kidneys showing scarring in lower pole of left kidney.

kidney is taken. If an ectopic or renal transplant kidney is imaged then the pelvic area needs to be included on acquisition.

Collimators used

- Low Energy High Resolution, or Low Energy General Purpose for very young children.

DYNAMIC RENAL SCANS (RENOGRAM)

Main indications

Assessment of renal function, obstructed kidney.

Radiopharmaceutical and rationale

^{99m}Tc-MAG3 (mercaptoacetyltriglycine):
- The radiopharmaceutical is excreted from the kidneys via tubular excretion.[4]

Procedure

- The patient is encouraged to drink plenty of fluids for an hour prior to the examination to ensure hydration.

- The patient is asked to micturate immediately prior to the examination.
- The patient should remove metal objects and have an empty bladder prior to the start of the scan.
- The patient lies supine.
- The gamma camera is positioned under the patient so the kidneys are in the field of view.
- The patient is injected intravenously.
- The patient is scanned immediately.
- Posterior images are acquired for 30 min; an injection of a diuretic may be used to indicate if the kidneys are obstructed.
- Time activity curves are acquired (Fig. 16.17).
- A post micturition scan may be acquired.

Collimators used

- Low Energy High Resolution or Low Energy General Purpose.

INDIRECT MICTURATING CYSTOGRAM

If a child is potty trained and can cooperate well then the acquisition of an indirect cystogram can

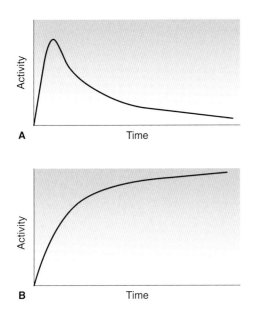

Figure 16.17 Kidney renogram curves. **A** Normal. **B** Obstructed.

occur. This demonstrates reflux, which can cause scarring to the kidneys. The child micturates into a bedpan whilst sitting against the gamma camera and time/activity curves can be drawn. If urine is refluxing back to the kidneys it will show on the curves. This examination avoids the need for catheterisation of the child. Adults can also have a cystogram in this way, although requests for adult patients are not a common occurrence.

PATIENT CARE AND ADVICE

PATIENT CARE PRIOR TO THE SCAN

Children and pregnant women are not normally allowed to accompany patients to the nuclear medicine department to prevent them receiving a radiation dose from other patients. They can enter if they need to have a scan, normally by prior arrangement with the department.

Patients are normally sent information leaflets in advance of their scan that explain the procedure and precautions to be taken afterwards. All patients who receive radiation should be given clear written advice which sets out the risks associated with ionising radiation and specifies how doses

resulting from their exposure during the scan can be restricted as far as reasonably possible so as to protect persons in contact with them (IR(ME)R 2000, see p. 14). Most patients have to avoid prolonged close contact with pregnant women and children for the rest of the day. These precautions may be longer for scans involving higher radiation doses or a radionuclide other than ^{99m}Tc.

Most patients have to wait for several hours between injection and scan and should be given clear instructions as to any precautions that apply during this period. The patient's ability to understand the precautions and comply with them is checked prior to injection of the radiopharmaceutical. The request form has to be justified by an ARSAC certificate holder, although this can be delegated under guidelines. The radiopharmaceutical can only be injected by a person who has had adequate training. This is normally a radiologist, nuclear medicine physician, radiographer or technologist. All female patients of reproductive age should be asked if they are pregnant or breastfeeding as they should not receive a radiopharmaceutical injection except under very special circumstances, which would need to be justified by the ARSAC certificate holder. For most examinations patients need to drink plenty of fluids throughout the day and empty their bladder frequently to reduce the radiation dose.

When a ward patient has a nuclear medicine scan information informing ward staff of radiation precautions and length of time that they apply should be provided.

PATIENT CARE DURING THE SCAN

Most nuclear medicine scans take about 30 minutes to run and the patient is unable to move during this time. Patients must be made as comfortable as possible during acquisition of the image because any movement means the procedure has to be repeated.

Patients are required to lie flat on the scanning table, with no more than one pillow under their head, in order to enable the gamma camera to be positioned as close as possible to their body. The scanning tables are very narrow and the armrests are normally hard Perspex (Fig. 16.18). The scan

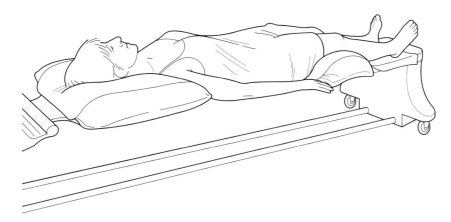

Figure 16.18 Gamma camera scanning table.

must start on an empty bladder, so patients are instructed to visit the toilet before the scan commences and then should be warned about the length of time they will have to spend on the scanning table. Metal objects such as coins and keys, which could cause artefacts, have to be removed from the patients before they get on the table. Patients usually keep their clothes on and do not change into gowns. The gamma camera rooms are air-conditioned and can feel cold to the patients, so blankets should be available to keep them warm. A pillow or knee support should be placed under the knees to increase comfort.

When the patient is lying comfortably on the scanning table a check should be made to make sure there are no tubes or lines hanging from the patient and that no parts of the patient's anatomy are likely to get caught when the camera or table moves. Music can be played during the scan to help patient relaxation; in some departments DVDs are available for the patients to watch during scan. The gamma camera has to come as close as possible to the patient, so the patient should be warned about this. It is useful to put your hand between the patient and the gamma camera head when moving it towards the patient, so the camera hits your hand before touching any part of the patient. For patient safety a member of staff

should always be present when the gamma camera is acquiring a scan.

When the scan has finished the patient is warned not to move until the table and camera have stopped moving. The table should be at its lowest level before the patient sits up and gets off. Some patients feel dizzy after getting up from lying flat, so they need time to get their bearings back.

After the scan the patients are advised about how and when they will receive the results of their scan. A check is made to ensure that each patient remembers any radiation precautions that still apply and how long they apply for.

PATIENT PATHWAYS

These pathways can be seen in Appendix 2.[5,6] These are simple generic pathways, which may differ from patient to patient depending on the imaging modalities available and the patient's condition. Nuclear medicine involvement in the pathway is in bold type.

References

1. The Ionising Radiations Regulations 1999 (SI 1999/3232). London: HMSO.

2. Administration of Radioactive Substances Advisory Committee. Notes for guidance on the clinical administration of radiopharmaceuticals and use of sealed radioactive sources. Oxford: Health Protection Agency; 2006.

3. Sampson C. Textbook of radiopharmacy; theory and practice, 3rd edn. Amsterdam: Gordon and Breach; 1999.

4. Sharp PF, Gemmell HG, Smith FW (eds). Practical nuclear medicine. Oxford: Oxford University Press; 1998.

5. Eisenberg R, Johnson N. Comprehensive radiographic pathology. St. Louis: Mosby; 2003.

6. Underwood J. (ed.) General and systematic pathology. London: Churchill Livingstone; 2004.

Recommended reading

Sharp P, Gemmell H, Murray A. Practical nuclear medicine. New York: Springer; 2005.

This is a clearly written book. It contains information on radionuclides, radiopharmaceuticals, equipment, radiation protection and imaging. It is the next step for students who require a more in-depth knowledge of nuclear medicine. It is easy to read and you can just read the chapter that interests you or the whole book.

Chapter 17

Introduction to ultrasound

Rita Phillips

CHAPTER CONTENTS

KEY POINTS

- Diagnostic ultrasound uses high frequency sound waves in the megahertz (MHz) range.
- Ultrasound is a form of non-ionising radiation.
- Sound waves are created by the piezoelectric effect.
- The sound waves are transmitted into the body and reflected back in varying amounts from an anatomical interface and these reflected waves are detected to produce an image.
- Modern ultrasound machines interpret the returning signals to generate images, which they send either to film or to a picture archiving communication system.
- Ultrasound transducers have different frequencies and are usually in the range of 1–20 MHz.
- The higher the frequency, the better the resolution, but the poorer the penetration.
- Ultrasound is a cross-sectional study and therefore each organ can be examined in several planes.
- Ultrasound is operator dependent and improper use of ultrasound techniques and equipment can lead to missed or misdiagnosis.
- In order to aid diagnosis, a full clinical and medical history must be available.
- Ultrasound studies include motion mode; spectral; colour and power Doppler; two-, three- and four-dimensional imaging.
- Although ultrasound has been in use for several decades with no proven evidence of damaging effects, high levels of ultrasound energy can cause bio effects in tissue; therefore prudent use of ultrasound is recommended.

- Ergonomics play an important part in minimising ultrasound work related disorders, especially affecting the upper limbs due to repeated movements, stretching and twisting.
- Training, quality assurance and audits are all important factors for maintaining high quality patient-focussed ultrasound examinations.

INTRODUCTION

Ultrasound was originally developed during World War I to track submarines as SONAR technology (Sound, Navigation And Ranging). Ultrasound was first used medically in the 1950s, with very early applications in fetal biometry; nowadays, it is used in just about every field of medicine. Furthermore, it is also now practised by a wide variety of professionals, in a multidisciplinary setting.

SOUND WAVES

Sound is a wave that is created by vibrating objects and propagated through a medium from one location to another, via particle interaction (Fig. 17.1). These particles move in a direction parallel to the direction of the wave; that is, longitudinally. Each individual particle pushes on its neighbouring particle and propels it in a forwards direction whilst restoring its original position at the end of the interaction. This backwards and forwards motion of particles in the direction of

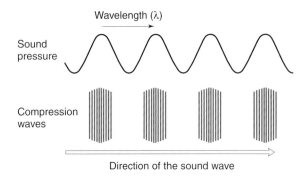

Figure 17.1 Sound waves.

the wave creates regions of high pressure within the medium, where the particles are compressed together (compressions), and also regions of low pressure, where the particles are spread apart (rarefactions). The wavelength of sound is the distance between two successive high pressure pulses or two successive low pressure pulses.

The frequency of a wave refers to how often the particles of the medium vibrate when a wave passes through it and is measured as the number of complete back-and-forth vibrations (cycles) of a particle of the medium per unit of time. The hertz (Hz) is a unit for frequency where 1 Hz is equivalent to one cycle per second. Humans can hear sound with frequencies of 20 to 20 000 cycles per second (i.e. 20–20 000 Hz).

ULTRASOUND

Ultrasound is high frequency sound beyond the hearing of the human ear. The frequencies of ultrasound required for diagnostic medical imaging are in the range 1–20 MHz. These frequencies can be obtained by using piezoelectric materials (particularly crystals). When an electric current is applied and reversed across a slice of one of these materials, the material contracts or expands. So a rapidly alternating electric field can cause a crystal to vibrate. These vibrations are then passed through any adjacent materials, or into the air as a longitudinal wave is produced – a sound wave (Fig. 17.2).

The piezoelectric effect also works in reverse. If the crystal is squeezed or stretched, an electric field is produced across it. So, if the ultrasound energy makes contact with the receiving crystal, it will cause the crystal to vibrate in and out and this will produce an alternating electric field. The resulting electrical signal can be amplified and processed in a number of ways. The piezoelectric effect occurs in a number of natural crystals, including quartz, but the most commonly used substance is a synthetic ceramic: lead zirconate titanate. The crystal is cut into a slice with a thickness equal to half a wavelength of the desired ultrasound frequency, as this thickness ensures most of the energy is emitted at the fundamental frequency.

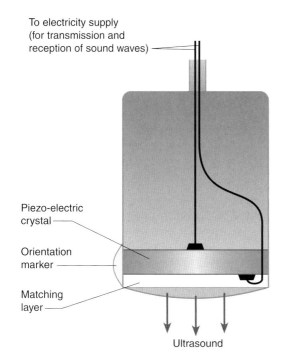

To electricity supply (for transmission and reception of sound waves)

Piezo-electric crystal

Orientation marker

Matching layer

Ultrasound

Figure 17.2 Sound production from a piezoelectric transducer.

Table 17.1   Speed of sound through various mediums

Medium	Speed (m s^{-1})
Air	330
Water	1497
Fat	1440
Blood	1570
Metal	3000–6000
Soft tissue	1540

Normally the transmitting and receiving crystals are built into the same hand-held unit, known as an ultrasonic transducer or probe. The transducer emits ultrasound in rapid pulses and also acts as a receiver most of the time.

It is important to note that the minimum interval between ultrasound pulses equals the time for the deepest echoes to return to the transducer, and the distance that each echo takes to return from the interface depends on the distance of the particular interface from the transducer and the speed of sound within that material. The thickness, size and location of various soft tissue structures in relation to the origin of the ultrasound beam are calculated at any point in time using this 'pulse echo technique'.

Equation for the calculation of the distance of tissues from a transducer:
Distance = Time × Speed of sound

The speed of sound itself varies from one material to another (Table 17.1) and is dependent on temperature, pressure and other factors.

Through electronic processing of the returning sound waves, a two-dimensional image can be created that provides information about the tissues and objects within the tissues. Real-time B-scans allow body structures that are moving to be investigated. This is done by allowing a rapid series of still pictures to be built up to capture the movement. The faster the frame rate, the quicker the image will be updated and the better the resolution of the image. More sophisticated systems have an array of transducers rather than just one pair of transmitter and detector.

Images can be then be displayed on a screen monitor (via what is known as a scan converter) and can be recorded on videotape, thermal paper, laser imaging or digitally on a picture archiving and communication system (PACs) or DVD. The thickness, size and location of various soft tissue structures in relation to the origin of the ultrasound beam are calculated at any point in time using this 'pulse echo technique'.

ACOUSTIC IMPEDANCE

The strength of the reflected sound wave depends on the difference in 'acoustic impedance' between adjacent structures. The acoustic impedance of a medium is related to its density and the speed of sound through that medium (Table 17.2). The greater the difference in acoustic impedance between two adjacent structures, the more sound will be reflected, refracted or absorbed at their boundary rather than transmitted.

Table 17.2 Typical acoustic impedance of various mediums found in the body

Medium	Acoustic impedance (in acoustic ohms)
Air	0.000429
Water	1.50
Blood	1.59
Fat	1.38
Muscle	1.70
Bone	6.50

Example

Air and bone have such very different impedances to those of fat, muscle or water that a beam of ultrasound wave meeting bone or air is almost entirely reflected, refracted or absorbed; consequently there will be no transmission of sound beyond this layer. Similarly, air and skin have very different acoustic impedances; therefore a coupling medium is needed to match the impedance of the crystal in the probe more closely to the impedance of the skin of the patient and thus allow transmission of sound through the skin surface. The most common coupling medium, acoustic gel, is applied on the patient's skin before an ultrasound examination. Coupling gel also has the advantage of reducing air bubbles between the skin surface and the transducer, thereby improving contact and minimising friction.

On the other hand, body layers such as fat, muscle and many body organs have very similar acoustic impedances, enabling most of the beam to pass from one layer into the next, with only a small fraction being reflected, and making this modality ideal for imaging soft tissue organs (Table 17.3).

ULTRASOUND ENERGY

There are two types of ultrasound energy used in diagnostics: continuous energy and pulsed energy.

1. Continuous sound energy uses a steady sound source and, when ultrasound is reflected from a moving surface, the frequency of the sound is altered slightly in a manner that depends on the speed of movement of the surface. This is due to the Doppler effect.
2. Pulsed sound energy is based on a pulse echo technique, whereby a pulse of sound is transmitted and then followed by a pause, during which time an echo has a chance to bounce off the target and return to the transducer. Pulsed ultrasound, because of its high frequency, can be aimed in a specific direction and obeys the laws of geometric optics with regard to reflection, transmission and refraction.

DOPPLER ULTRASOUND

The Doppler effect was discovered by Christian Andreas Doppler (1803–1853) and is now commonly used in ultrasound imaging to examine the movement of liquids, such as blood flow in arteries and veins, allowing the location of blockages to be determined precisely. It is also used in fetal echocardiograms (ECG) in detecting and listening to the fetal heartbeat. Pulsed wave Doppler can also be used to evaluate blood flow through different structures and measure the velocity of the blood flow.

TRANSDUCERS

Ultrasound transducers, also called probes, come in different shapes, sizes and frequencies to allow use in different scanning situations (Fig. 17.3). For example, in an obstetric or upper abdominal scan the transducer used is known as a 'convex-array' or curvilinear transducer. This contour allows the transducer to be moved across the abdomen whilst maintaining good contact with the abdominal surface and also giving the wide field of view needed to see the upper abdomen or the whole fetus. Examples of Doppler studies are spectral, colour and power Doppler.

Table 17.3   Different types of ultrasound scan

Type of scan	How echo is received	Example of scan
A mode	Amplitude mode Each layer producing a reflection shows up as a peak on the trace. The larger the echo, the higher the peak	Amplitude mode 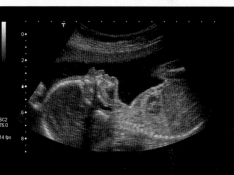
B mode	Brightness mode Each reflecting echo is registered as a bright spot; the larger the amplitude of the reflecting echoes, the brighter the spots	Musculoskeletal detail
M mode	Motion mode Moving echoes are recorded to give traces of fetal heart pulsations	Fetal pole (B mode) + waveform (M mode) 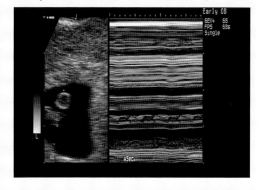

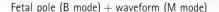

Figure 17.3 A selection of ultrasound probes.

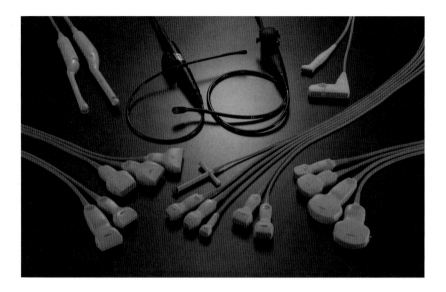

For thyroid, breast or musculoskeletal scans, a transducer with a flat surface – a 'linear-array' transducer – is commonly used.

In some applications, where the window to the organ of interest is small, transducers with a small footprint (i.e. the surface in contact with the patients) are used. These include:

- neonatal head scans – the fontanelles are used as a window
- inter-cavity scans – the transducer head is inserted into the vagina or rectum
- cardiac scans – the space between the ribs is used as a window.

FREQUENCY SELECTION

Higher frequency ultrasound waves have a shorter pulse waveform (wavelength), longer near field and less divergence in the far field; they allow better resolution of superficial structures. More energy, however, is absorbed and scattered by the soft tissues so that higher frequencies have less penetrating ability. On the other hand, low frequency ultrasound waves are longer in length and allow better penetration to image deeper organs. So the ultrasound operator has to weigh up the risk and benefit of selecting resolution as the expense of the penetration, depending on the organ being imaged.

Example

A low frequency transducer will be able to image structures as deep as 15–20 cm, but may not give as good a resolution and image quality as a higher frequency probe such as a 10 MHz or 12 MHz probe.

Typically, for general use of ultrasound in obstetrics and upper abdominal scans, a range of 3.5–6 MHz probe is suitable, and a high frequency transducer (7–12 MHz) can be used for scanning the thyroid gland, breast and testes. It can also be used to examine paediatric and neonatal patients.

SAFETY

A vast amount of research has been carried out in laboratories and animal studies to investigate the effect of using high intensity ultrasound. These studies have found that there are two main changes occurring within the body tissues:

- Heating effect, which can result in localised rise in tissue temperature (prolonged temperature rise, typically above 41°C, can cause damage to tissue cells).
- Cavitations effect can occur in the presence of very high ultrasound pressures, causing oscillation of microbubbles, which can result in the destruction of tissue cells.

It has been over 35 years since ultrasound was first used on pregnant women and some earlier studies found increased frequency of left handedness in boys, dyslexia, and low birth weights in babies who had had excessive prenatal scans. However, these results were not reproduced in larger later studies.

Nevertheless, the prudent use of ultrasound should be recommended. Guidelines on the safe use of ultrasound are available and these recommend working within the safe levels of primary regulated metrics such as TI (thermal index), a metric associated with the tissue heating bio-effect, and MI (mechanical index), a metric associated with the cavitation bio-effect.

Ultrasound power and scanning times should be kept 'as low as reasonably practicable' to achieve an adequate image for interpretation. This is the ALARP principle and all trained operators should adhere to it. It is also very important for the operator to assess the risk/benefit of the ultrasound examination to minimise the unnecessary exposure of patients to ultrasound.

ULTRASOUND MACHINES

Nowadays, advanced technology has enabled ultrasound machines to be smaller, more compact, more mobile and portable (Fig. 17.4). So ultrasound can be used in different settings – from departments with dedicated ultrasound rooms to bedside examinations where ultrasound can be used without moving the patient to another place. Wherever it is used, it important to select a machine that is fit for the purpose for which it is required (i.e. the needs of a department, particular clinic or practitioner).

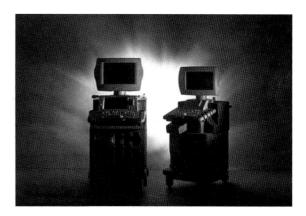

Figure 17.4 A range of ultrasound machines.

APPLICATION OF ULTRASOUND TECHNIQUE

Ultrasound is usually utilised as a first line investigation, due to its advantages, but may have to be complemented with other cross-sectional imaging studies (e.g. MRI or CT). Information can be obtained by using different imaging planes, such as sagittal, coronal and transverse (Box 17.1).

Box 17.1 Information gained by ultrasound examination

- Size of organ – e.g. of a kidney or aorta
- Volume measurements – e.g. as bladder volumes
- Morphological features – e.g. liver, fetal organs
- Wall outline – e.g. smooth, thick walled
- Internal architecture – e.g. cystic or solid
- Echogenicity/texture – e.g. simple or complex lesions
- Relation to adjoining structures – e.g. ectopic kidneys, pancreas
- Presence of free fluid – e.g. presence of ascites in the abdomen
- Haemodynamics

ADVANTAGES OF ULTRASOUND COMPARED WITH OTHER MODALITIES

- Ultrasound examinations are generally non-invasive and more acceptable to patients – the studies do not generally involve use of contrast and there is a lesser degree of discomfort compared to other cross sectional imaging modalities.
- Ultrasound methods are relatively inexpensive, quick and convenient – compared to techniques such as X-rays, CT, MRI scans. This makes it an ideal modality to monitor changes over a period of time; for example in tumour growth or a progressive disease. It is also very suitable as a screening tool in applications such as ovarian screening and screening for abdominal aortic aneurysm or fetal anomalies. The equipment can be made portable for convenience and the images can be stored electronically.
- Ultrasound does not involve ionising radiation – this makes it suitable for obstetrics and paediatric examinations.
- An ultrasound study is dynamic – this means movements and physiological changes can be observed to aid diagnosis.
- It has no known long-term side effects.

DISADVANTAGES OF ULTRASOUND COMPARED WITH OTHER MODALITIES

- It is highly dependent on the operator – as ultrasound examinations are interpreted during the scan, operators need to be highly skilled to obtain accurate images and then interpret them.
- Ultrasound cannot be used for examinations of areas of the body containing gas or bone – this means the method is of very limited use in diagnosing digestive or skeletal problems, such as bowel pathology, lung lesions, fractures and adult brains.
- Ultrasound is not specific in diagnosing all pathology – there may be many pathological conditions that can look the same on the image. Previous and current medical history of the patient is vital to enable accurate interpretation.
- Images are dependent on the characteristics of the patient – therefore it is not always possible to obtain diagnostic images from patients with high body mass indices as excessive fat layers can weaken the signal on transmission and reflection back to the transducer.

ROLE OF AN ULTRASOUND DEPARTMENT

- To provide first line investigations; e.g. in right upper quadrant pain to exclude biliary colic, renal colic, for pelvic pain to exclude ovarian cysts or ectopic pregnancies.
- To obtain additional information to aid diagnosis in cases of abnormal liver function tests, palpable lumps, pain.
- As a valuable tool in one-stop clinics (haematuria, one stop breast clinics, early assessments clinics).
- To speed up patient management and improve patient pathway in cases of definitive diagnosis.
- For reassurance purposes; e.g. during pregnancy.
- To screen for abnormalities such as ovarian cancer, aortic aneurysm and fetal anomalies.
- To provide a good monitoring/surveillance modality; for example, fetal well-being and aortic aneurysms.
- To provide a research tool to aid technological advances in this field and improve diagnostic efficiency of ultrasound.

PATIENT PREPARATION

The patient should eat and drink normally before and after the scan unless otherwise instructed; for example for gall bladder scans the patient will have to avoid fatty foods for 6 hours before the scan; for renal and bladder scans the patient will be required to attend with a full bladder. In obstetrics and gynaecology a full bladder may also be necessary to displace the bowel gas upwards and laterally to allow good visualisation of the pelvic structures. Usually patients are advised to carry on taking their usual medication.

The other important patient preparation is to obtain informed consent from the patient, by providing an explanation of the scan, who is going to do the scan, and when the results will be available. This is because in most cases the result can be available immediately and it is important to make the patient aware of this in case of bad news.

OPERATOR SKILLS IN ACQUIRING AND INTERPRETING AN ULTRASOUND IMAGE

There are many factors that affect the accuracy and safety of ultrasound; operator skills are probably the most important of these.

By using the correct techniques to allow adequate visualisation of the organ investigated, the operator can be sure that any potential pathology cannot be missed. Equally, knowledge of anatomy (especially cross-sectional anatomy), and understanding of physiology is vital to recognise physiological and pathological appearances that may be apparent on an ultrasound image.

Knowledge of ultrasound equipment technology is crucial to enable the sonographer to manipulate the controls on the ultrasound machine. By using the equipment appropriately the sonographer can ensure that the image obtained can be optimised to give the best possible quality for diagnosis.

The sonographer should be aware of artefacts, which are appearances that are falsely created by the reflection, refraction and absorption of the sound waves. These appearances can confuse the operator, leading to misdiagnosis. It is important for the operator not only to recognise but also to try to minimise them. Examples of these are mirror images and reverberation echoes.

Excellent interpersonal skills are needed to establish a good relationship with the patient, which enables the acquisition of adequate images for interpretation. In some cases counselling skills are necessary for the sonographer to support the patient initially in case of bad news, such as fetal abnormalities or fetal death.

COMMON APPLICATIONS OF ULTRASOUND

OBSTETRIC ULTRASOUND

Early pregnancy

Diagnosis and confirmation of on-going early pregnancy can be done by a high frequency trans vaginal scan. A gestation sac can be seen as early as 5 weeks of pregnancy (Fig. 17.5). It is very important to initially confirm the site of the pregnancy within the cavity of the uterus, thereby excluding the possibility of an ectopic pregnancy (although in very rare cases, an intra- and extrauterine pregnancy can occur together). A fetal pole and a visible heartbeat can be detectable by ultrasound by about 6–7 weeks. For women with vaginal bleeding an ultrasound scan is important to exclude miscarriage. Complicated conditions such as molar pregnancies (a pre-cancerous condition of the placental tissue) can also be detected in time for effective management. Multiple pregnancies can be excluded or confirmed, and the type of twins (identical or non-identical – 'chorionicity') can also be determined by ultrasound (Fig. 17.6).

Dating pregnancies

The establishment of correct gestational age and assessment of fetal size is very important for pregnancy management in terms of delivery and the timing of further tests; therefore ultrasound

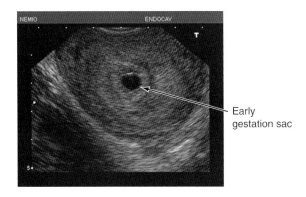

Early gestation sac

Figure 17.5 An early intrauterine gestation sac of approximately 5 weeks (3 weeks from conception).

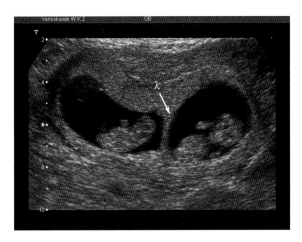

Figure 17.6 Multiple pregnancy with lambda sign indicating non-identical twins.

dating scans provide an accurate estimated date of delivery (EDD) by evaluating the fetal size. Fetal measurements (Table 17.4) include crown rump length (CRL), biparietal diameter (BPD), head circumference (HC) and femur length (FL). In later scans, the abdominal circumference (AC) is used in the assessment of fetal growth. Growth trends can be monitored by serial scans to exclude intrauterine growth retardation, or macrosomia in high-risk women (Fig. 17.7).

Diagnosis of fetal anomalies

The National Screening Committee recommends that every woman should be offered a routine

Table 17.4   Fetal measurements

Measurement	Example of scan
Crown rump length (CR length)	Bi-parietal diameter (head circumference, HC)
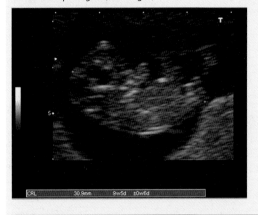	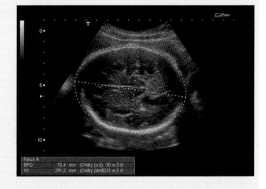
Femur length (FL)	Abdominal circumference (AC)
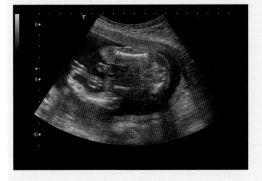	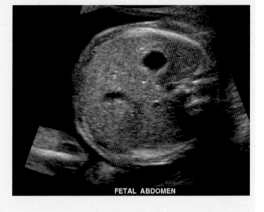

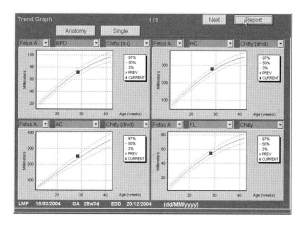

Figure 17.7 Fetal growth charts.

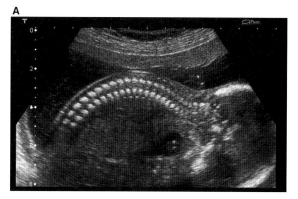

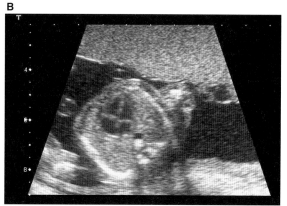

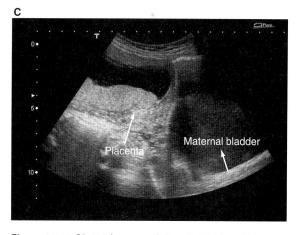

Figure 17.8 Obstetric scans. **A** Longitudinal section of fetal spine. **B** Cross section of fetal chest to show 4-chamber view of the heart. **C** A low lying placenta.

scan to allow her the choice to screen her baby for abnormalities. This scan is usually performed at about 18–20 weeks of pregnancy (Fig. 17.8). Although ultrasound is sensitive for the detection of a variety of fetal anomalies, such as spina bifida, skeletal dysplasia, abdominal hernias, renal problems, it cannot detect all abnormalities as some problems may either be too subtle to be seen on a scan or develop late in pregnancy. Some fetal organs may be more challenging to assess; for example the detection of certain heart defects in the fetus is made more difficult, owing to its size and movement. Doppler studies of the fetal heart can be useful in some cases.

The placenta can also be assessed for its site to exclude complications in later pregnancies, such as placenta praevia (see Fig. 17.8C). Amniotic fluid volumes (liquor) can be assessed to exclude excessive (polyhydramnios) or reduced (oligohydramnios) liquor volumes in cases of certain fetal abnormalities or growth disorders. Fetal presentations (breech, oblique) and fetal intrauterine death can also be confirmed. A pregnancy scan may also reveal other pathology, such as uterine fibroids and ovarian cysts.

Fetal chromosomal disorders

Ultrasound is not very sensitive in the detection of chromosomal abnormalities; the most promising feature so far that is used in the assessment of Down syndrome is fetal nuchal translucency (fluid area behind the fetal neck; Fig. 17.9). This measurement can be used alongside blood results, fetal age, and maternal age to determine the risk of Down syndrome. Invasive diagnostic tests such as amniocentesis (sampling the liquor); chorionic villus sampling (CVS; sampling the placenta) and

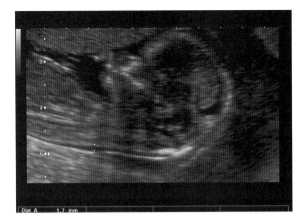

Figure 17.9 Nuchal translucency.

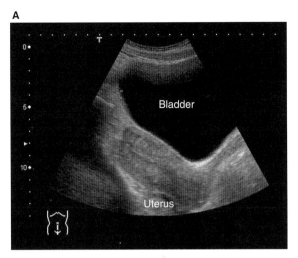

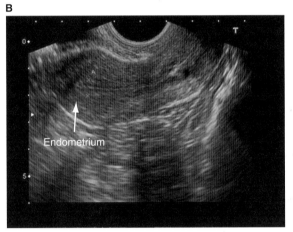

Figure 17.10 A Transabdominal image with full bladder and uterus. B Transvaginal uterus with endometrial measurement.

fetal blood sampling (from the umbilical cord) can be performed under ultrasound guidance to obtain fetal cells to determine the genetic composition (karyotype).

GYNAECOLOGICAL ULTRASOUND

Ultrasound is primarily used in the assessment of uterine and ovarian structures (Figs 17.10 and 17.11). The uterus can be examined to exclude normal uterine variants such as bicornuate or didelphic uterus, or pathologies in the presence of pelvic pain, abnormal vaginal bleeding or palpable masses within the pelvis. Pathologies such as fibroids, simple or complex ovarian cysts, endometrial polyps, tubo-ovarian abscess and suspected endometrial cancer can be detected by ultrasound. This modality is also very extensively used in the assessment and monitoring of patients with infertility, by monitoring and tracking follicular and endometrial development and determining correct timings for infertility procedures. The role of ultrasound in screening for ovarian cancer is still being researched, as the ultrasound appearances are sometimes very subtle to interpret in non-postmenopausal women.

ACUTE ABDOMINAL ULTRASOUND

In acute medicine, ultrasound is an ideal first line investigation (Figs 17.12–17.15); for example for right upper quadrant pain, biliary colic can be assessed by investigating the gall bladder and the bile ducts to exclude stones. In cases of renal colic, obstruction can be detected by the presence of pelvicalyceal dilatation and the presence of calculi, depending on their size. Acute pancreatitis and cholecystitis may well present with an oedematous appearances and wall thickening. Acute pelvic pain can be investigated to exclude ectopic pregnancy, ruptured ovarian cysts or inflammation caused by appendicitis. Pyrexia can be as a result of abscesses present within the abdomen or acute appendicitis, which ultrasound scans can confirm or exclude.

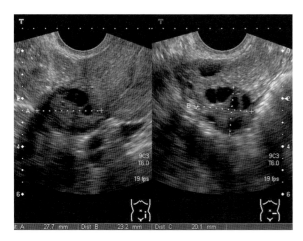

Figure 17.11 Ovary showing normal follicles.

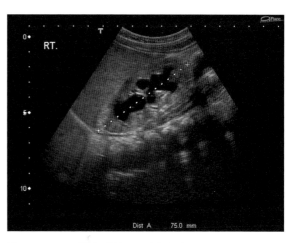

Figure 17.14 Right kidney with hydronephrosis.

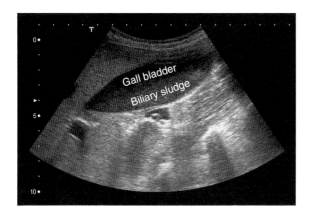

Figure 17.12 Gall bladder with sludge.

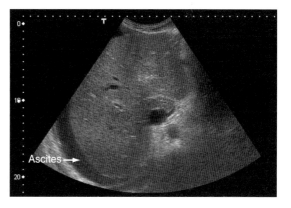

Figure 17.15 Ascites.

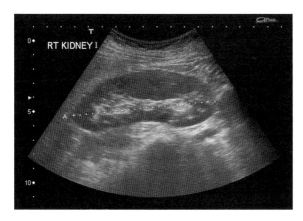

Figure 17.13 Normal right kidney.

In cases of blunt abdominal trauma, FAST scanning (Focussed Assessment with Sonography for Trauma), is used in some accident and emergency departments to determine any organ injury. A scan is performed to detect abnormal interabdominal fluid collections, which can be a result of haematomas and interabdominal bleeding.

NON-ACUTE ABDOMINAL ULTRASOUND

In the presence of abnormal liver function tests (LFTs), ultrasound can be used to assess the liver for obstructive jaundice and detect any focal lesions (e.g. metastasis, Fig. 17.16) or general

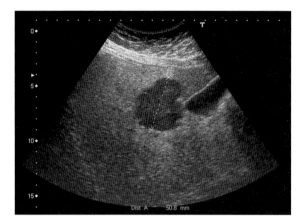

Figure 17.16 Liver metastasis.

diffuse disease such as cirrhosis. Hepato- or splenomegaly can be assessed by measurements and reference to the normal ranges. In urogenital cases, congenital renal abnormalities can be excluded, such as ectopic or horseshoe kidney, and the kidneys can be examined to exclude any focal benign or malignant lesions, stones or obstruction. Urinary bladder volumes can be calculated if required. Inflammatory conditions like acute or chronic cholecystitis and pancreatitis can be excluded with ultrasound. Ultrasound is also a useful screening tool for the detection of abdominal aortic aneurysm by measuring the diameter of the aorta (Fig. 17.17). Depending on the size of the aneurysm, the patients can either be monitored over a period of time for any

changes or referred for surgery. Ultrasound is an accepted tool to investigate and monitor patients after renal transplants to detect any signs of rejection.

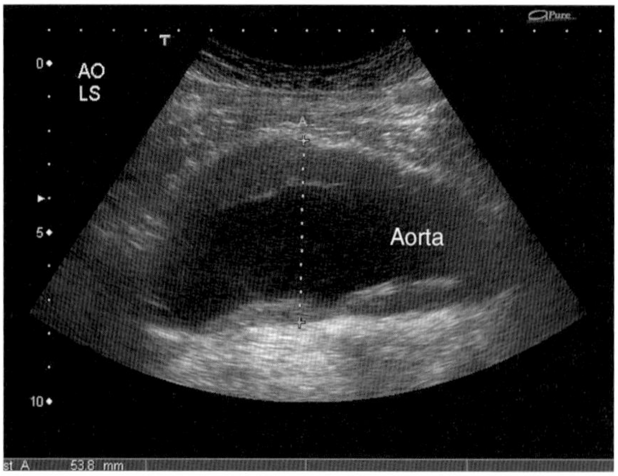

HEAD AND NECK ULTRASOUND

Ultrasound can be useful in cases of abnormal thyroid function tests in detecting palpable thyroid lumps, enlarged thyroids and non-functioning thyroids (Fig. 17.18). Pathology such as nodular goitres and cystic disease can be detected in cases of thyroid lumps; it is not always possible to distinguish between benign and malignant tumours. Parathyroid glands are difficult to see on an ultrasound scan unless there is enlargement present due to disease. Salivary glands (i.e. parotid, submandibular and sublingual glands) can also be assessed with ultrasound to exclude pathology such as inflammation, stones and benign or malignant tumours. Doppler colour flow studies, fine needle aspirations (FNAs) and biopsies under ultrasound control may be necessary for further evaluation.

BREAST ULTRASOUND

Ultrasound can provide information concerning the breasts and the axillary lymph nodes (Fig. 17.19). It acts as a complementary imaging modality to characterise lesions that are non-specific on a

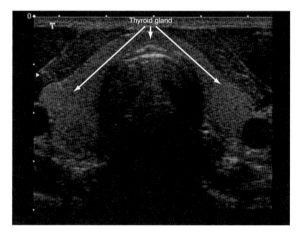

Figure 17.17 Longitudinal section of abdominal aortic aneurysm.

Figure 17.18 Thyroid.

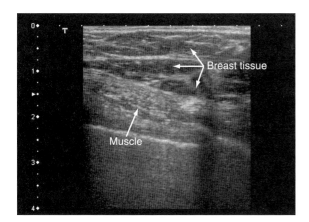

Figure 17.19 Ultrasound of the breast.

mammogram. It is also the method of choice over mammograms when examining patients with a breast prosthesis. It can detect benign breast changes such as adenomas and cystic disease. However, FNAs and biopsies are needed to confirm more sinister pathology such as breast carcinomas.

PAEDIATRIC/NEONATAL HEAD ULTRASOUND

This modality is ideally suited to this as it does not utilise ionising radiation and is relatively quick and easy to perform. The equipment does not appear as threatening to the patients as an X-ray tube or MRI/CT. The parents or guardians are able to sit and comfort the children while the scan is performed.

An experienced sonographer can detect paediatric and neonatal complications, such as developmental dysplasia of the hip (DDH), pyloric stenosis, intussusceptions, intracranial haemorrhage and hydrocephalus.

MUSCULOSKELETAL ULTRASOUND

With advanced ultrasound technology, such as high frequency probes and panoramic and extended fields of view, musculoskeletal ultrasound is emerging as a reliable modality to detect soft tissue masses such as Baker's cysts, abscesses and lipomas. Inflammatory processes in synovitis and bursitis can be confirmed by the presence of free fluid between the joint spaces. In sports medicine, trauma to the muscles, tendons and ligaments can be assessed for the degree of severity in order to aid treatment. Musculoskeletal ultrasound complements MRI in the evaluation of musculoskeletal abnormalities, as it can offer important information.

VASCULAR ULTRASOUND

Using the Doppler principle, blood flow can be assessed with ultrasound (Figs 17.20 and 17.21). Complications such as stenosis of a blood vessel (narrowing), thrombus (blood clot) and

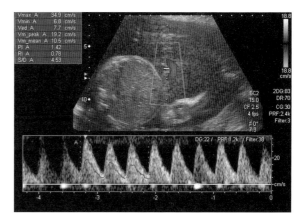

Figure 17.20 Doppler of fetal umbilical artery.

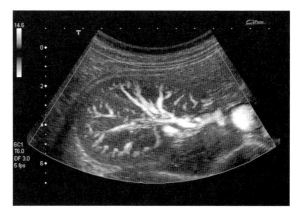

Figure 17.21 Colour flow images of the kidney.

associated haemodynamics can be easily assessed. It is also used to detect various other conditions such as ischaemic stroke, vascular occlusion and blood vessel malformation.

ECHOCARDIOGRAPHY

By using a transducer with a small footprint and scanning in between the ribs, scans can reveal information about the heart, such as the wall thickness, the heart chambers, the heart valves, their functions, abnormal heart rhythms, congenital defects and the presence of pericardial effusion. It is also possible to evaluate the blood flow.

ONE-STOP CLINICS

With improving patient pathways and care, one stop clinics have evolved to streamline patient experience and minimise time spent waiting for appointments and planning treatments. Ultrasound has an eminent place in these clinics because obvious problems can be diagnosed, and a treatment/follow up plan made, during one visit to the clinic.

Examples of one-stop clinics

- Early pregnancy
- Haematuria
- Symptomatic breast assessment
- Emergency gynaecology

INTERVENTIONAL PROCEDURES UNDER ULTRASOUND CONTROL

Because of the dynamic nature of the real-time ultrasound, FNAs and biopsies can be performed under ultrasound guidance and surveillance. The needle tip can be located and followed to ensure accurate placing and successful aspiration, biopsy or treatment of the area of interest, thus reducing the risk of complications.

ULTRASOUND CONTRAST STUDIES

Ultrasound contrast agents (USCAs) are non-toxic, gas-filled microbubbles that are injected intravenously and capable of crossing the pulmonary capillary bed after a peripheral injection. Doppler examinations are improved by using USCAs when studying deep and small vessels, vessels with low or slow flow, or vessels with a non-optimal insonation angle. Ultrasound contrast agents also enhance detection of flow within abnormal vessels, including tumour vascularisation and stenotic vessels, and provide better delineation of ischemic areas. Current research is focussing on the development of specific contrast imaging sequences that allow detection of tissue enhancement similar to that obtained with CT or MRI. Targeted agents, such as anticoagulants or cytotoxic compounds, could further widen USCA applications to specific delivery of active drugs.

INTRACAVITY ULTRASOUND

In some situations a clearer image can be obtained from a transducer that can be inserted within the body. These transducers are very small and can be inserted into the vagina, rectum or urethra to get better images of the pelvic organs, such as uterus, ovaries and prostate gland. Specially designed transducers can also be swallowed by the patient and these help to get a clearer image of the heart, as this lies just in front of the oesophagus. They can also be used during an operation to help guide the surgeon. Recent guidelines have advocated the use of ultrasound guidance in central venous line insertions.

3D ULTRASOUND

3D scans require special transducers and software to accumulate and render the images, and with advancing technology the rendering time has been reduced from minutes to seconds (Fig. 17.22). A good 3D image is often quite impressive and further 2D scans may be extracted from 3D blocks of scanned information. Volumetric

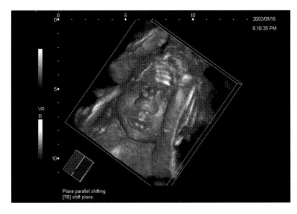

Figure 17.22 3D image.

measurements are more accurate and sonographers can appreciate the presence or absence of a certain abnormality in a 3D scan more easily than in a 2D one; for example a cleft lip. There is also the possibility, in obstetric ultrasound, of increasing psychological bonding between the parents and the unborn baby. The ability to obtain a good 3D picture is nevertheless still very much dependent on operator skill. Its greatest potential is still in research, and particularly in the study of fetal embryology.

THERAPEUTIC APPLICATIONS

Using lower frequencies than medical diagnostic ultrasound, for example from 250 to 2000 kHz, but significantly higher energies, benign and malignant tumours and other disorders can be treated via a process known as focussed ultrasound surgery (FUS) or high intensity focussed ultrasound (HIFU). The ultrasound beam is focussed on the diseased tissue, resulting in a significant rise in the temperature within the tissue. This will cause the destruction of the diseased tissue by coagulation necrosis. The treatment is often guided by MRI, as in magnetic resonance guided focussed ultrasound (MRgFUS). Other applications include ultrasound assisted target drug and gene delivery. This treatment can be combined with radiotherapy or chemotherapy. FUS can also be used to break up kidney stones by lithotripsy.

WORK-RELATED UPPER LIMB DISORDERS

An extended role, along with the demand for more ultrasound scans, has exacerbated the workload on sonographers. Ill-designed equipment and poor working conditions have resulted in sonographers suffering from work-related upper limb disorders (WRULD) such as repetitive stress injuries (RSI), neck, shoulder and back pains. Nowadays manufactures and employers are more aware of these risks and have designed various ways of minimising WRULD. There are specific guidelines to ensure that working conditions for sonographers are in place to prevent such disorders and maintain the workforce.

TRAINING AND QUALITY ASSURANCE

In the last twenty years, ultrasound practice has moved from being only available in hospital radiology departments to smaller setting such as clinics and private practices. This has an effect of decentralisation of ultrasound services. The acceptance and demand from the public has also increased dramatically, especially in the obstetrics field, and this, coupled with increased usage by various medical specialties and sub-specialties, means that the standards and quality of scans are becoming an emerging problem. Ultrasound practitioners must ensure that they are suitably trained and have achieved and maintain the necessary competency to carry out the scans. Local protocols have to be developed to ensure that practitioners work to the accepted level of practice for their knowledge and expertise and have the capability to recognise limitations in their own abilities and of the ultrasound equipment, in order to avoid litigation. National and international guidelines should be adhered to for the safe and accurate use of ultrasound. In addition, there must be quality assurance measures to monitor standards and performance, and competencies.

THE FUTURE OF ULTRASOUND

Ultrasound has established its role in modern medicine, and its future is ensured until an alternative imaging modality emerges that offers similar advantages of rapidity, accuracy and cheapness. With advancing computer and software technology, ultrasound machines will most likely become more sophisticated, with better image quality, and have more memory for storing data. Transducer probes may get smaller; more intracavity applications will be developed to gain better images of internal organs. 3D and 4D (real-time 3D) ultrasound will be more highly developed and become more popular. Wireless technology will minimise work-related disorders by enabling sonographers to control the ultrasound machine remotely and by voice activation. Ultrasound practices are destined to move further into every field of medicine, not only in diagnostic capabilities but also in the treatment of diseases.

Bibliography

Bates J. Practical gynaecological ultrasound, 2nd revised edn. Cambridge, UK: Cambridge University Press; 2006.

Bates JA. Abdominal ultrasound: how, why and when. London: Churchill Livingstone; 2004.

Bradley M, O'Donnell P (eds). Atlas of musculoskeletal ultrasound anatomy. London: Greenwich Medical Media; 2003.

Cardenosa G. Breast imaging. Baltimore: Lippincott Williams & Wilkins; 2000.

Chudleigh P, Thilaganathan B. Obstetric ultrasound: how, why and when, 2nd edn. London: Churchill Livingstone; 2004.

College of Radiographers. Occupational standards for diagnostic ultrasound: an abridged version. London: College of Radiographers; 1999.

De Bruyn R. Paediatric ultrasound: how, why, when. London: Churchill Livingstone; 2004.

Gaspari R. Emergency ultrasound; principles and practice. Philadelphia: Mosby; 2005.

Hoskins P. Diagnostic ultrasound physics and equipment. London: Greenwich Medical Media; 2002.

Kremkau FW. Diagnostic ultrasound: principles and instruments, 7th edn. Philadelphia: WB Saunders; 2005.

Kurjak A, Jackson D. Atlas of three- and four-dimensional sonography. London: Taylor and Francis, 2004.

Rumack CM, Wilson SR, Charboneau JM. Diagnostic ultrasound. Philadelphia: Mosby; 1998.

Sidhu P. Ultrasound of abdominal transplantation. St Louis: Thieme Publishing Group; 2002.

Tempkin BB. Ultrasound scanning: principles and protocols, 3rd edn. Philadelphia: WB Saunders; 2007.

Ter Haar G, Duck FA (eds). The safe use of ultrasound in medical diagnosis. London: British Institute of Radiology; 2000.

Thrush A. Peripheral vascular ultrasound: how, why and when. London: Greenwich Medical Media; 2000.

Twining P, McHugo JM, Pilling DW (eds). Textbook of fetal abnormalities. Edinburgh: Churchill Livingstone; 2006.

Zagzebski JA. Essentials of ultrasound physics. Philadelphia: Mosby; 1996.

Chapter **18**

Computed tomography

Sophia Beale and Catriona Todd

KEY POINTS

- Modern scanners are capable of imaging large volumes during one scan.
- System components include the scanner, the computer system, the image display system and remote work stations.
- Image reconstruction occurs in three stages: preprocessing, convolution and back projection.
- Artefacts are an important factor that will affect image quality.
- Patient care is essential throughout the entire examination.
- Contrast medium is used in computed tomography to enhance the image.

INTRODUCTION

The earliest types of computed tomography (CT) scanner were known as sequential scanners and acquired images a single slice at a time. This was because the gantry contained large high-tension power cables, and in order to prevent these cables becoming tangled after every 360° rotation, the X-ray tube had to reverse rotate back to the start point before the next slice could be acquired. These were known as first and second generation scanners.

The 1980s saw a significant advancement in technology with the introduction of slip rings, which eliminated the need for a high-tension cable supply to the X-ray tube and detectors and allowed the X-ray tube to rotate continuously in one direction around the patient. This is known as spiral or helical CT. Slip rings are 'electromechanical devices consisting of circular electrical conductive rings and brushes that transmit electrical energy across a rotating interface'.[1] Slip ring technology was first incorporated into the third generation scanners. The most common type of CT scanner in use today is the fourth generation scanner, incorporating a stationary circular ring of detectors and a large fan beam of X-rays.

The advantage of slip ring technology is continuous rotation of the X-ray tube, meaning it spirals around the patient as the table moves through the gantry, allowing a volume of data to be collected rather than individual slices. It also means that large volumes can be scanned in a single breath hold as a result of faster scan times.

SYSTEM COMPONENTS

System components for CT generally fall into four categories:

- Imaging system (also known as the scanner) – comprising the gantry and the patient couch.
- Computer system – where all the data is digitally analysed and processed.
- Image display system – usually situated in the control room with the console used for planning and carrying out the scans.
- Remote workstations – used for post-scan 3D image reconstruction and manipulation. Radiologists can also review thin slices.

IMAGING SYSTEM

Patient couch

The patient couch adjusts to a range of heights to allow patients to mount and dismount with ease. This also enables safe transfer of patients from beds or trolleys of varying heights. To enable coverage during scanning the patient couch also moves horizontally through the gantry, allowing the patient to be scanned from head to mid thigh without the need to reposition.

Gantry

The gantry is square with a circular opening. Staff are able to access the patient from both the front and the back of the gantry. The circular opening through which the patient couch travels is known as the 'aperture'; this is also the opening at which the patient is positioned for scanning. Most scanner apertures measure 70 cm in diameter, enabling access to the patient should it be needed. The gantry also has laser lights to aid patient positioning. An important feature of the CT gantry is the tilting range to aid positioning of patients and the variety of clinical examinations. The degree of tilt varies but on most scanners $+/- 30°$ is usually standard. For spiral scanning the tilt often has to be at $0°$ to enable reconstruction of images. Housed within the gantry are important system components, such as the high-tension generator and X-ray tube on a rotating scan frame, a ring of detectors, slip rings and collimators.

The high-tension generator and X-ray tube are connected via a short cable, allowing the generator to sit on a rotating frame with the X-ray tube and eliminating the need for long high-tension cables. Situated in front of the X-ray tube is a collimator (similar to those used on a conventional X-ray tube), which determines the slice thickness of the scan being performed and can be adjusted. Another collimator is also situated directly opposite the X-ray tube on the opposite side of the rotating frame. This is known as a post-scan collimator and its purpose is to eliminate the low energy scattered radiation emitted from the patient during the scan, enabling the scanner to produce sharper, more detailed images.

The detectors are situated on a stationary ring inside the gantry. They are designed to measure the attenuation of the transmitted X-rays from the patient and convert them into an electrical signal. The electrical signal is then amplified and analysed by the DAS (data acquisition system). The DAS is situated between the detector ring and the computer system.

The most common types of CT scanner in use today are multi-slice scanners, i.e. 16 and 64-slice scanners (Fig. 18.1). The number of slices refers to the number of rows of detectors contained within a gantry; for example a 64-slice scanner will contain 64 rows of detectors.

Slip rings are situated at the diameter of the gantry and contain wire brushes made from conductive material which carry the electrical supply required for the scanner to operate. Slip rings provide continuous rotation of the gantry through eliminating the need for long high-tension cables to the X-ray tube.

The CT gantry must be kept cool in order for the system components to operate efficiently. This can be either air or water-cooled. The scanning rooms are also air-conditioned to ensure the system does not overheat.

THE COMPUTER SYSTEM

A mini-computer controls the processing in a CT system. The computer and image processing systems work together and utilise fast processing of data and include a large storage capacity. The

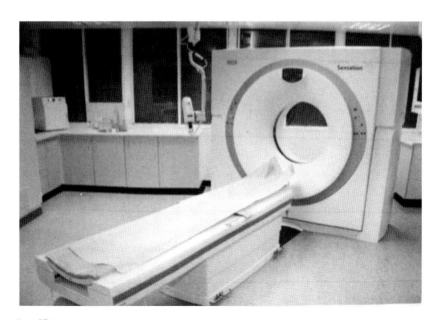

Figure 18.1 16 slice CT scanner.

computer system receives the numerical data from the DAS and, once the raw data is processed and the process of convolution and back projection have taken place, it assigns a grey scale to the numerical values (grey-scale images are easier for radiologists to interpret than numerical data). These numerical values are known as CT numbers or Hounsfield units (HU), named after Sir Godfrey Hounsfield (1919–2004). CT numbers are related to the linear attenuation coefficient of the tissues within the slice and therefore related to the attenuation of X-rays by the tissues. They are measured using the attenuation of water as a reference, with water assigned the value zero (0). The value for bone is +1000 and for air is −1000, with various soft-tissue types placed somewhere along the scale. These grey-scale images are then sent to the image display system within the scanning control room for the operator to visualise.

IMAGE DISPLAY

Most image display systems are flat screen colour monitors, although the images are displayed in grey-scale.

Most units will have preselected window widths and levels for each examination. These will be very similar on different make scanners, although not identical. Some examples are:

Lung	1500 and −500
Soft tissue chest	350 and 50

IMAGE RECONSTRUCTION

Once the scan has been performed the data collected by the detectors must be processed and displayed as an image. This process occurs in the image reconstruction system (IRS). There are three main stages to this process:

1. Preprocessing
   This is where the data is 'cleaned up' and made ready for reconstruction. These corrections are necessary due to inherent variations in the X-ray tube and detectors.

2. Convolution
   This is necessary to compensate for the blurring that occurs during the next stage of back projection.

3. Back projection
   During this stage the data is converted into a 2D axial image. A density is assigned to each pixel of this image. This is the grey scale, which allows different tissues to be identified.

The IRS is driven by high specification computer systems, which allow multiple reconstructions with different slice thickness, algorithms and pre-set viewing windows to be carried out for each set of acquired data. If the IRS is not functioning then, as a fail-safe the scanner will not function.

With the fast computing systems now available we are no longer limited to basic 2D axial images. Although many post-processing functions may be undertaken on the operator console a separate workstation now comes as standard with all scanners. Radiographers and radiologists can manipulate and view the data using multi-planar reformats (MPR), optimised filters and volume rendering techniques (VRT).

ARTEFACTS

Artefacts affect the quality of the CT images that we produce. A scan degraded by artefact can be much more difficult for the radiologist to interpret.

MOTION ARTEFACT

This is caused by the patient moving during scan acquisition. However, with the sub-second scanning available with the fourth generation scanners, artefacts due to breathing are much less of a problem now than previously. Indeed it is common practice to not suspend respiration for intubated patients during body scanning. Nevertheless, if a sequential scan technique is being used (e.g. high-resolution chest), this can still be a problem. Physical movement during the scan is minimised by ensuring the patient is comfortable, using immobilisation aids and by giving the patient full instructions on the examination.

PARTIAL VOLUME

Again, this is much less of a problem now with the widespread use of multi-slice scanners. Partial volumes occur when an object does not fill the entire slice thickness. During image reconstruction it can be difficult for the computer to separate the CT numbers allocated to each tissue type so an average value is given and the resultant object will be poorly visualised on the image. The easiest way to correct this is to use thin slices. A typical body CT scan will use 16×1.5 collimation; this data will then be reconstructed to 2 mm slices for the radiologist to report from. A second reconstruction will then be carried at 8 mm and this is what will be either transferred to the PACS system or filmed.

METAL ARTEFACT

The blocking of radiation from the detectors by the metal present causes metal artefacts. Metal artefacts will typically be seen as a star burst effect emanating from the metal (Fig. 18.2).

Steps should be taken to remove all external metal objects before scanning. For internal metal, selection of an appropriate algorithm can reduce the effect. Most scanners will also have a specific postprocessing VRT for minimising this even further (Fig. 18.3). This can prove useful when imaging patients after spinal fusion surgery to check the position of the pedicular screws.

ARCING

This artefact is the least common. It is seen as a random streak across one image. The scanner may also stop after this slice. This is caused by arcing in the X-ray tube and should be reported to the lead radiographer as it can indicate that the X-ray tube is reaching the end of its life.

PATIENT CARE

The vast majority of patients encountered will be mobile, self-caring outpatients.

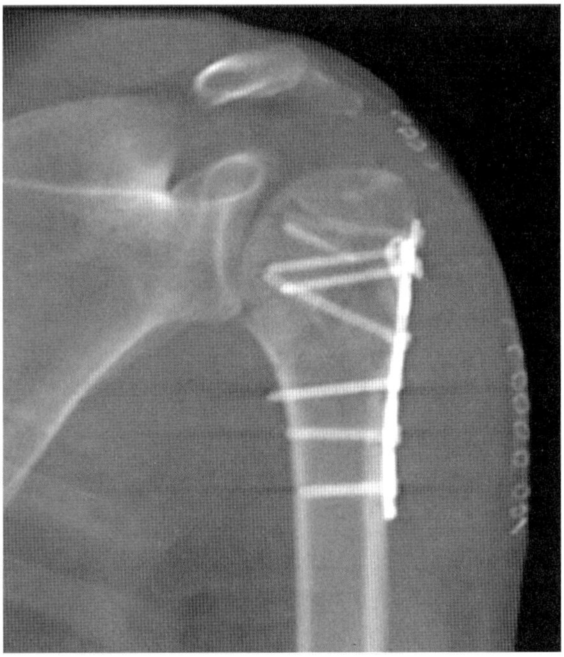

Figure 18.2 Metal artefact. Courtesy of Siemens Medical.

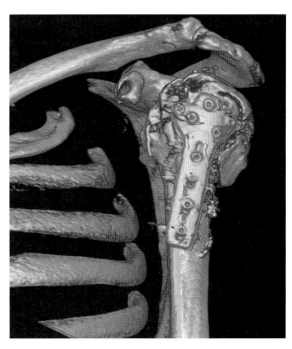

Figure 18.3 Post-processing volume rendering technique (VRT) to reduce metal artefact. Courtesy of Siemens Medical.

PRE-SCAN PREPARATION

Oral contrast

Depending on what type of scan a patient is having they made require oral contrast prior to the scan. Some departments will use positive contrast agents such as barium or gastrografin and others may use negative contrast agents such as water. Oral contrast agents can be administered at any time between 4 hours and 15 min prior to a scan commencing. This information is all dependent on individual departmental scanning protocols.

Pregnancy status

It is essential under the IR(ME)R guidelines that when scanning patients of childbearing age (commonly between the ages 12 and 55, but may vary), you must establish a pregnancy status (Fig. 18.4). This should apply to all scans in the region between the diaphragm and the knees.

Siting of a cannula

Some patients require a cannula for the introduction of contrast medium. The following points should be remembered:

- Ensure you are able to prepare an injection tray with all the required components.
- Be sensitive to needle phobic patients who may require extra care whilst the needle is being sited.
- Be aware if a patient is diabetic and has been fasting. This is because the blood sugar levels will be low and so the patient will be prone to hypoglycaemic attacks.
- Change patients into gowns where appropriate.
- Remove essential jewellery only.

SCAN ROOM CARE

- Owing to the vertical movements of the table, minimal assistance is required for patients.
- Make use of accessories such as straps and cushions to maintain patient comfort throughout the scan.

- Always give clear instructions and ensure that they are understood. This may mean practising the required breathing technique.
- As well as oral recorded instructions some scanners have a lighting system to indicate the breathing phase, which is of value for patients who are hard of hearing.
- Intravenous contrast may be administered by a pump injection or hand injection. Patients should be warned that they might experience feelings of warmth throughout their body and a metallic taste in their mouth.
- Rarely a patient will react to contrast (Fig. 18.5). This can range from vomiting through to anaphylactic shock. Basic life support procedures should be practised and essential equipment should be to hand at all times.
- Recognise reactions and take appropriate action; for example, patients may only notice urticaria when they are getting dressed and they may draw attention to this.

SCAN PROCEDURE

Under IR(ME)R guidelines CT scan requests are vetted and justified by a radiologist who will determine the type of scan protocol required. Once this has occurred then the scan procedure can begin.

Each time a patient is scanned a series of events happens. It is very important that the patient's details are registered on the scanner console before the examination commences to avoid irradiating a patient incorrectly. When entering patient details the patient's position within the gantry is required (i.e. 'head first – supine, feet first – supine, or head first – prone'). By doing this the scanner will image the patient and orientate the images as though the scan has been performed in the supine position.

Each examination has a set of protocols and these must always be followed to ensure the correct positioning of the patient from the start of the examination. This will include:

- Patient position – head first or feet first, supine or prone.
- Centring point – this will be determined by the patient's position.

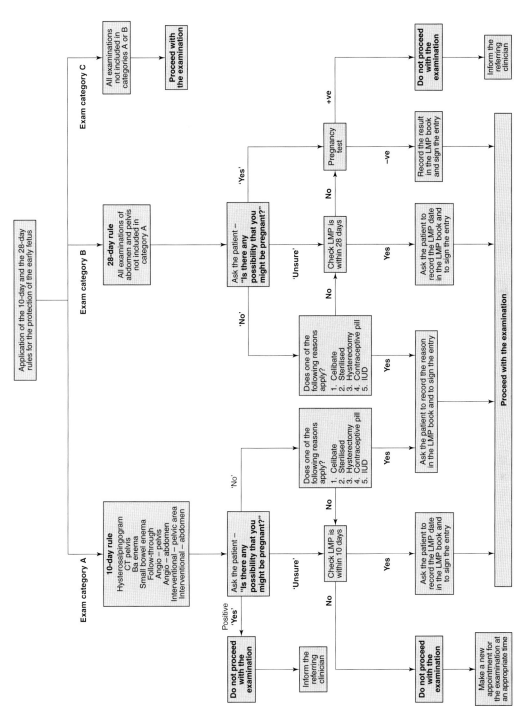

Figure 18.4 'Last menstrual period' (LMP) check procedure prior to examination. Courtesy of Charing Cross Hospital Radiological Services Unit.

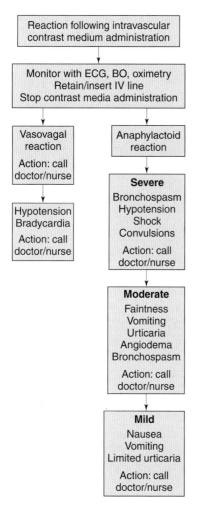

Figure 18.5 Reactions to contrast medium. Adapted from Charing Cross Hospital, with permission.

- Placing of any accessory equipment – e.g. drains, pumps, and oxygen cylinders.
- Breathing instructions – if these are part of the required scan, they must be explained to the patient before the scan starts. (It is important to ensure that the patient understands the breathing instructions, whether these are verbal or visually indicated by the scanner gantry.)

Once the patient is in the desired position it is essential to use the infrared lights positioned on the gantry to obtain the correct centring point according to the departmental protocol. If a thorax or abdominal scan is to be performed,

ensure that artefacts are placed away from the scan area and that the patient's arms are placed above the head or in a position so as not to cause unnecessary artefacts on the images. Some scanners provide immobilisation bands to ensure the patient is comfortable and still. Check that these are not at risk of getting caught in the scanner table as it moves through the gantry. Once this is established and the patient is in a position in the gantry ready to start the scan, switch the infrared lights off, if they do not automatically do this, to avoid damage to the patient's eyes.

Localiser/topogram/scout/scanogram

The above terms are those used by the different manufacturers of CT scanners. This is the initial image produced and has the appearance of an X-ray image. As this scan happens the table will move slowly through the gantry, the patient using breathing instructions if required. This image may appear as an AP (anteroposterior) view or a lateral view. Its purpose is to allow the operator to determine the start and end position on the patient's body of the required scan area (e.g. start – apices of the lungs; finish – bottom of the liver). The positioning device is either displayed as a transparent block for the slices or a block with a series of lines indicating the slices.

Slice thickness

This is determined by the scan protocol, which you select from a menu within the scanner. The menu is often separated into body parts with subsections for specific scans, such as 'lung cancer protocol' or staging scans.

Scan

With the modern multi-slice scanners available today a typical scan will take on average 25–30 seconds with breath-holds usually lasting no longer than 30 seconds. Whilst the scanner is performing the scan, the scan table will move through the gantry and the reconstructed images will appear on the monitor. This process occurs extremely quickly. It is advisable to watch the patient during the scan, especially if intravenous contrast is being administered via a pump injector, to ensure that the contrast appears to be flowing correctly and that the patient does not have an immediate reaction to the contrast. If post-scan reconstructions are required these can be performed once the patient has left the scan room or while you are removing the patient from the table. At this stage patient care is important; therefore, if it is required that scans are checked by a radiologist before the patient leaves, ensure you make the patient comfortable by lowering the patient's arms to a natural position and giving information on what is happening. If the patient has had a scan with intravenous contrast and is leaving the department to go home, ensure you correctly remove any cannula in the patient's arm by applying pressure to the area and then dispose of the sharp into a sharps bin.

POST-SCAN CARE

- The CTDI (CT Dose Index) must be recorded in the scanner logbook or saved onto the PACS record.
- Ensure that diabetic patients are fit to travel home alone and that they have brought something with them to eat.

PROTOCOLS

At the core of every CT department are the scanning protocols. These are agreed with the consultant radiologist, lead radiographer and the radiation safety advisor. These protocols must conform to the IR(ME)R regulations and they are designed to give maximum diagnostic information with the least radiation possible. Protocols will vary from one department to another and within departments from one machine to another.

References

1. Brunett CJ, et al. CT design considerations and specifications. Picker International; 1990.

Recommended reading

Seeram E. Computed tomography: physical principles, clinical applications, and quality control, 2nd edn. London: WB Saunders; 2001.

This text provides discussion of all aspects of CT physics to include multislice applications.

Jackson S, Thomas R. Cross-sectional imaging made easy. Oxford: Churchill Livingstone; 2004.

This is a clear text providing information on all aspects of cross-sectional imaging to include CT. This text also covers common CT diagnoses.

Chapter **19**

Magnetic resonance imaging

Juliet C. Semple

KEY POINTS

- MRI works because of the Larmor equation which states that $\omega = \gamma \times B_0$, where ω is the precessional frequency of a proton, γ is the gyromagnetic ratio and B_0 is the strength of the magnetic field.
- The three main types of MRI magnet are superconducting, resistive and permanent.
- A radiofrequency (RF) coil picks up the MRI signal generated.
- The two main types of MRI pulse sequence are spin echoes and gradient echoes
- The main sorts of image weighting are called T1, T2 and proton density.
- The quality of the MRI images produced depends a lot on the signal-to-noise ratio and spatial resolution.
- MRI images are prone to many different types of artefact.
- The contrast agent used in MRI is called gadolinium.
- Safety is paramount in an MRI unit.
- MRI is continually developing and there are many new advanced techniques.

INTRODUCTION

An MRI (magnetic resonance imaging) scanner is found in most hospitals today. It is an extremely valuable investigative tool and is an essential piece of equipment in a modern radiology department. The MRI scanner can produce high quality diagnostic images of almost any part of the human body.

In June 1970 a medical doctor called Raymond Damadian used the technique of nuclear magnetic resonance (now called MRI) to differentiate healthy from cancerous tissue in mice. In March 1973, Paul Lauterbur, a professor of Chemistry at the State University of New York at Stony Brook published a paper in Nature showing that by using magnetic resonance (MR) it was possible to build up two dimensional pictures of structures that could not be visualised with other methods. Professor Sir Peter Mansfield from the department of physics at Nottingham University showed how MR signals could be mathematically analysed, which made it possible to develop a useful imaging technique. In the late 1970s and early 1980s a number of groups in the USA and UK, together with manufacturers, showed promising results of MRI in vivo. The first commercial MR scanner in Europe (from Picker Ltd.) was installed in 1983 in Manchester.

TYPES OF MAGNET

There are many types of MRI magnet and a multitude of manufacturers who make them.

> T (or tesla) is the SI unit of magnetic flux density or magnetic induction.

This unit is used to describe the magnetic field strength of the MRI scanner. Another term you may hear is gauss. There are 10 000 gauss in 1 tesla. To give you an idea of how strong the magnetic field is in an MRI scanner, the Earth's magnetic field is 0.5 gauss, whereas an MRI scanner in a hospital is commonly 15 000 gauss.

There are two types of magnet used in an MRI scanner: electromagnets and permanent magnets.

Electromagnets can be either superconducting or resistive.

SUPERCONDUCTING MAGNETS

Superconducting magnets are the most frequently used type in hospitals. This type of magnet has a field strength of 0.5 T or upwards (1.5 T MRI scanners are normally used in a modern MRI department although 3 T scanners are becoming more common). These superconducting magnets need liquid helium to cool them. The magnetic field is always present with these scanners (24 hours a day, 7 days a week, and 365 days a year); in other words, it is present when the scanner is not scanning. The only way to stop the magnetic field is to remove the liquid helium from the system. In an emergency situation this can be done by 'quenching' the magnet – at the press of a button the helium is released from the system through a venting pipe to the outside world, resulting in a loss of the magnetic field.

RESISTIVE MAGNETS

Resistive magnets are electrically powered and therefore can be turned off. They have a field strength of up to 0.6 T.

PERMANENT MAGNETS

Permanent magnets have a field strength up to 0.3 T and also have a permanent magnetic field.

MRI SCANNING UNIT

The MRI scanning unit may well be a separate unit to the radiology department. It will consist of the MRI scanning room which houses the MRI scanner, the MRI control room where the console that controls the scanner is located and the MRI plant room which contains the electronics and equipment that make the scanner work. The entire unit will be behind locked doors as safety is paramount in an MRI environment.

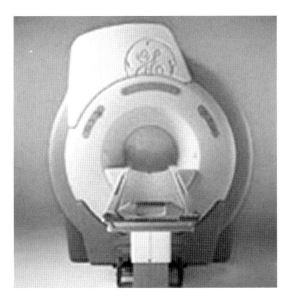

Figure 19.1 A closed MRI system. With permission of GE Healthcare.

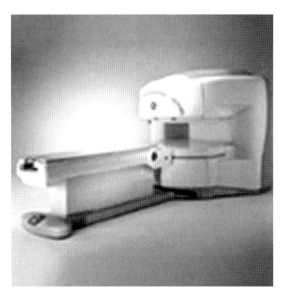

Figure 19.2 An open MRI system. With permission of GE Healthcare.

TYPES OF SCANNER

Scanners can be closed or open. Closed systems are the most commonly used (Fig. 19.1). These scanners are tube shaped and, although called a closed system, have an opening at each end. This tube is called the bore. On a modern 1.5 T system the bore is likely to have a diameter in the region of 50–60 cm.

Open systems are not tube shaped and tend to be more open, as the name implies (Fig. 19.2). They use two doughnut shaped magnets that are placed above and below the patient.

THE PHYSICS BIT

If a piece of card is placed over a bar magnet and then sprinkled with some iron filings, the filings line up with the magnetic field lines running from the north pole of the magnet to the south pole of the magnet (Fig. 19.3). The MRI scanner is just the same (however, the magnet is a lot stronger). The magnetic field lines run down the centre of the bore and extend around the sides of the

scanner in the same pattern as the iron filings described above (Fig. 19.4).

When the patient is placed into the scanner the magnetic field aligns all the hydrogen protons in his body in the same direction as the main magnetic field and they precess like a spinning top. The human body is made up of approximately 72% water, and as water is H_2O there are a lot of hydrogen protons in the body. This is what makes MRI such a good diagnostic tool.

A radiofrequency or an additional magnetic field/gradient is applied to flip these protons from the longitudinal plane to the transverse plane. Then the protons are allowed to relax back

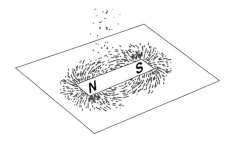

Figure 19.3 Magnetic field with iron filings.

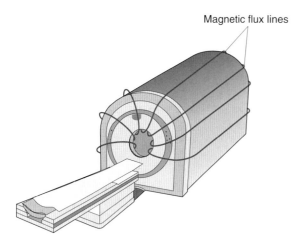

Figure 19.4 Scanner flux lines.

to the longitudinal plane. When they relax back they emit a small radio signal. This signal is picked up in an antenna or coil. Different tissues emit different intensities of signal and, with some clever computational analysis, we can differentiate these different intensities and their position and therefore produce a picture. This follows the Larmor equation.

The Larmor equation states that

$$\omega = \gamma \times B_0$$

where

ω is the precessional frequency of a proton
γ is the gyromagnetic ratio
B_0 is the strength of the magnetic field.

The frequency is measured in MHz (megahertz). The gyromagnetic ratio is a constant for each proton and the strength of the magnetic field is measured in tesla. So if the gyromagnetic ratio of hydrogen is 42.56 MHz, and if we were using a 1.5 T scanner, we could work out the precessional frequency of hydrogen as follows:

$$\omega = \gamma \times B_0$$
$$\omega = 42.56 \times 1.5$$
$$\omega = 63.84 \text{ MHz}$$

THE COILS

As mentioned previously, when the protons relax back they emit a signal that we pick up in a coil. These coils are called radiofrequency coils. The biggest coil of all is the MRI scanner itself. The scanner is made up of thousands of niobium–titanium coils wrapped around the bore. These coils produce the main magnetic field.

It is possible to do an MRI scan using the main magnetic field/coil but in practice smaller coils are used that plug into the scanner. There are coils for most body parts; a brain/head coil, a spine coil, a flex coil (for wrapping around small body areas), a torso coil, and a knee coil. There are also many specialised coils, like breast coils, neurovascular coils, TMJ (temporomandibular joint) coils and shoulder coils. If the MRI scanner is based in a specialist hospital, the coils will be specialised for the scanner's workload; moreover, each coil differs functionally:

- Receive only coils – these use the main magnetic field to excite the protons and then the receive coil, as its name suggests, receives the signal.
- Transmit/receive coils – these transmit a radiofrequency (RF) pulse and then receive the signal back.
- Phased array coils – these have an array of elements that can pick up the signal. MRI radiographers can select which elements they wish to use to get the best pictures possible. It also means that the entire spine can be scanned without putting the patient on a separate coil.

MRI PULSE SEQUENCES

In MRI scanning there are different types of pulse sequence. The two main types are:

- spin echo sequences
- gradient echo sequences.

There are then many types of sequence within the two main types. Some of the more common spin echo sequences are fast/turbo spin echo (FSE/TSE), fluid attenuated inversion recovery (FLAIR) and short TI inversion recovery (STIR). Gradient echo sequences include steady state free precession (SSFP), spoiled gradient echo and coherent gradient echo. All of these pulse sequences take minutes to achieve. In MRI there is also a very fast sequence (a matter of seconds) called echo planer imaging or EPI. EPI scans can be spin echo or gradient echo sequences.

During a scan the hydrogen protons are flipped over and allowed to relax back. The resulting signal from this relaxation is picked up in the coil and generates a picture. The way these protons flip over varies from sequence to sequence. A variety of different radiofrequency (RF) pulses and magnetic gradients are applied at various points in time and at different angles to create the pulse sequence. The basic principles of each sequence will be discussed below.

SPIN ECHO (SE) SEQUENCE

A 180 ° pulse follows a 90 ° pulse and then the signal is generated (Fig. 19.5).

FAST SPIN ECHO (FSE/TSE) SEQUENCE

A 90 ° pulse is followed by a series of pulses (normally a 180 ° pulse), with a signal being generated after each 180 ° pulse (Fig. 19.6). The number of 180 ° pulses is called the 'echo train length' (ETL).

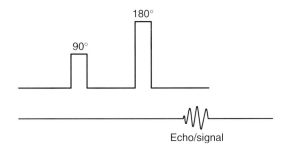

Figure 19.5 Spin echo.

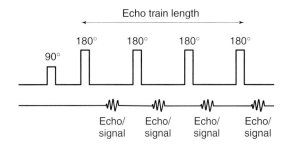

Figure 19.6 Fast spin echo.

FLUID ATTENUATED INVERSION RECOVERY (FLAIR) AND SHORT TI INVERSION RECOVERY (STIR) SEQUENCES

A 180 ° inverting pulse is applied before the 90 ° pulse (Fig. 19.7).

GRADIENT ECHO (GE) SEQUENCE

Gradient echo scans are very different to a spin echo sequence. A smaller RF pulse produces a small flip angle of less than 90 ° and, instead of another RF pulse, a magnetic gradient is then applied (Fig. 19.8).

PULSE SEQUENCE FACTORS

- TE (or echo time) is the time from the 90 ° pulse to the peak signal being generated in the coil. It is measured in milliseconds (ms).

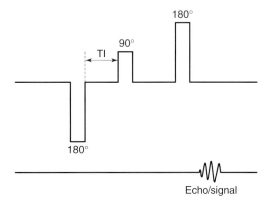

Figure 19.7 Inversion recovery.

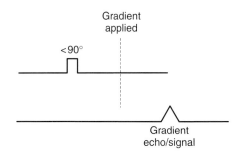

Figure 19.8 Gradient echo.

- TR (or repetition time) is the time from the application of one RF pulse to the application of the next RF pulse. It is also measured in ms.
- TI (or inversion time) is the time between the 90 ° inversion pulse to the 90 ° pulse and is measured in ms.
- Flip angle is a small RF pulse.

These times are input into the scanner to create the pulse sequence. By changing the times for these factors we can produce images with different 'weightings'. Weighting of an image determines the signal intensity of different tissues.

IMAGE WEIGHTING

The main image weightings you will use in MRI are T1, T2 and proton density (PD). Spin echo and gradient echo sequences can be T1, T2 or PD.

T1 WEIGHTED SPIN ECHO OVERVIEW

T1 weighted scans use a short TE and a short TR. Short TE is defined as less than 35 ms and a short TR as less than 800 ms. These figures vary between scanners and field strengths but the figures quoted are a good rule of thumb.
    A T1 SE sequence, for example, could be achieved with a TE of 15 ms and a TR of 600 ms.

T2 WEIGHTED SPIN ECHO OVERVIEW

T2 weighted scans use a long TE and a long TR. A long TE is defined as more than 80 ms and a long TR as over 2000 ms.

So a T2 SE sequence, for example, could be achieved with a TE of 102 ms and a TR of 3000 ms.

PD WEIGHTED SPIN ECHO OVERVIEW

PD weighted scans use a short TE and a long TR. So an example of these parameters would be a TE of 20 ms and a TR of 3000 ms.

T1 WEIGHTED GRADIENT ECHO OVERVIEW

In the T1 GE sequence, flip angles are used as well as setting the TE and TR. To obtain a T1 weighted GE scan, a large flip angle in the order of 70–110 ° is used, plus a short TE of 5–10 ms and a short TR of less than 750 ms.

T2 WEIGHTED GRADIENT ECHO OVERVIEW

When discussing a T2 weighted GE scan it is referred to as T2* not T2. A T2* GE scan uses a small flip angle of 5–20 °, a long TE of 15–25 ms and a long TR of more than 100 ms.

PD WEIGHTED GRADIENT ECHO OVERVIEW

To obtain a PD weighted GE scan, a small flip angle in the order of 5–20 ° is used, plus a short TE of 5–10 ms and a long TR of more than 100 ms.

INTERPRETING IMAGES

Different tissues relax back at different speeds (fat for example is a lot quicker than water) so, depending on when in time the echo/signal is observed, different densities will appear on an image for the different tissues.

For example, on a T1 SE weighted scan, fat looks bright white and water dark black – so the fat in the scalp is seen as a bright area and the ventricles of the brain, which contain cerebrospinal fluid (CSF), look dark because CSF is a fluid like water (Fig. 19.9). On the T2 FSE weighted scan the opposite is seen – the fat is now darker and the fluid bright (Fig. 19.10). A PD scan looks at just the density of hydrogen protons and produces a very grey image that effectively is a proton density map (Fig. 19.11).

By knowing what different tissues are made up of and how they look on different image weightings a diagnosis can be made. For example, a scan of a patient's brain may demonstrate a lump or possibly a tumour, but how does the radiologist know what the lump is? Well, what does it look like on T1 and T2?

The pathology shown in Figure 19.12 looks bright on T2 and dark on T1 so implies the lesion is made primarily of fluid. This is the case and the radiologist can suggest an arachnoid cyst as the likely diagnosis. So the radiologist can make accurate diagnoses knowing how different

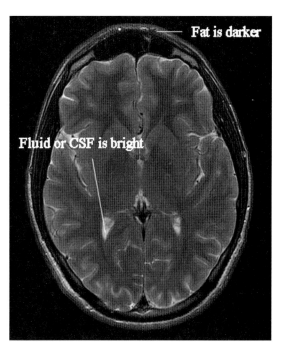

Figure 19.10 T2 brain.

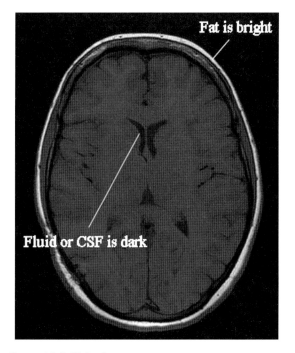

Figure 19.9 T1 brain.

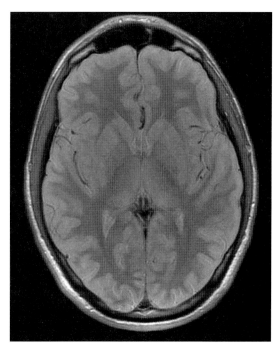

Figure 19.11 PD brain.

A

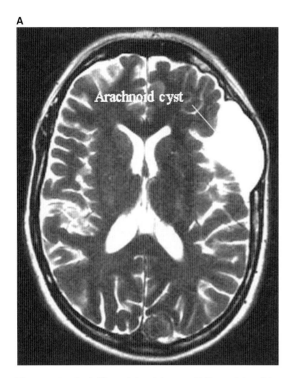

B

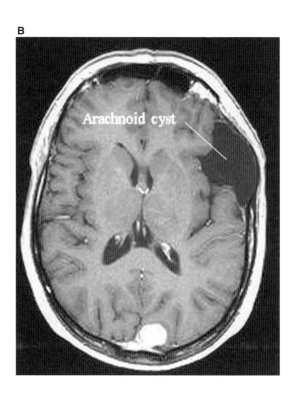

Figure 19.12 A T2 weighted image. B T1 weighted image.

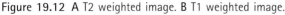

tissues and pathologies look on different image weightings.

SIGNAL-TO-NOISE RATIO

Signal-to-noise ratio (SNR) is the ratio of the amplitude of the signal received to the average amplitude of the noise. SNR is affected by the scanner hardware, the field strength of the scanner, the pulse sequences employed, the choice of radiofrequency coil and the parameters set by the operator. Good image quality is determined by good parameter selection, utilisation of the most appropriate coil and utilising the scanner capabilities. MRI scanning is one big parameter juggling and trade-off exercise. Parameters can be set that would produce a scan of exceptional quality but would take 20 minutes to run, by which time the patient would probably have moved. Parameters can also be set that ask too much of the system and create poor or, even worse, undiagnostic images.

FACTORS AFFECTING THE SNR

- Field of view (FOV) – the larger the FOV, the more signal generated, so increasing the SNR (Fig. 19.13).
- Matrix size – scans can be performed with varying matrix sizes. The matrix is the frequency encoding multiplied by the phase encoding. Examples could be 256×256 or 512×512. The 512×512 matrix will have fewer protons in each voxel (the 3D equivalent of a pixel) than the 256×256 matrix scan so therefore has less SNR (Fig. 19.14).
- Slice width – the smaller or thinner the slice, the smaller the signal generated, thereby reducing the SNR (Fig. 19.15).
- NEX – NEX means number of excitations (how many times the protons are excited in a slice). The more times the protons are excited the better the SNR (Fig. 19.16).

A

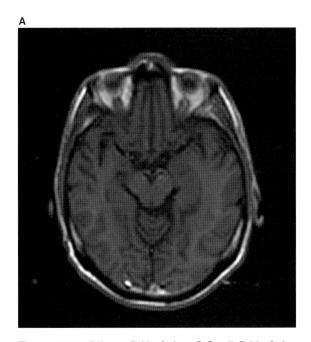

Figure 19.13 A Large field of view. B Small field of view.

A

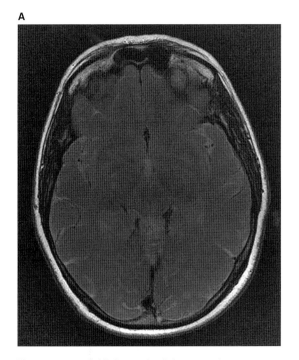

B

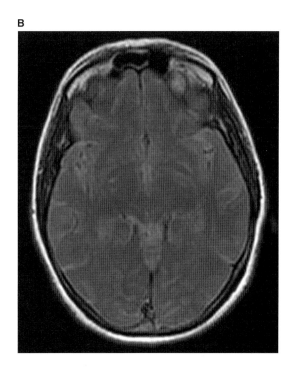

Figure 19.14 A High matrix. B Low matrix.

A
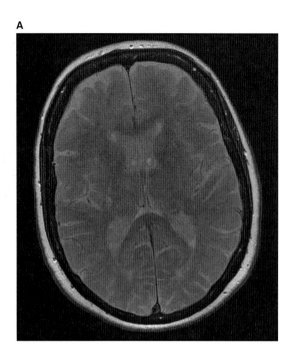

B
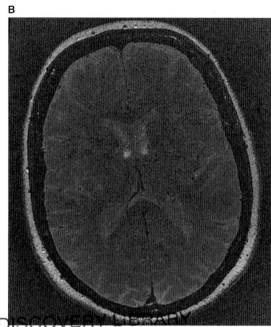

Figure 19.15 A Thick slice width. B Thin slice width.

A
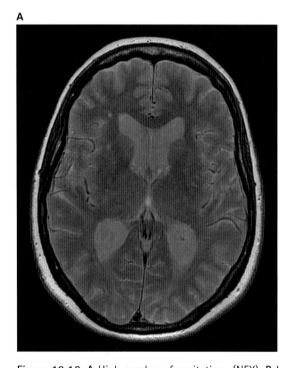

B
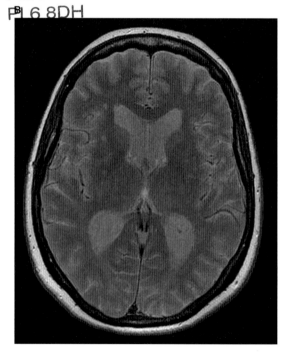

Figure 19.16 A High number of excitations (NEX). B Low NEX.

A

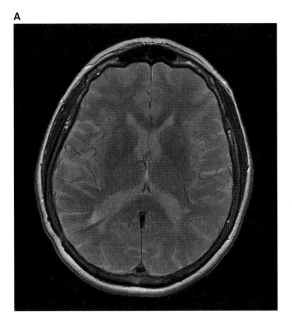

B

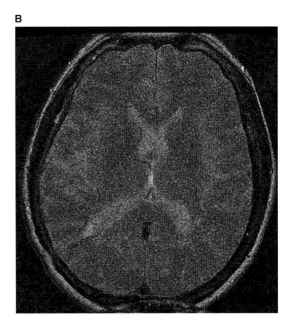

Figure **19.17 A** 8-channel brain coil. **B** Body coil (the main magnetic field).

- Coil choice – the most suitable coil for the body part under examination needs to be selected (Fig. 19.17). Ideally, it needs to be as close to the area of interest as possible and cover the area under examination. Most modern MRI scanners now use multichannel coils, which increase the SNR.
- Sequence parameters – TR, TE and flip angle affect SNR. Spin echo sequences tend to have a better SNR than gradient echo sequences. Increasing the TR increases the SNR. Decreasing the TE increases the SNR.
- Bandwidth – the receive bandwidth is the range of frequencies sampled by the readout gradient (Fig. 19.18). As bandwidth increases, SNR decreases.

SPATIAL RESOLUTION

Spatial resolution is the ability to differentiate between two points as separate and distinct in the image. Good spatial resolution is needed to produce good quality images. Thin slices, high matrices and small FOVs are required in order to achieve good spatial resolution.

ARTEFACTS

As with most imaging modalities MRI is not exempt from the problem of artefacts, and probably has more to contend with than other modalities.

PHASE WRAP

Phase wrap is when an area of anatomy outside of the field of view is mapped (or wraps) inside the image. This occurs along the phase encoding direction. Changing the phase encoding direction or using the 'no phase wrap' option on the

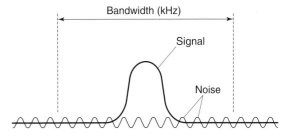

Figure **19.18** Bandwidth.

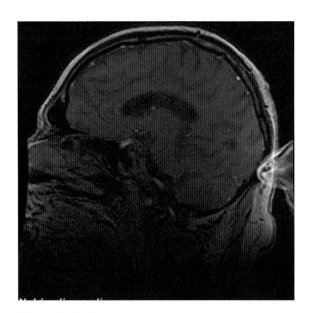

Figure 19.19 Phase wrap.

scanner can remedy this. In Figure 19.19 the nose is wrapped around the image and is now on the back of the head, not the front.

PHASE MISMAPPING

Phase mismapping is when an area of anatomy moves along a gradient during the scan. Examples would be eyes moving during a brain scan, swallowing during a neck scan and the chest wall moving during a scan of the thorax. The artefact produced is called ghosting and always occurs along the phase encoding direction. Selecting the correct axis for the phase encoding can, however, reduce it.

Another remedy is to use a saturation band to nullify the signal from the moving anatomy. For example, when imaging the lumbar spine an artefact can occur across the spinal cord from the moving contents of the abdomen. If a presaturation pulse/band is placed in front of the spinal column covering the abdominal contents, the artefact on the image is reduced (Fig. 19.20).

CHEMICAL SHIFT ARTEFACT

Chemical shift artefact is caused by the different precessional frequencies of fat and water. Precessional frequency is proportional to the strength of the main magnetic field. At low field strengths the difference between the precessional frequencies is not great, but at high field strengths the difference is enough to cause chemical shift artefact. An example is shown in Figure 19.21.

To reduce this artefact the biggest receive bandwidth should be used in conjunction with the smallest field of view possible.

CROSS–TALK

Cross-talk, or cross-excitation, occurs when the RF excitation pulse in an adjacent slice excites protons in the slice being scanned. To reduce the effects of this artefact it is best to keep a gap between slices of about 10% and try not to cross slices. An example of cross-talk is shown in Figure 19.22; the dark band across the image is where the cross-excitation has occurred.

MAGNETIC SUSCEPTIBILITY ARTEFACT

Magnetic susceptibility artefact is caused by the ability of a substance to become magnetised. The degree to which it becomes magnetised results in a difference in phase and precessional frequency and there is signal loss or void on the image. This primarily happens with metal. A patient who has a metal implant in the area being scanned will have images with magnetic susceptibility artefact. If at all possible the metal should be removed, but in the case of a metal prosthesis fixed within the body the only option is to choose pulse sequences that are less susceptible to this type of artefact. In general, SE sequences are less susceptible than GE sequences. An example of signal void or magnetic susceptibility is shown in Figure 19.23; there are black signal voids where this patient's hips should be due to his bilateral hip replacements causing magnetic susceptibility artefact.

A

B

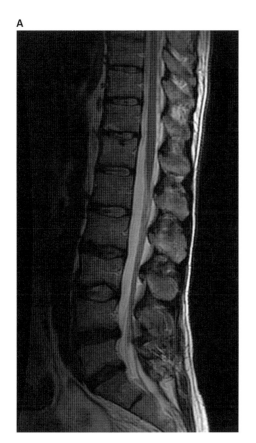

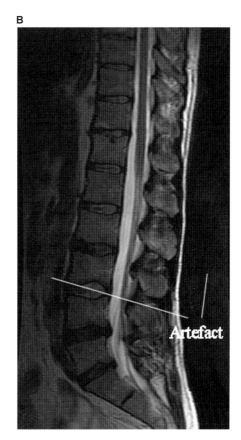

Figure 19.20 **A** With saturation band. **B** Without saturation band.

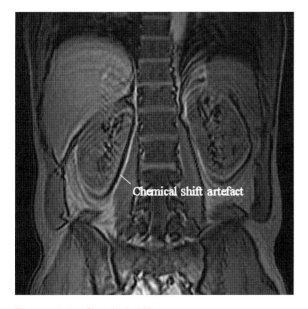

Figure 19.21 Chemical shift.

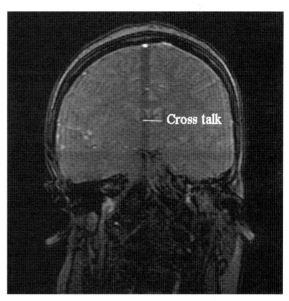

Figure 19.22 Cross-talk.

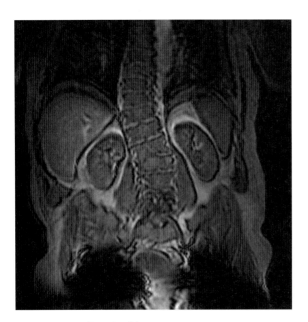

Figure 19.23 Signal void.

ZIPPER ARTEFACT

Zipper artefact is caused by extraneous RF entering the scan room. It results in a line across the image that looks like a zip, hence the name. It is caused by a gap in the RF cage that shields the MRI scan room. As long as the RF cage is intact this artefact should not be seen.

MRI CONTRAST AGENTS

In common with most imaging modalities, extra information can be gained by the administration of a contrast agent. In MRI a contrast media called gadolinium is used. Gadolinium is one of the 'rare earth' metals known as lanthanoids. The gadolinium is bound to a chelate called DTPA and Gd-DTPA or gadopentetate is formed. This is a water-soluble contrast agent that is commonly used in MRI. It is relatively safe to use, with a low anaphylactic risk and few other side effects, but as with all contrast media the radiographer should be aware of potential adverse affects and have the appropriate training to deal with these if they were to occur.

The administration of gadolinium affects the T1 recovery of tissue and shortens its T1 recovery time. On T1 weighted scans areas of contrast enhancement will appear bright white on the image. Contrast agents are taken up by tissues with an enriched blood supply (e.g. tumours and sites of infection). Some pathology has very characteristic patterns of contrast enhancement; for example, brain abscesses ring enhance and meningiomas tend to have uniform enhancement. The administration of contrast can therefore aid the radiologist with making a diagnosis. Because some tissues appear bright on a T1 weighted scan without the administration of gadolinium (e.g. fat) a T1 weighted scan is performed pre and post the administration of the contrast. The pre contrast image can then be compared to the post contrast image to see which tissues are really enhancing (Fig. 19.24).

MRI SAFETY

The most important issue when undertaking MRI scanning is MRI safety. This point cannot be emphasised enough. To reiterate, the magnetic field is present 24 hours a day, 7 days a week, 365 days a year, even when the scanner is not performing a scan and is silent. All personnel and patients entering the MRI scan area should complete an MRI safety questionnaire. Every MRI unit will have their own safety form but it will cover the same main safety issues (Fig. 19.25). Most MRI safety issues relate to the main magnetic field and the time varying magnetic field (the switching of gradients and RF pulses during scanning).

PROJECTILE EFFECT

On a modern 1.5 T MRI system the strength of the magnet will accelerate a ferromagnetic object to 40 mph. Just think of the damage even a 1 p coin could make if it hit an individual at 40 mph; the result of an oxygen cylinder hitting at 40 mph would probably be fatal. This is called the projectile or missile effect.

METAL OBJECT REMOVAL

All metal objects need to be removed from everybody (including radiographers, patients and

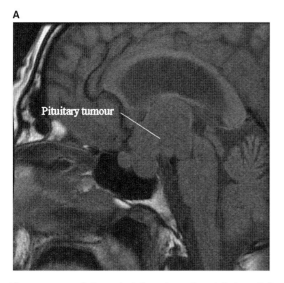
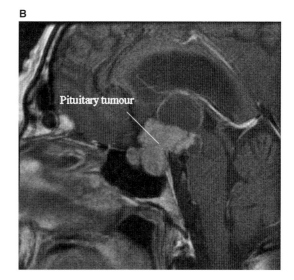

Figure 19.24 **A** Pre-administration of gadolinium. **B** Post-administration of gadolinium.

Figure 19.25 MRI safety form.

MAGNETIC RESONANCE IMAGING (MRI) SAFETY QUESTIONNAIRE

YOUR NAME _____ Date Of Birth-____/____/_____

	Please answer all the questions very carefully. They are designed to identify items which may either interfere with the scan or are potentially hazardous in a strong magnetic field. If you have any questions please ask.	Yes	No
1	Have you had an MRI scan before?		
2	Do you have or have you ever had a cardiac pacemaker?(**If yes please contact MRI Dept**)		
3	*Have you ever had any surgery to your* (a) heart or chest?		
	(b) head or brain? e.g. aneurysm clips or programmable hydrocephalus shunt.		
	(c) eyes?		
	(d) ears?		
4	Do you have any metal plates, screws or joint replacements?		
5	Do you have any electronic, mechanical or metal implants in any part of your body?		
6	Have you had any surgery in the last 8 weeks? (**If yes please contact MRI Dept**)		
7	Have you **ever** had any incidents to your face or eyes where metal splinters have entered at high speed (e.g. while drilling or grinding)? Please tick **Yes** even if these have been removed at an eye hospital. (**If yes please contact MRI Dept**)		
8	Have you had any incidents where bullets, shrapnel or other pieces of metal have entered your body?		
9	Do you suffer from diabetes, blackouts or epilepsy?		
10	*Do you have any of the following?* (a) Removable dentures containing metal.		
	(b) A hearing aid		
	(c) Body piercing		
	(d) Jewellery		
	(e) An artificial limb, calliper or corset.		
	(f) A transdermal patch?		
	(g) Permanent cosmetics (e.g. eyeliner)		
	(h) Tattoos		
11	*For females of child bearing age* a) Are you pregnant?		
	b) Are you breast feeding?		

Before your scan you must remove all metal objects you are wearing or have in your pockets.
e.g: jewellery   watches   keys   credit cards
body piercing,   hair clips   hearing aids   coins

I confirm that I have been asked the above questions and the information is correct to the best of my knowledge.

Signature of Patient   _____   Weight_____

Signature of Radiographer   _____   Date_____

doctors) before entering the MRI scan room. This includes coins, keys, scissors, stethoscopes, hair clips, cigarette lighters, etc. The list is endless, so the safest thing is to remove everything; some units even require all patients to wear only a hospital gown to stop anything metal being accidentally overlooked. Other objects like bankcards or mobile phones need to be removed because although they might not be attracted to the magnet the magnetic strip on the cards will be wiped and the components of the phone ruined.

IMPLANTS

Implants that should not be exposed to a high magnetic field

- Pacemaker
- Cochlear implant
- Aneurysm clip
- Some heart valves
- Neurostimulators

Anyone (patient or staff) who has any of the preceding implants should never enter the MRI scan room. Death could result due to the failure of the implant.

INTRAOCCULAR FOREIGN BODIES

It is also necessary before entering the scan room to check for intraoccular foreign bodies, usually caused from high speed welding, grinding or metalwork. Even a small amount of metal in the eye can be pulled by the magnetic field and result in damage to the eye or, even worse, blindness. Patients who need to undergo an MRI and have a previous history of metal going into their eye can be screened with an orbital X-ray; if the X-ray is clear then an MRI scan can be performed. It is also necessary to check for shrapnel or bullets. These are not always a contraindication

for MRI but the extent and site of the injury need to be fully assessed before entering the scan room.

OTHER IMPLANTS

Most MRI centres will also check for other metal implants/prostheses. Anything that can be removed should be, even if it is not magnetic. Metal can heat up sufficiently during an MRI scan (because of the current induced in it) to cause burns. Jewellery should be removed before undertaking a scan. Also, if the metal is in the area of interest it will cause signal void/magnetic susceptibility artefact on the images. It is safe to have a scan with most orthopaedic implants (e.g. a hip replacement) but most MRI centres tend to wait 8 weeks after surgery before scanning.

PREGNANCY AND BREASTFEEDING

MRI does not use ionising radiation and essentially there are no biological affects. Routinely, most centres will not scan patients in the first trimester of pregnancy; however, if the gain outweighs the very low risks a scan will be performed. The pregnant patient should make her own decision. Most centres would not administer gadolinium to the pregnant patient. It is worth noting that gadolinium passes across the breast into breast milk, so if a patient who is breast-feeding requires a scan they need to express breast milk prior to the examination and refrain from breast-feeding for at least 24 hours.

IMPLANT SAFETY SHEETS

The main advice if there is uncertainty as to whether someone or something is safe to go into an MRI scan room is DON'T go into the scanner without seeking further advice. Most manufacturers of implants produce safety sheets that state their suitability for MRI scanning. The ultimate responsibility regarding who and what goes into the MRI scan room rests with the MRI radiographer.

NOISE

Having an MRI scan is a very noisy procedure. The magnetic field itself is silent, and when the scanner is not scanning a soft 'chirping' sound in the scan room is heard, which is the compressor pumping the liquid helium around the scanner. However, when the scanner is performing a scan the noise is literally deafening. The noise is the magnetic gradients switching very quickly. All patients and personnel who remain in the scan room have to wear ear protection. Earplugs are perfectly adequate for the job but most modern scanners have a stereo system attached to some MRI compatible headphones so the patient can listen to music whilst also protecting their ears.

SPECIFIC ABSORPTION RATE

RF can heat tissues within the patient. There are limits to the heating of tissues. The specific absorption rate (SAR) is measured in watts kg^{-1} and is how much heat the tissue can dissipate. Levels are set to protect the patient, and most modern scanners will not let these levels be exceeded. However, the scanner can only work this out by the patient's weight so it is important that an accurate weight is recorded when registering patient details into the scanner.

INDUCING CURRENT IN LOOPS

Any looped wire or lead in a moving/switching magnetic field can have current induced in it. This current is enough to make the wire or lead heat up and burn the patient. It is important that leads or wires (e.g. MRI compatible ECG leads) do not touch the patients' skin directly and are not coiled up. A small piece of gauze or a foam pad can be placed between the lead and the skin to avoid contact.

OTHER SAFETY CONSIDERATIONS

MRI compatible trolleys and wheelchairs that are not magnetic and are suitable for use in the scan room can be purchased. Also, most modern scanners have either undockable tables or tabletops that allow you to transfer the patient from a non-compatible bed or chair onto the scanner table outside the scan room and then move them into the scan room. A sick patient may need to be monitored or have drugs administered during the scan. Remember, equipment cannot go into the scan room unless it is MRI compatible. Various companies make compatible anaesthetic and monitoring equipment but it is very expensive. Some units prefer to use conventional equipment outside the scan room with extra long leads and connections. General anaesthetic scans are possible in the MRI scanner but are not to be undertaken lightly. Experienced personnel, the correct equipment and strict policies should be in place to ensure patient safety at all times. MRI scanners can be very isolated departments and the patient is remote to the radiographers and doctors.

The MRI scan unit should be locked and only trained personnel given either the key or code to the door. Anyone else entering the unit should be screened fully before being allowed to enter and should be supervised at all times.

QUENCHING OF THE MAGNET

If the worst happens and a metal object does enter the scan room, is stuck to the magnet and cannot be pulled off, the only way to extricate it is to remove the main magnetic field. To do this the magnet has to be quenched. There is a button in every MRI scanner to quench it. It is usually underneath a protective cover so that it does not get pressed by accident. When the quench button is pressed it very quickly releases all the helium in the scanner. It should be vented through a pipe from the scanner to the outside world. The magnetic field will then collapse so the object can be removed from the scanner. The release of the helium can also cause problems; for example, if there is a blockage in the pipe, the helium will enter the scan room, suffocating anyone inside – all MRI units should be fitted with an oxygen sensor that will set off an alarm if such an event happens. On hearing the alarm all personnel should be evacuated from the scan room. Quenching is something that should only be done in an emergency or life-threatening situation because the magnet can be damaged due to the heat generated in the coils and the cost of replacing tens of thousands of litres of liquid helium is expensive.

QUALITY ASSURANCE

MRI scanners, like all pieces of radiology equipment, need to have Quality Assurance or QA tests performed on them regularly. Different units will perform different tests specific to their unit but the most common test is an SNR test. This can be performed on a phantom, which is a plastic ball filled with fluid. Ideally this test should be done weekly on each coil the unit possesses.

ADVANCED TECHNIQUES

There are many advanced techniques that can be performed on an MRI scanner. A few of these are

- diffusion
- perfusion
- angiography (contrast enhanced and non-contrast enhanced)
- functional MRI (or fMRI)
- spectroscopy.

ADVANTAGES AND DISADVANTAGES OF MRI

ADVANTAGES

- Excellent soft tissue detail.
- Does not use ionising radiation.
- Multiplaner (can scan in all planes without moving the patient).

DISADVANTAGES

- Long scan times.
- Expensive.
- Not safe/suitable for all patients.
- Claustrophobic for some patients.

Bibliography

Marieb EN. Human anatomy and physiology, 3rd edn. California: Benjamin/Cummings; 1995.
Moses KP et al. Atlas of clinical gross anatomy. Philadelphia: Elsevier Mosby; 2005.
Thibodeau GA, Patton KT. Anatomy and physiology, 5th edn. Missouri: Elsevier Mosby; 2003.
Van Wynsberghe D, Noback CR, Carola R. Human anatomy and physiology, 3rd edn. New York: McGraw-Hill; 1995.
Waugh A, Grant A. Ross and Wilson: Anatomy and physiology in health and illness, 9th edn. Edinburgh: Elsevier; 2002.

Recommended reading

Westbrook C, Kaut Roth C, Talbot J. MRI in practice, 3rd edn. Oxford: Blackwell Publishing; 2005.

This text provides a clear introduction to MRI. The text is well laid out with clear diagrams.

Westbrook C. MRI at a glance. Oxford: Blackwell Science; 2002.

This provides clear, concise information on MRI physics.

McRobbie DW, Moore E, Graves M, Prince M. MRI from picture to proton, 2nd edn. Cambridge: Cambridge University Press; 2007.

This text approaches the theory as it is encountered when working in an MRI department from the image initially through to the physics at the very end.

Waugh A, Grant A. Ross and Wilson: Anatomy and physiology in health and illness, 9th edn. Edinburgh: Elsevier; 2002.

This text is currently used by first-year students on our radiography programme, as the overall content provides just the right depth in detail, and it has a good reader-friendly structure with clear illustrations.

Chapter **20**

Anatomy and physiology

Aarthi Ramlaul

KEY POINTS

- The respiratory system functions as a series of air passages through which air enters the lungs and travels to the alveoli where gaseous exchange occurs.
- Respiration consists of active inspiration and passive expiration.
- The cardiovascular system is a closed network of blood vessels that carry oxygenated blood to all body tissues and transport deoxygenated blood away from body tissues to the lungs for excretion, with the exception of the pulmonary vessels.
- Blood is composed of a liquid plasma and formed elements consisting of red and white blood cells as well as platelets.
- Blood is the 'life' of body cells and tissues as it carries vital life-sustaining oxygen and nutrients.
- The skeletal system is made up of the axial and appendicular skeleton.
- This skeleton provides a supportive and protective framework for the body, which together with muscles gives the body its ability to carry out a wide range of movements.
- A joint is where two or more bones meet. Muscles acting across joints provide the mechanism by which movement takes place.
- The nervous system is the body's network of communication that receives, interprets and relays messages to and from the brain.

- The functional unit of the nervous system is the nerve cell or neuron.
- The spinal cord is a long tract of fibres that provides a 'road' through which impulses can travel.
- The alimentary tract extends from the mouth to the anus.
- Food taken into the mouth is swallowed (ingested); digested by mechanical movements and chemical enzymes; its nutrients are absorbed and the left over waste eliminated.
- The liver, gall bladder and pancreas are accessory organs of digestion.
- The nephron forms the functional unit of the kidney to filter waste material from the blood and eliminate this as urine.
- The kidneys play an important role in regulating the electrolyte balance of the body.
- The kidneys produce rennin which helps to regulate blood pressure levels.
- The endocrine system plays a role in maintaining homeostasis by the action of chemical messengers called hormones.
- Hormone release is regulated by the hypothalamus via a feedback mechanism of communication.

INTRODUCTION

This chapter provides an overview of the aspects of anatomy and physiology that are relevant to radiographic practice. Developmental anatomy has been excluded from this chapter. Anatomy described has been based on the normal average adult male/female, and wherever possible and appropriate normal variations have been mentioned.

SKELETAL SYSTEM

The skeletal system is made up of bones and joints that work together with muscles and ligaments to provide a framework for the body (Fig. 20.1).

The skeleton is divided into two parts.

- Axial skeleton:
  - skull and facial bones
  - vertebrae
  - sternum and ribs.
- Appendicular skeleton:
  - upper limb including the shoulder girdle
  - lower limb including the pelvic girdle.

BONES

Bone is hardest of all connective tissue found in the human body and is formed by a process of ossification which takes place in two ways. The first is intramembranous ossification, where connective tissue is replaced by calcium phosphate, and this occurs in the skull. The second is intracartilaginous ossification, where hyaline cartilage is replaced by calcium phosphate, and this occurs almost throughout the skeleton.

Bone tissue comprises spongy/cancellous or compact bone. Microscopic structure of bone consists of Haversian systems arranged in concentric circles of lamellae (layers), which surround the Haversian canals. Each Haversian canal contains blood and lymphatic vessels and nerves. In compact bone, these Haversian systems and lamellae are packed closely together with very little space between them. In spongy bone there are fewer Haversian systems and the Haversian canals are larger with bigger gaps between the lamellae. These spaces help to reduce the weight of the bone. Bone marrow, consisting of both yellow and red marrow, fills the spaces created by the gaps.

Bone tissue is dependent on nutrients such as calcium, phosphorous and vitamins C and D for growth and repair. Exercise affects the growth and repair of bone and muscle by stimulating blood supply and circulation.

General structure and appearance

Bone has an outer covering called the periosteum, which is a tough outer membrane made up of fibrous tissue and containing blood vessels. The

Figure 20.1 The human skeleton – anterior view.

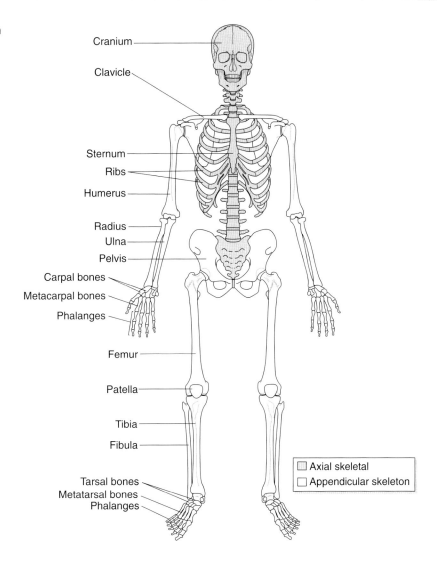

Cranium
Clavicle
Sternum
Ribs
Humerus
Radius
Ulna
Pelvis
Carpal bones
Metacarpal bones
Phalanges
Femur
Patella
Tibia
Fibula
Tarsal bones
Metatarsal bones
Phalanges

☐ Axial skeletal
☐ Appendicular skeleton

cortex is made up of compact tissue and lies directly below the periosteum. The inner layer of is made of spongy or cancellous bone, which is softer, compared to the tough outer cortex. Lastly, the innermost part of the bone is formed from 'fatty' yellow bone marrow, which contains a few white blood cells, and red marrow containing red blood cells.

Functions of bone

- Provide a framework of support and protection of the body's soft organs.
- Enable a range of movement, together with muscles, to provide stability and mobility.
- Provide storage for certain nutrients; e.g. calcium and phosphorous.
- Produce red blood cells (erythropoiesis). Bone marrow is an important site for this.

Bones are classified into the following types (Table 20.1):

- long
- short
- flat
- irregular
- sesamoid.

Table 20.1   Classification of bone

Shape	Description	Location in the body
Long bones	Length is greater than width	Upper limb (humerus, radius and ulna) Lower limb (femur, tibia and fibula)
Short bones	Equal in length, breadth and thickness	Wrist (carpal bones), ankle (tarsal bones)
Flat bones	Usually more curved and thin than flat; e.g. the curved bones of the skull protect the brain	Skull, chest (scapula, ribs, sternum), pelvis
Irregular bones	These do not have any of the above-mentioned shapes, hence 'irregular'	Axial skeleton, both shoulder and pelvic girdle and vertebrae
Sesamoid bones	Small bones that are found embedded in certain tendons connecting muscle to bone	Knee (the commonest sesamoid bone is the patella), but may also be seen on images of the hand, wrist and foot)

Plain film radiography is still the first line of investigation following injury or trauma to the bones and joints. If there appears to be ligamentous or tendon involvement then CT, MRI or ultrasound may be requested for further diagnoses, management and treatment. However, successful interpretation can usually be made by carefully evaluating the images in terms of bony and soft tissue appearances, e.g. tissue swelling, size of joint spaces, position of fat pad and cortical markings.

JOINTS

A joint forms at a point where two bones and cartilages meet or where adjacent bones and cartilages are joined. Although bone gives the body protective structure and muscles provide the ability to move, it is actually the joints that provide the mechanism by which movement takes place. Radiographic contrast can sometimes be injected into a joint space (e.g. in the glenoid cavity of the shoulder) to visualise any underlying pathology. This procedure is known as an arthrogram.

Classification

A joint can be classified according to the range of movement it provides or by its articular surface structure. All joints in the body can be classified as shown in Table 20.2; however, certain areas of the body may have a combination of two joints; for example the temporomandibular joint (TMJ) comprises gliding and pivot joints.

CARDIOVASCULAR SYSTEM

This system forms the transport network for the body.

Anatomical components of the cardiovascular system

- Heart.
- Blood vessels – the means of transport.
- Blood – the medium of transport. Blood forms part of the circulatory system as well as having a function in homeostasis. It also contributes to the cardiovascular system as a whole.
- Lymph and lymph vessels – an extension of the cardiovascular system.

Table 20.2   Classification of joints

Type of joint	Structure	Description of movement, with examples
Fibrous	• Do not have joint cavities • Mostly immovable although some have slight movement	• Sutures of skull – fibrous tissue is fused in adults and immovable, but has some movement in the fetus and in children • Bones held together by ligaments (e.g. radius/ulna and tibia/fibula) have a limited twisting movement • Roots of teeth in gums (where a 'peg fits into a socket') are mostly immovable but may have very slight movement
Cartilaginous	• Bones are joined by a hyaline cartilage • Mostly slightly movable • Some immovable	• Cartilage forms a disc-like cover over bone (e.g. symphysis pubis and intervertebral joints), giving slight movement • Some cartilage forms temporary joints (e.g. epiphyseal plates of long bones), which are immovable so that the bones can grow well
Synovial	Have lubricated articular cartilage between bones giving smooth, free movement in a range of directions	• Hinge joints – give movement of flexion and extension; e.g. elbow; knee; ankle and interphalangeal joints • Pivot joints – give movement of supination; pronation and rotation; e.g. atlantoaxial joint; proximal radioulnar joint and distal tibiofibular joint • Condyloid (ellipsoid) joints – are modified ball and socket joints that give movement of flexion; extension; abduction; adduction and circumduction; e.g. most metacarpophalangeal joints • Gliding joints – give movement of limited gliding action; e.g. acromioclavicular joint; articular processes of vertebrae and between some carpal and tarsal bones • Saddle joints – give movement of abduction, adduction, opposition and reposition; e.g. carpometacarpal joint of thumb (between the trapezium and first metacarpal) • Ball and socket joints – give movement of flexion; extension; internal, external and lateral rotation; abduction, adduction and circumduction; e.g. hip and shoulder joints

THE HEART

The heart is a muscle that acts as a pump and provides the energy and force to keep blood circulating throughout the body. Blood is circulated via a closed transport system; that is, oxygenated blood leaves the heart via arteries, passes through a tiny network of capillaries where transfer of oxygen and nutrients take place, and then deoxygenated blood returns to the heart via the veins.

Size, shape and location

The heart is conical in shape and, under normal circumstances, about the size of its owner's clenched fist. It is located anteriorly in the centre of the thorax, with about two-thirds of its bulk lying towards the left of the sternal margin. The tip of the 'cone' is called the apex and the flat portion is called the base. The base, normally found at the level of T5–T8, faces forwards and downwards to the left, ending in the apex. The apex lies at the level of the fifth intercostal space on the left midclavicular line (Fig. 20.2).

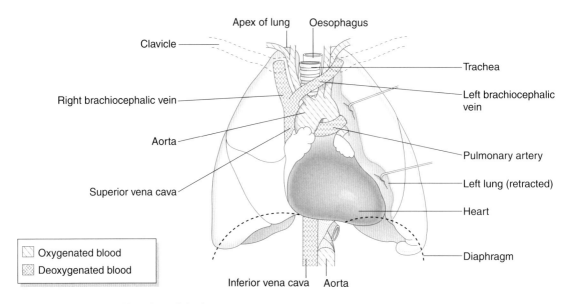

Figure 20.2 Position and location of the heart.

Occasionally patients may present with dextrocardia, a condition where the heart and great vessels originate with the same structure but opposite in direction (i.e. the apex lies towards the right side of the thorax rather than the left). This is a normal variant and is usually discovered as an incidental finding when the patient presents for a chest examination for an unrelated symptom.

Structure

The heart and the great vessels are surrounded and supported by a protective covering called the pericardium. The pericardium is a fibroserous sac that is attached to the sternum, diaphragm and great vessels by connective tissue.

The heart wall is made up of three layers of tissue (Fig. 20.3):

- pericardium
- myocardium
- endocardium.

The pericardium consists of two layers of tissue. The outer layer is a tough fibrous layer that serves to protect the heart wall and secure its position within the thorax. The inner layer is a serous layer. This serous pericardium is further

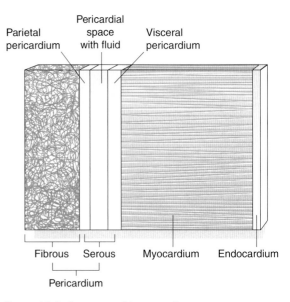

Figure 20.3 Structure of heart wall.

divided into an outer parietal layer, which forms the inner lining of the fibrous pericardium, and an inner visceral layer that forms the outer covering of the heart (also known as epicardium). Between these layers is a potential space, called the pericardial cavity. This contains serous fluid, which allows for flexibility in the movement of the heart during contraction and relaxation phases (heartbeats), thus reducing friction during these movements.

The myocardium is a thick layer of cardiac muscle lying between the pericardium and the inner endocardium. It has two layers of cardiac muscle arranged in a spiral form and it is this muscular arrangement that gives the heart its squeezing ability.

The endocardium is a thin fibrous layer made up of endothelial cells and connective tissue. It lines the inner surface of the heart walls and continues as the inner lining of the great vessels that emerge and leave from the heart.

Blood supply to heart wall is via the left and right coronary arteries and venous return is via the coronary sinus and cardiac veins.

Chambers of the heart

The heart is divided into left and right halves by a muscular septum. Each half has an upper atrium and a lower ventricle (Fig. 20.4). The atria are separated from each other by an interatrial septum and the ventricles are separated from each other by the interventricular septum. The atria are linked to the ventricles by atrioventricular valves. In a normal heart, blood flows from atria to ventricles and not the reverse. Figure 20.5 shows the sequence of events during the cardiac cycle.

Pumping action of the heart

The heart's own inherent autorhythmic cells act as a pacemaker to initiate and maintain the beating and pumping actions of the heart. These cells are also responsible for conducting these impulses throughout the cardiac muscle, thus creating an action in the path in which it travels (Fig. 20.6). Because the ventricles are responsible for sending blood out of the heart, the pressure in the ventricles is greater than the pressure in

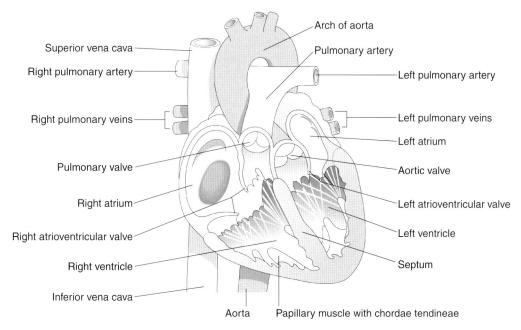

Figure 20.4 Chambers of the heart.

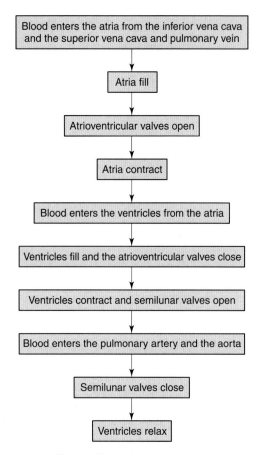

Figure 20.5 The cardiac cycle.

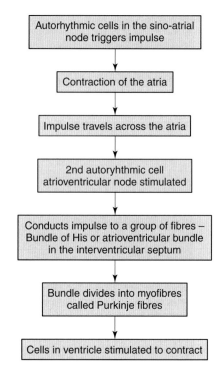

Figure 20.6 The pathway of electrical impulses through the heart.

the atria. The normal rhythm of a heart beat can be seen on an ECG (electrocardiograph) trace (see Fig. 20.7).

BLOOD VESSELS

Blood flows in the body in a closed system of circulation. The great vessels that come from the ventricles of the heart are the pulmonary artery and the aorta.

The pulmonary artery carries deoxygenated blood from the right ventricle to the lungs and after gaseous exchange takes place, oxygenated blood is then transported back to the heart via four pulmonary veins which empty into the left atrium. The pulmonary artery is the only artery in the body to carry deoxygenated blood and the pulmonary veins are the only veins in the body

to carry oxygenated blood. This is known as the pulmonary circulation.

The aorta and other arteries carry oxygenated blood to the body (Fig. 20.8) and have thicker walls to withstand the high pressure at which blood is pumped into them. The closer the artery is to the heart, the thicker the walls of the artery. Arteries and veins can be demonstrated radiographically by using contrast media (e.g. in angiography and venography).

Surrounding musculature exerts positive pressure on veins and this helps to force the blood through the veins and towards the heart. In addition, veins have thin walls due to their relatively low internal pressure and small flaps that act as valves to prevent the backflow of blood.

BLOOD

Blood is the 'life' of the body. It is a viscous tissue made up of liquid plasma and a combination of formed elements (blood cells). The plasma helps

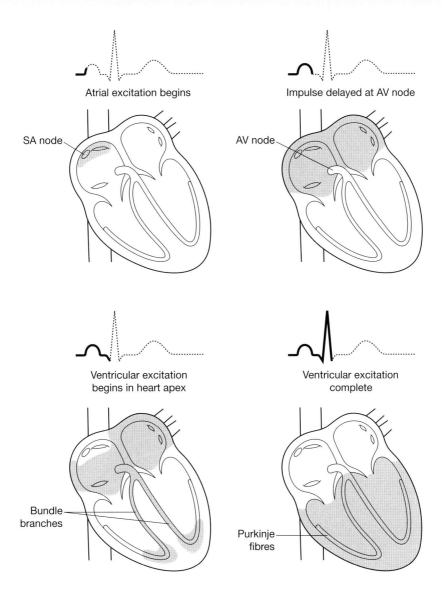

Atrial excitation begins

SA node

Impulse delayed at AV node

AV node

Ventricular excitation
begins in heart apex

Bundle
branches

Ventricular excitation
complete

Purkinje
fibres

Figure 20.7 ECG trace.

the body to maintain its normal state of hydration by responding to change in the internal environment via osmosis.

The formed elements are red blood cells (erythrocytes), a combination of different types of white blood cells (leucocytes) and blood platelets (thrombocytes).

These blood cells have different functions (Table 20.3). Together they serve to:

- maintain a healthy circulation by delivering oxygen, nutrients and useful substances to cells and tissues throughout the body
- play a role in homeostasis by regulating body temperature, initiating blood clotting to stop bleeding, and maintaining the pH (acid–base) balance of body fluids
- protect against harmful invasion of microorganisms.

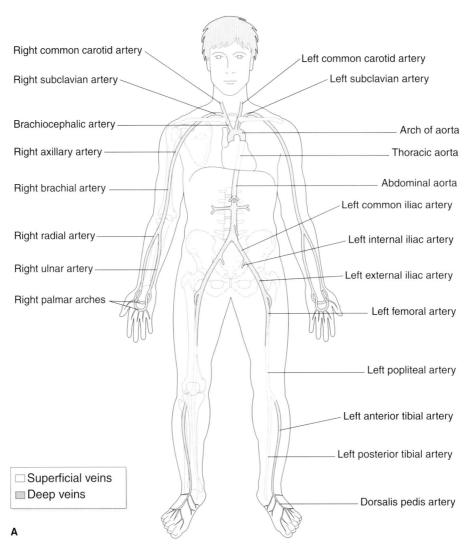

Right common carotid artery

Right subclavian artery

Brachiocephalic artery

Right axillary artery

Right brachial artery

Right radial artery

Right ulnar artery

Right palmar arches

Left common carotid artery

Left subclavian artery

Arch of aorta

Thoracic aorta

Abdominal aorta

Left common iliac artery

Left internal iliac artery

Left external iliac artery

Left femoral artery

Left popliteal artery

Left anterior tibial artery

Left posterior tibial artery

Dorsalis pedis artery

☐ Superficial veins
▨ Deep veins

A

Figure 20.8 Systemic circulation.

LYMPH AND LYMPH VESSELS

- Lymph is formed when fluid; proteins and certain substances (known as interstitial fluid) are forced out from the capillary bed, flow into surrounding tissues and gradually accumulate. This fluid is then collected by lymphatic capillaries and transported through the lymphatic system until it is returned to the bloodstream.

- Lymph vessels travel up towards the thoracic cavity to form lymphatic ducts, which then empty into the left subclavian vein, thus returning the fluid back into the bloodstream. The largest lymphatic vessel is the thoracic duct, which begins with a dilated portion called the cisterna chyli within the abdomen.
- Lymph nodes are small nodules that are found along the lymph vessels and these filter foreign particles that have entered the vessels. Examples of lymphoid tissue (glands) are the tonsils, spleen

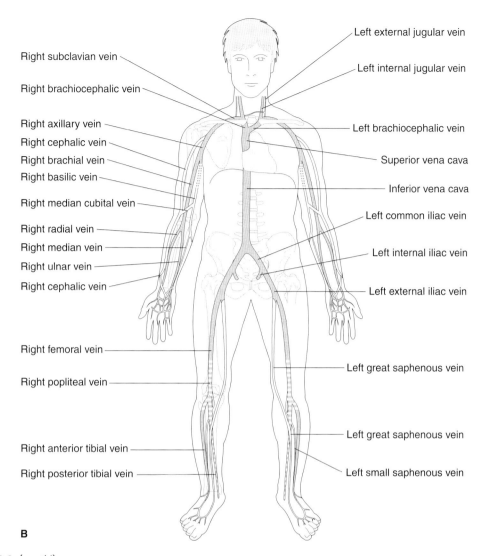

Right subclavian vein

Right brachiocephalic vein

Right axillary vein
Right cephalic vein
Right brachial vein
Right basilic vein

Right median cubital vein

Right radial vein
Right median vein
Right ulnar vein

Right cephalic vein

Right femoral vein

Right popliteal vein

Right anterior tibial vein

Right posterior tibial vein

Left external jugular vein

Left internal jugular vein

Left brachiocephalic vein

Superior vena cava

Inferior vena cava

Left common iliac vein

Left internal iliac vein

Left external iliac vein

Left great saphenous vein

Left great saphenous vein

Left small saphenous vein

B

Figure 20.8 (cont'd)

Table 20.3	Blood cells and their function
Blood cell	**Function**
Erythrocytes (red blood cells)	Contain haemoglobin (iron-containing pigment attached to a globular protein) for absorption and transport of oxygen from the lungs to cells and tissues
Leucocytes (white blood cells)	Provides immunity for the body by protecting against harmful invasion by disease-causing microorganisms – removes these, and debris from dead or damaged cells, from the blood.
Thrombocytes (blood platelets)	Responsible for clotting of the blood

and thymus gland whose function is to contribute to the body's defence by filtering body fluid and destroying foreign substances and by forming antibodies to aid immunity.

RESPIRATORY SYSTEM

The thorax is probably the most frequently imaged body part in radiology departments today because a single chest X-ray is sometimes sufficient to make a diagnosis and determine the overall health of a patient. The mechanism of breathing (inspiration and expiration) occurs within this system. It functions as a series of passages through which air travels from the outside (atmosphere) to the inside (lungs). In addition, this system contributes to wider ranging functions of voice production, coughing and sneezing.

Anatomical components of the respiratory tract are:

- Nose
- Pharynx
- Larynx
- Trachea
- Bronchi and bronchioles
- Lungs

NOSE

The nose has two external nostrils through which air enters. As the air enters it is warmed, filtered and moistened by the mucous membranes lining the nasal cavity. The mucous membranes have a constant supply of blood, which provide the warmth. The nasal cavity also serves as the centre of smell and has large air chambers for sound production.

Surrounding the nasal cavity is the hard palate, which forms the floor inferiorly, and the soft palate, which separates it from the oropharynx posteriorly. Leading into the nasal cavity, through small foramina, are a series of air spaces in the facial bones called the paranasal, maxillary, ethmoid, frontal and sphenoidal sinuses. These sinuses add a rich, full-bodied tone to the voice.

Sinuses are air filled; however, once infection sets in radiographs of the sinuses may be needed to demonstrate air-fluid levels that are especially prominent in the maxillary sinuses during an infection.

In addition, the nasolacrimal duct is connected from each eye to the nasal cavity and this drains excess tears into the nasal cavity.

PHARYNX

The pharynx is between the nasal cavity and the trachea and oesophagus, and therefore serves as a passage for both air and food. The pharynx has three parts: the nasopharynx (superior), oropharynx (middle) and the laryngopharynx (inferior).

When patients arrive at the department for postnasal space radiographs, this is the area that is being requested.

The nasopharynx has two auditory air passages (Eustachian tubes/pharyngotympanic tubes) that open into it. These air passages serve to balance out the air pressure on both sides of the tympanic membrane (the eardrums).

LARYNX

The larynx, or voice box, is composed of cartilages, the most important of which are the thyroid, cricoid and the epiglottis (Fig. 20.9). The thyroid

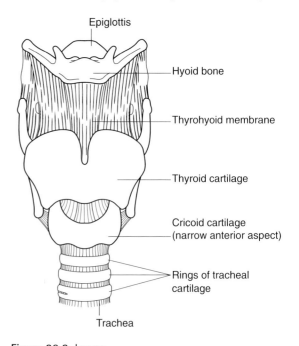

Figure 20.9 Larynx.

cartilage is situated at the level of approximately C5 (fifth cervical vertebra) but may extend roughly to about the level of T1 (first thoracic vertebra). It is made up of two segments of cartilages that form an angle anteriorly and is therefore prominently visible.

Just below the thyroid is the cricoid membrane, at the level of C5–C6. This is an important landmark as it forms the point of insertion for an airway in an emergency cricothyroidectomy.

The epiglottis is a flap-like appendage of cartilage that acts as a 'doorway', allowing air to pass through into the respiratory tract from the pharynx by blocking off the oesophagus and, conversely, allowing food to pass into the oesophagus by blocking off the upper pharynx.

TRACHEA

This is the continuation of the respiratory tract that is composed of C-shaped cartilaginous rings and extends from the larynx (around the level of C5) down to the upper lungs where it bifurcates into a left and a right main bronchus (Fig. 20.10).

These incomplete cartilaginous rings help support the trachea. The trachea's inner surface is lined with ciliated columnar epithelial tissue that traps dust and other particles that have passed down from the nasal cavity. If the particles are large, a coughing reflex is initiated to expel the foreign body.

BRONCHI AND BRONCHIOLES

The trachea branches into the left and right main bronchi at the level of the carina, normally around the level of T4–T5. The right main bronchus has a larger diameter and enters the lung at a more acute angle than the left. As a result, any inhaled foreign particles may get lodged here rather than in the left bronchus.

Each bronchus then branches further into smaller branches or secondary bronchioles and these further subdivide into much smaller branches of terminal bronchioles. These continue to branch and end in respiratory bronchioles. These respiratory bronchioles, in turn, then branch into alveolar ducts, which form the pathway to the

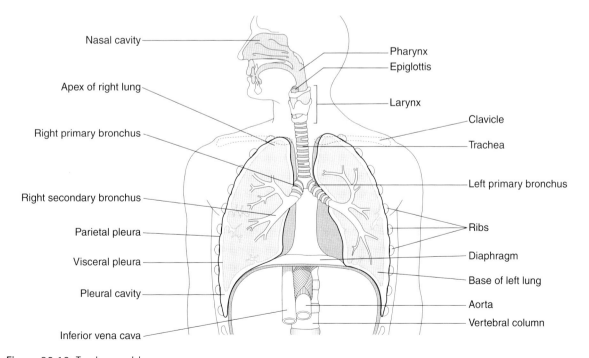

Figure 20.10 Trachea and lungs.

alveolar air sacs. Gaseous exchange takes place in the alveolar air sacs or alveoli, which form the functional unit of the lung. The alveoli are thin walled and lined with special excretory cells that produce a substance called surfactant. Surfactant serves to lubricate the lining of the alveoli to keep the walls inflated and thus reduce surface tension during the phases of gaseous exchange, when expansion and contraction of the alveoli occur.

LUNGS

Lungs are composed of alveolar air cells that are capable of expanding and contracting in order to perform their functions.

The two lobes are asymmetrical in shape with the left lobe being longer and slightly narrower in size due the heart's position on the left mediastinal border. The position of the liver on the right side elevates the right lung and gives it a higher and larger size. The hilum is present on the medial surface of each lung; structures such as the bronchioles and pulmonary vasculature enter and leave through this.

Each lung is divided into lobes, which are separated by fissures. These fissures are often prominent and can be seen on radiographs. A pleural membrane surrounds each lung. This pleural membrane has a potential cavity, the pleural cavity, which contains a serous fluid that allows expansion and relaxation of the lungs and reduces friction. The pressure in the pleural cavity is lower than the external atmospheric pressure and this helps in the breathing.

Each lung rests on the dome shaped band of muscle called the diaphragm – a very important musculotendinous structure that supports the lungs and plays a vital role in breathing. The diaphragm also separates the abdomen from the thoracic cavity.

On a chest radiograph, it is important to ensure that the costophrenic angles of the diaphragm are included and visible on the image to aid diagnoses.

INSPIRATION AND EXPIRATION

Breathing in and out is facilitated by the action of muscles. Diaphragmatic and intercostal muscle movements help the thorax increase and decrease in size, thus allowing for movement of air into and out of the lungs.

During inspiration (active phase) the diaphragm contracts and moves downwards, increasing depth; the intercostal muscles contract and extend sideways from rib to rib, increasing the width, and the pressure within the thoracic cavity decreases; air is drawn in from high pressure (outside) to low pressure (inside) the lungs.

During expiration (passive phase) the diaphragmatic and intercostal muscles relax; the thoracic cavity is reduced in size; pressure increases and air flows out of the lungs.

When air enters the lungs it travels until it reaches the alveolar air sacs. Gaseous exchange takes place by oxygen moving across the alveolar capillary membrane into the blood stream and carbon dioxide moving from the blood stream across the membrane, by diffusion, to be expelled. This alveolar capillary membrane interface must be structurally thin for effective gaseous exchange to occur. If the membrane becomes thicker, owing to the changes that occur during certain clinical conditions, then gaseous exchange is not effective and air trapping within the alveolar air sacs occurs, which causes lung fields on radiographs to appear overinflated and darker.

Look out for bronchiole 'tree' appearances on chest radiographs and compare lung appearance on images taken on good inspiration with that of those taken on poor inspiration (Fig. 20.11). To evaluate a good inspiratory radiograph, approximately six anterior ribs or ten posterior ribs should be visible on a posteroanterior (PA) chest radiograph.

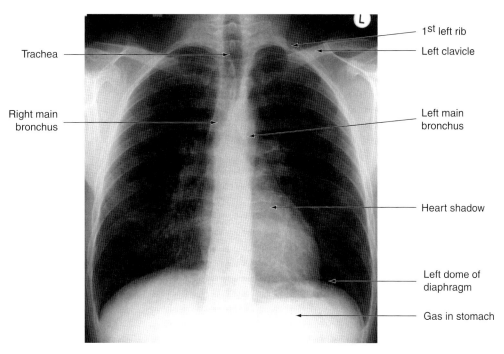

Trachea

1st left rib

Left clavicle

Right main bronchus

Left main bronchus

Heart shadow

Left dome of diaphragm

Gas in stomach

Figure 20.11 Chest radiograph.

DIGESTIVE SYSTEM

The digestive system functions to allow food to be taken into the mouth, swallowed (ingested), digested, absorbed and eliminated.

Various components make up this vast and varied tract and they will be discussed in the manner in which they represent anatomically. At this point the tract can be divided into two regions: that part of the digestive tract that lies above the diaphragm (upper tract) and then the part that lies below the diaphragm (lower tract or gastrointestinal tract) (Fig. 20.12). In addition, there are accessory organs associated with digestion; that is, the liver, gall bladder and pancreas.

Internal anatomy

The wall of the tract has the same basic structure throughout its length, although cell differentiation occurs in places in order to perform specific functions. These are mentioned wherever appropriate. The basic structure consists of the following four layers:

- mucus membrane (mucosa)
- sub-mucus membrane (submucosa)
- muscular layer (consisting of longitudinal and circular muscles)
- serous layer (serosa) containing vascular and lymphatic supply.

UPPER DIGESTIVE TRACT

This is made up of the following components:

- mouth or buccal cavity
- salivary glands
- pharynx
- oesophagus.

Mouth/buccal cavity

This is the oral cavity that is found at the very beginning of the digestive tract, through which food enters. The mouth is lined by mucus secreting stratified epithelial cells. Its anterior and lateral boundaries are the lips and cheeks, respectively.

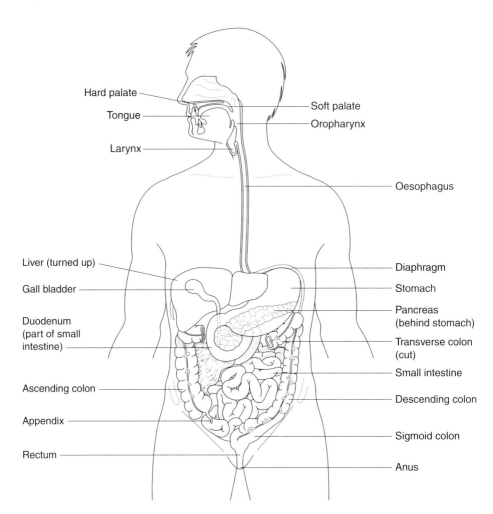

Figure 20.12 The digestive tract.

These help to keep the food in the mouth and have a role in speech.

Superiorly lies the hard and soft palate; inferiorly is the floor of the mouth and tongue. The hard palate forms a rigid surface for the tongue to press against during chewing. The soft palate lies posterior to the hard palate and during swallowing it rises to close off the nasopharynx, preventing fluid from entering into it. Beyond this the soft palate is continuous with the pharynx.

The tongue is a muscular organ attached to the hyoid bone inferiorly. The soft layer of tissue that attaches the tongue to the floor of the mouth is called the frenulum. The superior surface of the tongue contains small finger like projections called papillae which contain nerve endings for taste. Nerve supply to the tongue is via the hypoglossal nerve for voluntary movement; taste sensations are via the facial and glossopharyngeal nerves. The tongue has a very rich blood supply and injury can therefore cause extensive bleeding. Blood supply is via the lingual branch of the carotid artery and venous drainage is via the lingual vein to the internal jugular vein.

Salivary glands

1. Parotid (paired) – the largest salivary gland, found on either side of face just below each external auditory meatus. Each has its own

duct, the parotid duct, that opens into the mouth at about the level of the 2nd upper molar tooth.

2. Submandibular (paired) – found on each side of face just under the angle of the mandible. Each gland has a duct, the submandibular duct, that opens on either side of the frenulum of the tongue.

3. Sublingual (unpaired) – these are found just under the mucous membrane lining the floor of the mouth, anterior to the submandibular glands. Each gland has many tiny ducts, which pierce the mucous membrane, and pours onto the floor of the mouth.

Each gland (Fig. 20.13) is surrounded by a fibrous outer capsule and is lined with mucous-secreting cells. The secretions are called saliva, which is made up of water, mineral salts, a digestive enzyme called salivary amylase, mucous, lyso-somes (to remove/repair/replace injured cells), immunoglobulins (protection against microorganisms) and certain blood clotting factors. Secretions are controlled by the autonomic nervous system. The presence of food in the mouth triggers a reflex secretion of saliva. In addition, sight, smell or even the thought of food may have the same effect.

Pharynx

This is a funnel-shaped structure that contributes to both the digestive and respiratory tract (Fig. 20.14). Once food leaves the mouth it enters the pharynx. As discussed in the respiratory system, the pharynx continues inferiorly as the oesophagus. The epiglottis acts as a gate allowing food to enter the oesophagus by closing off the entrance to the trachea. The digestive function of the pharynx is to aid swallowing together with the effort of the muscles associated with the tongue, hyoid and soft palate.

Oesophagus

This is a long tube connecting the pharynx to the stomach. It is located just anterior to the vertebral column and posterior to the trachea. Once food leaves the pharynx it enters the oesophagus and is moved along by wave-like movements called peristalsis.

At its lower end the oesophagus has a band of smooth muscle that acts as a sphincter, which functions to let food pass into the stomach as well as preventing gastric contents from being refluxed back into the oesophagus. If the sphincter does not function properly, it could allow the acidic

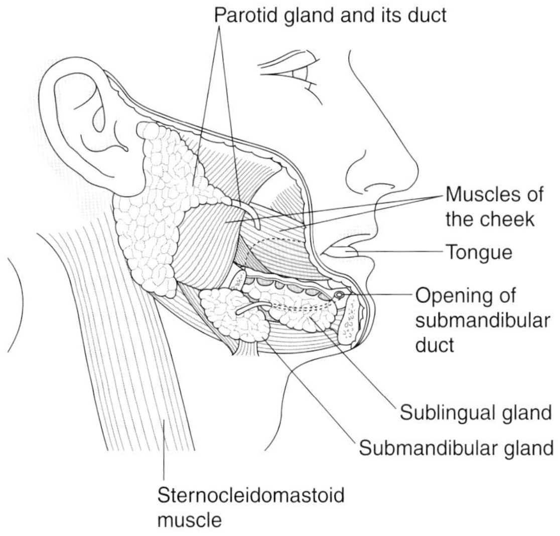

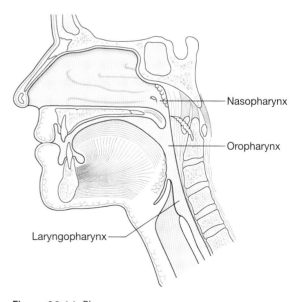

Figure 20.13 Salivary glands.

Figure 20.14 Pharynx.

gastric contents to move up the oesophagus causing a burning sensation, commonly referred to as heartburn.

LOWER DIGESTIVE TRACT (GASTROINTESTINAL TRACT)

This is made up of the following components:

- stomach
- small intestine
- large intestine

Plus the following accessory organs:

- liver and gall bladder
- pancreas.

Stomach

The stomach is a sac-like structure that can be located under the left hemi-diaphragm and functions to store food and aid in mechanical and chemical digestion (Fig. 20.15). Food enters the stomach from the oesophagus via the cardiac sphincter.

The stomach is anatomically divided into four regions: the cardiac, fundus, body and antrum. The lining of the stomach has folds, called rugae, and consists of columnar epithelial cells containing

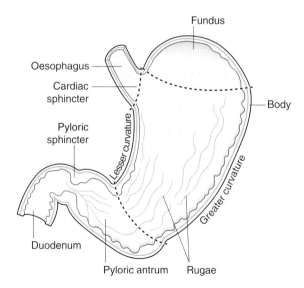

Figure 20.15 Stomach.

gastric pits which house the gastric glands. The outer layer of the stomach consist of muscular fibres arranged in circular and longitudinal fashion to facilitate the breakdown and churning of food required during mechanical digestion. Whilst the muscles provide the movement to aid mechanical digestion, the gastric enzymes (water, salts, mucus, hydrochloric acid (HCl) and pepsinogens) secreted by the gastric glands provide the chemical digestion. Once adequately churned, the food is then propelled towards the duodenum via the pyloric sphincter.

Small intestine

This is a narrow tube that is about 6 m long and divided into three parts:

- duodenum
- jejunum
- ileum.

Duodenum

This structure is easily identified as having a characteristic 'C'-shape and forms the proximal part of the small intestine. The duodenum has two openings on its internal surface. These are for receiving the digestive secretions of the gall bladder and pancreas. The duodenum produces its own digestive juices which, together with bile and pancreatic juice, further aid in digestion of the food. The lining of the duodenum has mucus-secreting goblet cells which swell and protect the duodenum from gastric acid entering with the food.

Jejunum and ileum

These parts form the second and third portions of the small intestine and continue from the duodenum to end at the caecum. Most of the nutrients from digested food are absorbed in this part of the small intestine. The mucosal lining has little protrusions called villi; these contain a rich blood and lymph supply, which helps the absorption of useful substances from the food. Between the villi are intestinal glands which produce enzymes and intestinal juice for further digestion as food moves along in the small intestine by peristalsis (Table 20.4).

Table 20.4   Digestive enzymes

Part of digestive tract	Enzyme
Mouth or buccal cavity salivary glands	Salivary amylase
Stomach	Gastric enzymes – pepsin, gastric amylase and gastric lipase
Small intestine	Intestinal enzymes – sucrase, lipase, maltase and lactase, and receives bile and pancreatic digestive secretions
Pancreas	Pancreatic enzymes – trypsinogens, pancreatic amylase and lipase

Large intestine or colon

This part of the tract extends from the terminal ileum to the anus. It is made up of various segments:

- Caecum – the first part of large bowel into which the terminal ileum empties.
- Appendix – the small appendage that is attached to the caecum. Food can become trapped in the appendix, which can then become infected by bacterial invasion. Inflammation of the appendix is known as appendicitis.
- Ascending colon – this travels upwards towards the liver and then curves medially forming the hepatic flexure.
- Transverse colon – this part of the larger intestine travels almost transversely to curve inferiorly at the spleen forming the splenic flexure.
- Descending colon – this part travels downwards until it makes a 'S'-shaped curve to form the sigmoid colon.
- Rectum – the most distal part of the large colon.
- Anus – the external opening for expelling faeces.

Food entering the large colon has already been stripped of its useful nutrients and the remainder is ready for excretion as waste. The colon has bacteria, which solidify faeces and causes flatulence. The bacteria are important in the formation of vitamin K for blood clotting. The lining of the colon contains mucous cells, which secrete mucus to neutralise the pH of the faeces as well as helping it to move towards the anus. The faeces are then expelled out of the body by internal and external anal sphincters.

The external surface has large bulges, called haustra. These haustral patterns are important during imaging and diagnoses, as their absence denotes pathology in the region.

ACCESSORY DIGESTIVE ORGANS

The accessory digestive organs are depicted in Figure 20.16.

Liver and gall bladder

The liver is a large wedge-shaped structure, which lies in the upper right quadrant of the abdomen, just under the right hemi-diaphragm. It is roughly divided into left and right lobes, which are separated by a ligament called the falciform ligament. This ligament forms an important landmark when imaging the liver during ultrasound examinations.

The liver has various functions in metabolism, blood cell production and digestion. It produces a pigment called bile, which is housed in a specialised sac called the gall bladder. Bile is secreted via the bile duct directly into the duodenum where it breaks down or emulsifies fats, thus aiding enzyme action by digestive enzymes.

Sometimes small calcifications resembling little stones form in the gall bladder and can be seen on a radiograph; these are called gallstones. Imaging of the gall bladder can be via ultrasound or by performing a cholecystogram. The liver is easily imaged using ultrasound, CT or MRI modalities.

Pancreas

The pancreas lies posterior to the stomach in the retroperitoneal space and acts as both an endocrine (see Endocrine system, p. 283) and exocrine gland. Its exocrine function is to produce digestive juices (pancreatic juices) and enzymes that are transported via the pancreatic duct to empty into the duodenum to help in digestion.

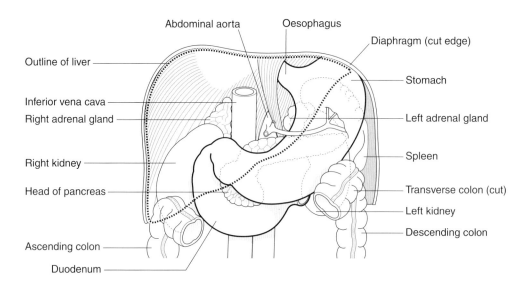

Figure 20.16 Accessory organs of digestion.

UROGENITAL SYSTEM

The urinary system (Fig. 20.17) comprises the following:

- kidneys
- ureters
- bladder
- urethra – male and female.

KIDNEYS

The human body has two kidneys, which are situated in the retroperitoneal aspect of the abdomen. Each kidney is about 10 cm long and about 5 cm wide and lies between the levels of T12 and L3. Because of their location, they are partly protected by the ribcage. The left kidney lies just inferior to the spleen, and makes brief contact with it; the right kidney lies in contact with the large, right lobe of the liver, making an impression on the liver's visceral surface. Because of this position, the right kidney lies lower than the left kidney.

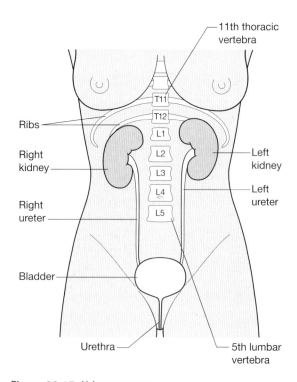

Figure 20.17 Urinary system.

The position of the kidneys in the abdomen is important for accurate radiographic technique required during intravenous urogram procedures (IVUs) (Fig. 20.18).

External anatomy

Each kidney is bean shaped, with a convex lateral border and a concave medial border. The medial border is called the hilum and it is here that blood vessels, nerves and ureter enter and leave the kidney.

Three layers of tissue surround the kidney and protect it from mechanical injury and infections. The innermost layer is a fibrous layer called the renal capsule; the middle layer is a 'fat' layer called the adipose capsule; and the outermost layer is a dense connective tissue layer called the renal fascia. The renal fascia provides attachment for the adrenal glands (small pyramid-shaped endocrine glands situated above each kidney) as well as attaching the kidneys to the posterior abdominal wall. The connective tissue of this layer also provides the flexibility needed by the kidneys during breathing movements.

Internal anatomy

There are three distinct areas on the internal surface of the kidney: a cortex, a medulla and a renal pelvis (Fig. 20.19). The cortex forms the outermost part of the internal structure of the kidney, whilst the middle portion is called the medulla and contains cone-shaped tissue called medullary pyramids. On a longitudinal section these pyramids appear to have stripes or striations. This is because they are composed of urine-collecting tubules arranged in a parallel manner. The pyramids have 'finger like' projections called papillae, which empty into the minor calyces. The renal pelvis is found medially and is the dilated portion of the ureter, which has two divisions known as the major and minor calyces. The minor calyces act as cups to collect the urine from the collecting

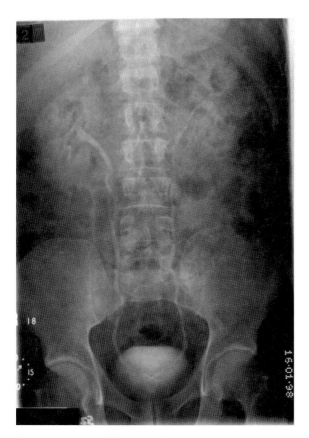

Figure 20.18 An IVU image demonstrating the urinary system.

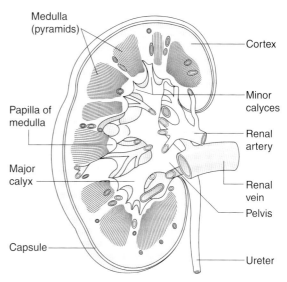

Figure 20.19 Longitudinal section of the kidney.

tubules of the pyramids and propels it, with the help of its smooth muscle containing layer, towards the pelvis. The pelvis acts as a reservoir to collect the urine and then transport it to the bladder for excretion.

Filtration, formation and flow of urine

Kidneys function to regulate the water, nutrient and electrolyte balance of the body. The component responsible for this activity is a microscopic, blood-filtering and functional unit called the nephron (Fig. 20.20). The nephron is associated with many renal tubules. These structures filter the blood and form urine. Collecting ducts then collect the urine, which is emptied into the minor calyx of the renal pelvis.

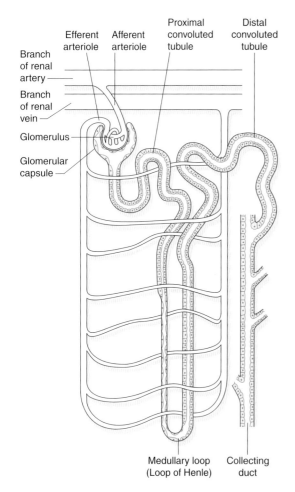

Figure 20.20 Structure of a nephron.

Each nephron is made up of a bundle of capillaries called the glomerulus, which is surrounded by a cup-shaped structure called the glomerular capsule. Together these two structures constitute the renal corpuscle and are associated with renal tubules.

Blood enters the glomerulus and is filtered. The filtrate then passes through the porous (fenestrated) epithelium of the glomerus into the glomerular capsule. From the glomerular capsule the fluid then flows into the proximal part of the renal tubule called the proximal convoluted tubule. The fluid then flows into a part of the tubule that resembles a hairpin, called the Loop of Henle; it continues to flow towards the distal part of the tubule called the distal convoluted tubule and finally into the collecting duct as urine.

When the fluid enters the glomerulus as a filtrate, it contains plasma, useful ions, blood cells and nutrients. These constituents of the filtrate are then absorbed as a result of the filtrate flowing through the renal tubule, and the fluid that remains at the distal end of the tubule empties into the collecting ducts and is now called urine.

Urine is generally a clear–pale yellow colour of watery fluid that has a slightly acidic pH due to the presence of urea, sodium, potassium, phosphate and sulphate ions, uric acid and creatinine.

Functions of the kidney

- Filtration of waste materials out of the blood, by reabsorbing useful nutrients (e.g. protein, glucose, minerals and water) back into the blood stream and filtering out the undesirable remainder.
- Plays a role in maintaining a balance in levels of electrolytes such as sodium, potassium and phosphorous.
- Produces hormones (e.g. rennin) that help to regulate blood pressure as well as water retention to prevent dehydration.
- Produces erythropoietin for the synthesis of red blood cells.
- Helps the body to absorb calcium by synthesis of vitamin D in its active form.

URETERS

Urine is transported into the ureters via the renal pelvis. The ureters transport the urine from the kidneys to the bladder. The ureters do not lie vertically in structure; instead they travel down along the posterior peritoneal wall and curve medially before entering the posterior bladder wall in an oblique manner. This morphology helps prevent the backflow of urine from the bladder into the ureters.

Because of the morphology, a slight filling defect sometimes occurs during an intravenous urogram (IVU) procedure when the patient lies supine. To help this, a prone position may be used for a few minutes, as well as compression.

BLADDER

The urinary bladder is a muscular bag that collects and stores urine until micturation occurs. It is located just posterior to the symphysis pubis and this forms an important anatomical landmark for accurate radiographic technique required for a 'bladder view'. The posterior walls of the bladder have three openings, known as the trigone, for both ureters and the urethra.

URETHRA

The urethra is a muscular tube that transports the urine from the bladder to the exterior. The urethra has sphincters that control the flow of urine and prevents urine leakage. The location and structure of the urethra differs in males and females (Fig. 20.21).

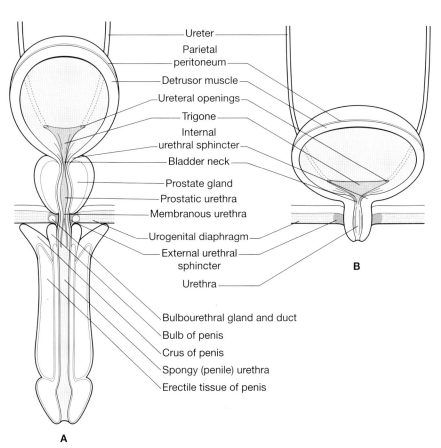

Ureter
Parietal peritoneum
Detrusor muscle
Ureteral openings
Trigone
Internal urethral sphincter
Bladder neck
Prostate gland
Prostatic urethra
Membranous urethra
Urogenital diaphragm
External urethral sphincter
Urethra
Bulbourethral gland and duct
Bulb of penis
Crus of penis
Spongy (penile) urethra
Erectile tissue of penis

A

B

Figure 20.21 A Male urethra. B Female urethra.

Male urethra

- Has a length of about 20 cm.
- Is divided into three segments: the prostatic urethra, which passes within the prostate gland (hence its name), the membranous urethra and the spongy urethra.
- The urethral opening is located distally on the tip of the penis.
- It serves two functions:
  - it has urinary function in expelling urine from the bladder to the exterior.
  - it has a reproductive function in carrying sperm from the reproductive ducts and glands, which it ejaculates during sexual intercourse. The sphincter located at the junction of the urethra and bladder controls the expulsion of urine during ejaculation.

Female urethra

- Has a length of about 3–4 cm.
- The urethral opening is located anterior to the vaginal and anal opening; and because of its short length and close proximity to the anal canal, infections of the urinary tract via the urethra is more common in females than in males.

MICTURITION

This is the action of urination or emptying of the bladder. Fullness of the bladder is perceived by the nervous system and by the impulses of the parasympathetic nerve pathways. Sometimes certain stressors can inhibit normal micturition and incontinence or urine retention can occur.

Incontinence is the inability to voluntarily control urination. Urine retention occurs when there is an inability to voluntarily urinate or micturate. Micturating cystourethrogram (MCUG) procedures may be necessary in some cases.

NERVOUS SYSTEM

The nervous system is a communication network, which, together with the endocrine system, controls body functions and maintains homeostasis.

This network is actually a vast organisation of nervous tissue collecting, interpreting and responding to changes that affect the body from within and from external elements.

The nervous system is divided into the central nervous system (CNS) and the peripheral nervous system (PNS). The CNS is made up of the brain and spinal cord and the PNS is made up of all the nerves outside the brain and spinal cord; that is, the peripheral nerves.

For the purposes of learning about the nervous system relevant to practice, only the following sections are going to be discussed in this chapter.

- Nervous tissue – brief structure and physiology
- CNS
  Brain
  - meninges
  - cerebrum
  - cerebellum
  - brain stem
  - ventricles and cerebrospinal fluid (CSF)
  - blood–brain barrier
  Spinal cord
- PNS
  Somatic nervous system
  Autonomic nervous system
  - sympathetic
  - parasympathetic.

NERVOUS TISSUE

Nerve cells are called neurons. These neurons are structurally supported by a connective tissue called neuroglial cells. A neuron's structure consists of a cell body, an axon and a few dendrites. If these axons are bound together, they are called a nerve bundle or simply 'nerves'. These nerve cells may be myelinated (covered by a sheath of specialised cells) or unmyelinated and function to initiate a nerve impulse and conduct this impulse from one neuron to another. This takes place by means of a synapse – a junction where the axon terminal of one neuron meets the dendrite terminals of another neuron. Synapses can be either chemical or electrical. In a chemical synapse the two neurons transmit signals via a chemical substance called a neurotransmitter. In an electrical synapse the impulse is conveyed directly from one cell to the other.

Axons and dendrites make up the white matter of the nervous system. Dendrites function to receive an impulse and direct it towards the cell body of the neuron. The axon functions to conduct this impulse away from the cell along its path of conduction. There are two types of nerve:

- sensory/afferent nerves
- motor/efferent nerves.

Sensory nerves receive stimulus from the sensory receptors on dendrites of neurons and pass these impulses onwards to the brain and spinal cord. Motor nerves arise in the CNS and respond to this impulse by causing an action in the muscles or organs of the body.

CENTRAL NERVOUS SYSTEM

Brain

The brain is a large mass of white and grey matter that would slump and sag if it was not supported by the cranium and meninges (Fig. 20.22). The cranium is the skull vault that surrounds the brain and protects it from injury.

Meninges

Directly surrounding the brain are the meninges (Fig. 20.23). These layers of tissue protect the brain and, together with the CSF, act as shock absorbers to prevent injury. There are three meningeal layers:

- Dura mater – the outermost layer that has two parts. The outer layer lines the cranium and the inner layer forms a protective covering for the brain. Between these two layers there is a potential space.
- Arachnoid mater – this forms the middle layer and the space between the arachnoid and the dura mater is called the subdural space.
- Pia mater – this forms the innermost layer, has a rich capillary blood supply and directly covers the brain. The space between the arachnoid and the pia mater is called the subarachnoid space. CSF flows within this space and totally immerses the brain.

Cerebrum

This is the largest part of the brain. The obvious features of the cerebrum are two large hemispheres of convoluted, wiggly folds of tissue called gyri that are separated by deep grooves called sulci. These convolutions increase the surface area of the cortex of the cerebrum.

The two hemispheres form the left and the right lobes. The lobes are made up of grey matter on the outer cortex and the inner layers are made up of

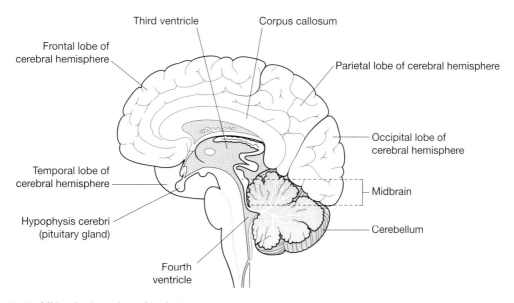

Figure 20.22 Midsagittal section of brain.

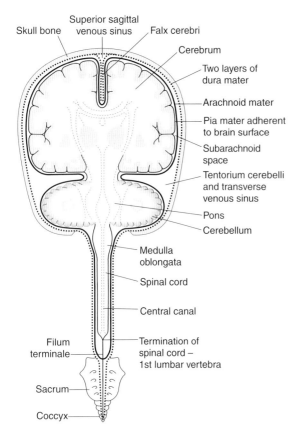

Figure 20.23 Cranial meninges.

white matter. The cerebrum consists of nerve tracts for communication between the lobes. The lobes are connected to each other by a dense bundle of nerve fibres called the corpus callosum. This relays impulses between the left and right lobes.

Each lobe is divided, by deep fissures, into smaller lobes which correspond with the part of cranium they lie under:

- Frontal – involved in motor control of voluntary movements, behaviour and emotion.
- Parietal – involved in general senses and taste.
- Temporal – involved in hearing, equilibrium and memory.
- Occipital – responsible for vision and forms of expression.

Functions of the left and right cerebral lobes

Both lobes are involved in different conscious actions, though in some people their roles can be reversed.

- Left lobe – this is active in speech, writing, calculation, language comprehension and analytical thought processes.
- Right lobe – this is active in general thought processes, appreciation of spatial awareness and conceptual non-verbal ideas.

L for Logic; R for cReativity

The Left brain sorts out parts of things and the Right brain sees the whole picture.

Cerebellum

The second largest part of the brain, the cerebellum lies inferior to the cerebrum and is separated from it by the central fissure. It is made up of left and right hemispheres separated by a central vermis. It is composed of an outer cortex made up of grey matter, with white matter in the inner layers. The inner white matter is made up of long and short tracts. These short tracts conduct impulses from neuron cell bodies on the outer cortex to the inner area. The long tracts conduct nerve impulses to and from the cerebellum itself.

Function of cerebellum

- Balance and coordination of muscular movements.
- Body posture and positions.
- Precision and timing of body movements.
- Proprioception.

Brain stem

The brain stem is the 'stalk' of the brain that acts a bridge and connects the cerebrum to the spinal cord. It is made up of three parts: the midbrain, pons and medulla oblongata.

The brain stem consists of long tracts of ascending and descending pathways that conduct impulses from the body to the cerebrum and from the cerebrum to the rest of the body. It houses an important structure called the reticular formation that controls the vital life-sustaining role of maintaining respiration and cardiac activity. It is also responsible for regulating consciousness and levels of 'awareness'. The reticular fibres desensitise the repetitive sounds and create levels of awareness for 'important' sounds.

A popular example of this awareness for certain sounds is when a mother, even whilst in deep sleep, wakes at the sound of her baby or sick child, yet the sound of a constant buzz in traffic is not heard at all.

Overall functions of the brain stem
- Involved with visual reflexes – i.e. movement of eyes; focussing of lens and dilation of pupils.
- Controls certain respiratory functions – i.e. regulates breathing.
- Serves as a message relay station from the medulla oblongata to the cerebrum.
- Regulates heart rate, respiratory rate, constriction/dilation of blood vessels, blood pressure, swallowing, vomiting, sneezing and coughing.

Ventricles and cerebrospinal fluid (CSF)

The ventricles are cavities within the brain that are filled with CSF (Fig. 20.24). These cavities are

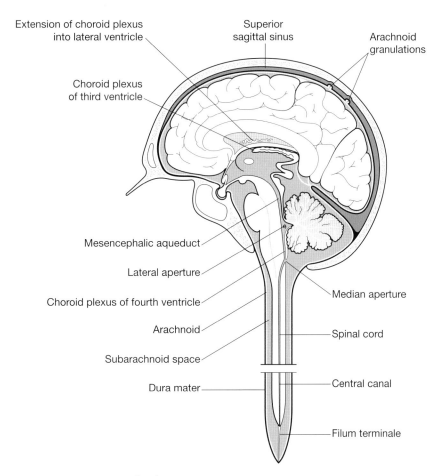

Figure 20.24 Flow of cerebrospinal fluid (CSF).

lined with cuboidal epithelial cells (called ependymal cells) that make contact with the pia mater at various points along its surface to form blood vessel network structures known as choroid plexuses.

CSF is formed at the choroid plexus due to the semipermeability of the capillary network. CSF is made up of water, small amounts of minerals, ions, white blood cells and organic compounds.

Blood–brain barrier

This is a network of semipermeable membranes that acts as a barrier, selectively preventing access to certain substances (e.g. certain drugs) whilst allowing other substances such as oxygen and essential nutrients to enter freely.

Astrocytes are a special type of neuroglial cell that support the nerve cells of the CNS but do not conduct impulses. A layer of astrocytes is found just inside the pia mater covering the brain. The blood–brain barrier is made up of this layer of astrocytes in addition to the capillary wall surrounding the pia mater. The choroid plexuses are considered to be part of the blood–brain barrier.

Blood supply to the brain

Blood supply to the brain is via the two internal carotid arteries and the arterial circle (circle of Willis), which exists between the internal carotids and the vertebral arteries.

Spinal cord

This is an elongated structure that is held together by dural ligaments and supported and surrounded by the meninges and CSF. The spinal cord is made up of tracts that form the connecting link between the brain and the rest of the body and is the centre for coordination of reflex action. It ascends superiorly from just below the foramen magnum to about the level of L1–L2 inferiorly.

Lumbar puncture procedures involve an injection into the subarachnoid space below the level of L2 so as to avoid injury to the spinal cord. In addition, injections into the epidural space (between the dura mater and the periosteum) are used to create a 'caudal block', as used sometimes during childbirth.

From the spinal cord, 31 pairs of spinal nerves emerge (Fig. 20.25). There are 8 pairs of cervical nerves, 12 pairs of thoracic nerves, 5 pairs of lumbar nerves, 5 pairs of sacral nerves and 1 pair of coccygeal nerves.

PERIPHERAL NERVOUS SYSTEM (PNS)

The PNS is made up of sensory and motor pathways that allow the brain and the spinal cord to communicate with the rest of the body. In addition to the spinal nerves, it comprises 12 pairs of cranial nerves.

It is divided into the somatic nervous system and the visceral nervous system.

Somatic nervous system

This is composed of both sensory and motor pathways. The sensory pathway receives impulses such as touch, pain and heat as conscious perceptions. Impulses from the mouth, skeletal muscles and joints, nose, etc., are relayed via cranial and spinal nerves and are perceived at an unconscious level. The motor pathway of the somatic system is composed of motor neurons, which conduct impulses from the CNS to the skeletal muscle, enabling the muscles to voluntarily 'act' or contract.

Visceral nervous system

This is also composed of sensory and motor pathways. The sensory pathway receives impulses from sensory receptors of visceral systems

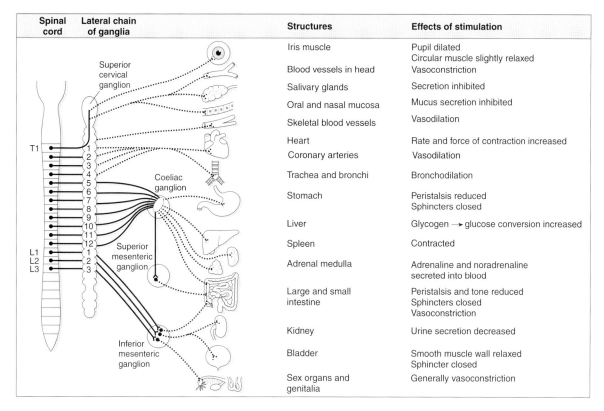

Spinal cord	Lateral chain of ganglia	Structures	Effects of stimulation
		Iris muscle	Pupil dilated Circular muscle slightly relaxed
		Blood vessels in head	Vasoconstriction
		Salivary glands	Secretion inhibited
		Oral and nasal mucosa	Mucus secretion inhibited
		Skeletal blood vessels	Vasodilation
		Heart	Rate and force of contraction increased
		Coronary arteries	Vasodilation
		Trachea and bronchi	Bronchodilation
		Stomach	Peristalsis reduced Sphincters closed
		Liver	Glycogen → glucose conversion increased
		Spleen	Contracted
		Adrenal medulla	Adrenaline and noradrenaline secreted into blood
		Large and small intestine	Peristalsis and tone reduced Sphincters closed Vasoconstriction
		Kidney	Urine secretion decreased
		Bladder	Smooth muscle wall relaxed Sphincter closed
		Sex organs and genitalia	Generally vasoconstriction

Figure 20.25 Spinal cord and spinal nerves.

(e.g. cardiovascular, digestive and urinary). These impulses are perceived on an unconscious level; however, some impulses are conveyed on a conscious level – e.g. pain, taste and feeling of fullness of the bladder.

The motor pathway of the visceral nervous system is known as the autonomic nervous system.

Autonomic nervous system

These are the motor pathways that respond to impulses from the visceral nervous system and secretions from endocrine and exocrine glands of the body. This system can be divided into two parts whose responses are generally antagonistic (i.e. have the opposite effect) to each other, although they function together to promote homeostasis. They are:

- Sympathetic nervous system.
- Parasympathetic nervous system.

Nerve fibres from these systems innervate visceral organs and they tend to have the opposite effect to each other. For example the sympathetic division would constrict an artery whilst the parasympathetic division would dilate the artery. However, there are instances where both systems are stimulated to have the same effect (e.g. production of saliva).

The parasympathetic division functions to 'conserve' energy by slowing the heart rate and blood pressure and stimulating excretion of waste products, whereas the sympathetic division is involved in action and activity, thereby increasing heart rate and blood pressure.

ENDOCRINE SYSTEM

It has been mentioned before that the endocrine system together with the nervous system controls body activities and maintains homeostasis. Whereas the action of the nervous system is rapid, with immediate but shorter-lived responses, the response of the endocrine system is slower but the effects are longer lasting. The nervous system influences bodily activities by means of chemical messengers known as neurotransmitters. The endocrine system influences metabolic activities of body cells by means of chemical messengers better known as *hormones*. Organs or glands that can be classified into exocrine and endocrine structures secrete these chemical messengers.

HORMONES

Hormones are chemical substances that act as messengers at their target organs. The message they carry acts as a stimulus to their target or inhibits an action at their target. Overall, hormones help to control bodily activities and bring about a balance within the internal body environment to maintain homeostasis. Hormones act by binding to target cells that receive the impulse. Depending on the nature of the hormone, the target receptor cells may bind and receive the stimulus either on the membrane surface of target cells or within the cellular matrix or cytoplasm of the cells.

Hormones are derived from two different sources.

- Peptide hormones – are formed from amino acid (protein) chains and are water-soluble. These hormones bind to receptor cells on the membrane surface in order to be absorbed, as they are unable to penetrate the membrane surface due to being water-soluble.
- Lipid hormones (better known as steroids) – are derived from cholesterol and are fat-soluble, making them permeable (able to diffuse through a membrane) and therefore allowing them to bind to receptor cells within the cytoplasm of target cells to be absorbed.

Examples of hormones, their gland or organ of origin and functions are listed in Table 20.5. Hormone stimulation, release and inhibition are controlled via a feedback mechanism. This method of control is used by the endocrine system to regulate the amount of secretion required. Feedback may be positive or negative.

- Positive feedback – presence of a substance relays a message to the gland of origin to secrete more of the substance.
- Negative feedback – presence of a hormone in the blood has reached its required level, a message is 'sent' to the gland of origin to slow down or stop secreting any more of the substance.

Control of hormone secretion is regulated by the hypothalamus via the feedback mechanism (Fig. 20.26).

ENDOCRINE ORGANS AND GLANDS

As already mentioned, organs and glands can be classified as being either exocrine or endocrine.

- Exocrine glands – the distinctive feature about these glands is that they possess ducts that act as an outlet for releasing their secretions. Examples of these are the sweat glands, which have ducts that empty directly onto the skin's surface to cool the skin, or the salivary glands that empty directly into the mouth to help begin chemical digestion of food. It must be mentioned, though, that the secretions from exocrine organs/glands are not hormones but that certain exocrine organs/glands also have endocrine properties, e.g. the pancreas, the gonads.
- Endocrine glands (Fig. 20.27) – these glands are structurally different in that they empty their secretions directly into blood or lymph (the organs/glands they arise from have good vascular supply and lymphatic drainage).

Table 20.5 Endocrine glands, hormones and functions

Organ/gland	Hormone	Functions
Hypothalamus		Has nerve cells that control the pituitary by producing neurochemicals that either stimulate or suppress the secretions from the pituitary. Acts as a primary link between the nervous system (brain) and endocrine system (mainly the pituitary)
	Antidiuretic hormone (ADH)	Regulates the body's fluid balance
	Oxytocin	Stimulates contraction of uterine muscles during childbirth; ejection of milk during lactation
Pituitary gland (hypophysis)		The most important endocrine gland because its responses control the action of some of the other endocrine glands
Anterior pituitary or adenohypophysis	Growth hormone (GH)	Bone, muscle and body tissue growth
	Prolactin (PRL)	Activates milk production in the mammary glands during pregnancy
	Thyroid stimulating hormone (TSH)	Stimulates the thyroid gland to produce thyroid hormones
	Adrenocorticotropic hormone (ACTH)	Stimulates the adrenal glands to produce hormones
	Follicle stimulating hormone (FSH) – also known as gonadotropin	Regulates the functions of the ovaries and testes, including the production and secretion of oestrogen and progesterone
Posterior pituitary or neurohypophysis	Does not produce its own hormones	Receives and stores the neurohormones ADH and oxytocin (see below) from the hypothalamus
Thyroid gland	Thyroxine triiodothyronine	Affect almost every cell in the body by regulating the metabolic rates of carbohydrates, proteins and fat; increase heat production as energy for use by the body; stimulate oxygen take-up by the body (except the brain), important role in skeletal muscle growth and development of the nervous system in children.
	Calcitonin	Decreases the level of calcium in the blood when the levels are high
Parathyroid gland	Parathyroid hormone (PTH)	Increases the level of calcium in the blood when the levels are low
Adrenal glands		
Adrenal cortex	Secretion of corticosteroids:	
	Glucocorticoids	Regulate glucose levels and metabolism of food; acts as an anti-inflammatory agent for immunity; affects growth and development and provides resistance to physical and emotional stress
	Mineralocorticoids	Regulate water and ion balance in the body together with the enzyme renin, produced by the kidneys (see below), and angiotensin (produced in the liver)
	Gonadocorticoids	These have a small effect on onset of puberty and sexual development

Continued

Table 20.5 Endocrine glands, hormones and functions—cont'd

Organ/gland	Hormone	Functions
Adrenal medulla		
	Epinephrine (adrenalin)	During stress these hormones produce the 'fright, fight or flight' response in the body by causing the body to act quickly; e.g. increases heart rate and blood pressure; dilating blood vessels, etc.
		Given as an intravenous injection during allergic reactions; e.g. reactions to iodine during radiographic procedures, and has the greater effect on the heart and metabolism
	Norepinephrine (noradrenalin)	Acts as neurotransmitter as part of the nervous system and has the greater effect on the blood vessels
Pancreas (islets of Langerhans)	Insulin	Lowers blood nutrient levels when they are high, especially glucose
	Glucagon	Increase blood glucose levels when they are low by converting glycogen to glucose
		Levels of both insulin and glucogon are regulated by somatostatin that is produced by the hypothalamus
Gonads	Testosterone	Stimulates the production of sperm; maintains growth of sexual organs and development of sexual behaviour; stimulates growth changes associated with puberty; e.g. facial and pubic hair, deepening of voice, etc.
	Oestrogen	Regulates menstrual cycle, development of mammary glands and female sexual characteristics
Others		
Kidneys	Renin	Influences blood pressure; sodium–water balance and volume
	Erythropoietin	Stimulates bone marrow to produce red blood cells
Pineal gland	Melatonin	Helps to regulate the sleep–wake cycle
Thymus	Thymosin	Helps in the development of T lymphocytes (also known as T cells) for immunity
Heart	Atrial natriuretic peptide (ANP)	Helps in the regulation of blood pressure
Digestive tract	Secretin	Neutralises gastric acid
	Cholecystokinin	Activates contraction of the gall bladder to secrete bile
Placenta	Oestrogen, progesterone and chorionic gonadotropin	Occurs during pregnancy to help maintain pregnancy
Prostate and throughout the body	Prostaglandins	Regulate blood pressure, digestive secretions; aid immunity by providing an anti-inflammatory response
Blood cells (basophils)	Histamine	Provides a response during an allergic or inflammatory process (e.g. causes bronchoconstriction); is reversed by the action of antihistamines

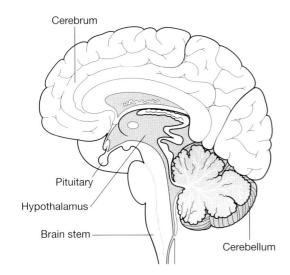

Figure 20.26 Hypothalamus and hypophysis (pituitary gland).

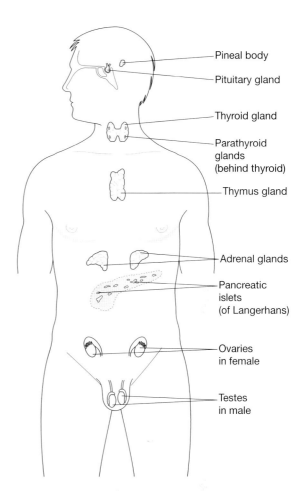

Figure 20.27 Endocrine glands of the body.

Recommended reading

Waugh A, Grant A. Ross and Wilson: Anatomy and physiology in health and illness, 9th edn. London: Elsevier; 2002.

This text is ideal for further information on anatomy and physiology as the overall content provides just the right depth in detail and has a good, reader friendly structure with clear illustrations.

Chapter **21**

Pathology

Stuart Grange

KEY POINTS

- Pathology is the study of disease.
- The purpose of medical imaging is to demonstrate the presence or absence of disease, so it is important for imaging practitioners to have some understanding of the types they might encounter.
- Many diseases share common pathological processes relating to the causation and progression of the illness.
- Understanding these general concepts in pathology can aid in the understanding of diseases specific to particular regions of the body.

INTRODUCTION

This chapter provides an overview of pathology relevant to radiography. Pathology is a complex subject – it is only possible to cover some fundamental ideas in this chapter.

An overview of the pathology of the following systems are included:

- Skeletal
- Cardiovascular
- Respiratory
- Digestive
- Urinary
- Nervous.

INFECTION

Infection occurs when microorganisms multiply in tissues where they are normally absent or present in only small numbers. Those that cause disease are described as *pathogenic* (Table 21.1). The types of microorganism involved in infection include bacteria, viruses, yeast, fungi and protozoa.

INFLAMMATION

Inflammation is a physiological process that may occur in response to infection, damage or some other disruption of the normal tissue structure. Inflammation is beneficial where it assists in the destruction or isolation of invading organisms; however, it is also possible for harmful effects to result from it. Inflamed tissue may be broken down by the release of digestive enzymes from cells of the immune system, such as neutrophils and macrophages. The swelling associated with inflammation may be harmful if it causes compression of the tissue around it. For example, inflammation in the respiratory tract may result in airway obstruction, or in the brain may result in increased intracranial pressure and impaired blood flow.

Table 21.1 Examples of pathogenic microorganism

Disease	Organism and type	Effect
Tuberculosis (TB)	*Mycobacterium tuberculosis* (bacterial)	Pulmonary or other organ infection resulting in chronic inflammation and tissue destruction
Cholera	*Vibrio cholera* (bacterial)	Severe diarrhoea
Pneumonia	*Streptococcus pneumoniae* and others (bacterial)	Pulmonary inflammation with fever
Osteomyelitis	*Staphylococcus aureus* and others (bacterial)	Often chronic bone infection resulting in pain and swelling
Gangrene	*Clostridium perfringens* (bacterial)	Severe tissue destruction resulting in tissue death and putrefaction
Acquired immune deficiency syndrome (AIDS)	Human immunodeficiency virus (HIV)	Destruction of T lymphocytes resulting in increased susceptibility to infection and development of rare tumours; e.g. Kaposi's sarcoma
Influenza	Influenza virus	Severe respiratory tract infection. Potentially fatal depending on the strain
Squamous epithelial tumours	Human papilloma virus	Malignant transformation of infected squamous epithelium, especially in the cervix
Viral hepatitis	Hepatitis B virus and others	Liver inflammation and potentially fatal
Pneumonia	*Pneumocystis carinii* (fungus)	Another cause of pneumonia, particularly in the immunocompromised; e.g. AIDS
Aspergillosis	*Aspergillus fumigatus* (fungus)	Chronic lung infection
Thrush	*Candida albicans* (yeast)	Mucous membrane lesions
Malaria	*Plasmodium* (protozoa)	Fever, anaemia, liver, spleen and lymph node enlargement. Potentially fatal

Inflammation may be of rapid (acute) or slow (chronic) onset.

ACUTE INFLAMMATION

Acute inflammation displays typical features:

- Warmth and redness – results from increased blood flow to the area, known as hyperaemia.
- Swelling – occurs because of infiltration of proteins and fluid from the blood into the extracellular spaces as a result of increased permeability of the blood vessel walls. The accumulated protein rich fluid is called exudate. Cells of the immune system, mainly neutrophils and macrophages, also migrate into the tissues from the blood to destroy infecting organisms or digest damaged tissue.
- Pain – occurs as a result of stretching of the tissues and the release of chemical mediators of acute inflammation.

Causes of acute inflammation include:

- infection
- physical – trauma, radiation, burns or frostbite
- immunological – hypersensitivity to a substance
- chemical – corrosive or poisonous
- tissue death (necrosis).

CHRONIC INFLAMMATION

Chronic inflammation differs from acute inflammation in the cell types present (fewer neutrophils and more lymphocytes) and the increased amount of granulation tissue (new capillaries and fibrous tissue) formed.

Causes of chronic inflammation include:

- infection – especially where the organism is resistant to killing by immune cells, e.g. tuberculosis, leprosy
- necrotic fat or bone
- foreign bodies or particles – implants or mineral dust and fibres
- autoimmune diseases
- specific diseases of unknown cause, e.g. ulcerative colitis
- as a consequence of repeated acute inflammation, e.g. cholecystitis.

CONSEQUENCES OF INFLAMMATION

There are a variety of potential outcomes for inflamed tissue.

Resolution

The most favourable outcome of inflammation is repair of the damaged or infected tissue, with restitution of function and minimal scarring. Some tissues are much better able to repair themselves than others. For example, bone and other connective tissues can usually repair themselves completely, but the central nervous system cannot.

Suppuration

Infection by certain organisms produces large amounts of pus. Pus is a mixture of tissue debris, living and dead bacteria and neutrophils. A collection of pus may become 'walled off' by an outer fibrous coat. This is referred to as an abscess. Sometimes a channel called a sinus opens up between the abscess and the skin surface, or the between the abscess and a hollow organ – a fistula.

Ulceration

The surface tissue of an organ is lost and replaced by inflammatory tissue, forming a crater. If the ulcer is in the wall of a hollow organ it is susceptible to perforation; for example a duodenal ulcer.

Fibrosis

Scar tissue may be formed from inflamed tissue, particularly where there has been a large amount of tissue destruction, or the exudate, and debris cannot be removed. This may lead to distortion of the organ shape, or adhesions between one organ and another.

CARCINOGENESIS

Tissues that are growing or that have to replace cells lost or damaged as part of their normal function will show rapid cell division; in other tissues cell division will be very slow. In both cases the process is highly coordinated to ensure that the tissue is renewed in a way appropriate to its

Box 21.1   Types of tumour

Carcinoma	A cancer of epithelial tissue origin. Often prefixed by the type of epithelium; e.g squamous cell carcinoma; transitional cell carcinoma.
Sarcoma	A cancer of connective tissue origin. Often prefixed by the type of connective tissue; e.g osteosarcoma; chondrosarcoma.
Teratoma	A cancer of germ cell tissue origin; e.g. testicular.
Lymphoma	A cancer of lymphoid tissue origin.
Adenoma	A tumour of glandular epithelium.
Papilloma	A tumour of non-glandular epithelium.
Adenocarcinoma	A cancer of glandular epithelium.
Melanoma	A cancer of pigment producing cells found in the skin.
Glioma	A cancer of neuroglia in the central nervous system.

function. Sometimes this careful coordination is lost and a cell may begin to divide more frequently than normal. As a result a mass of abnormal tissue may form which may be referred to as a *neoplasm* or *tumour*. The transformation of normal tissues or benign tumours into cancer is called *carcinogenesis*. Box 21.1 explains some of the terminology relating to tumours.

CANCER INCIDENCE

Cancer incidence increases with age (Fig. 21.1). The transformation of a normal cell into a cell that will form a tumour is primarily a genetic event, but this may be triggered by environmental factors. Cells from older people have had more time to experience the environmental factors that can lead to carcinogenesis and this may explain the increasing incidence with age. Table 21.2 gives details of some commonly seen cancers.

TUMOUR BEHAVIOUR

Benign tumours

- Slow-growing masses.
- Have well-defined margins.
- Do not invade adjacent tissues or spread to other parts of the body.

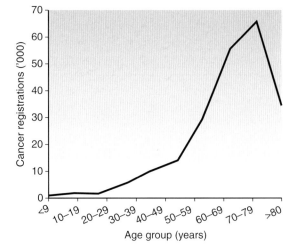

Figure 21.1 Incidence of cancer in different age groups in the UK.

- Cause problems by compressing adjacent structures.
- Those arising from endocrine organs may result in the over-secretion of a hormone.

Malignant tumours

- Have poorly defined margins.
- Invade adjacent organs and structures.
- Are typified by their tendency to spread throughout the body (metastasis), which they

Table 21.2 Description of some commonly seen cancers

Organ	Tissue of origin	Causes	Secondary spread	Prognosis
Lung	Mainly bronchus	Predominantly smoking	Bone, liver, brain, lymph nodes	Very poor
Bladder	Epithelial lining of bladder	Industrial chemicals; smoking	Liver, lungs, bone, adrenals	Poor if metastasis has occurred
Colorectal	Glandular epithelium lining the bowel	Linked to increased intake of saturated animals fats and poor intake of dietary fibre	Liver, lymph nodes	Poor if not diagnosed early
Breast	Milk producing lobules and ducts	Linked to genetic factors and exposure of breast tissue to oestrogen	Bone, liver, brain, lymph nodes	Generally poor if not diagnosed early
Prostate	Glandular epithelium of the prostate	Linked to age-related hormonal changes	Bone, liver, lungs, lymph nodes	A number of effective treatments prolong life, but cure is not common

do either by the lymphatic channels or through the blood.

The grading and staging of malignant tumours

The prognosis of a person's cancer is determined by both its grade and its stage. Grade refers to how well differentiated the tumour cells are; that is, how much like the tissue of origin they are. Poorly differentiated cells that have lost the particular characteristics of the organ from which they arise tend to form more aggressive tumours. Stage is determined by the size of the primary tumour and the degree of spread to local or remote organs and lymph nodes. Table 21.3 explains the staging scheme used for breast cancer.

CANCER TREATMENT

Cancer treatment is usually simpler when the tumour is confined to a discrete area, and may be removable by surgery. Infiltration of adjacent tissues or metastasis may require radiotherapy or systemic treatments such as chemotherapy.

SKELETAL SYSTEM

The skeleton consists of 206 bones connected by mobile and fixed joints. Bone is living tissue and is susceptible to disease like any other.

DELAYED FRACTURE HEALING

The speed of fracture healing is highly variable, depending on their complexity and the age of patient, but an uncomplicated fracture in a child may show complete healing within 8 weeks. On occasions the normal process of reunification of bone fragments may be delayed or not occur at all. The following factors may be responsible:

- Excessive movement at the fracture site.
- Extensive damage leading to bone necrosis.
- Poor intrinsic blood supply.
- Interruption of blood supply.

Table 21.3 The main staging systems used to assess the extent of spread of breast carcinomas

Stage	Extent of spread
International classification	
I	Lump with slight tethering to skin, but node negative
II	Lump with lymph node metastasis or skin tethering
III	Tumour which is extensively adherent to skin and/or underlying muscles, or ulcerating or lymph nodes are fixed
IV	Distant metastases
TNM	
T_1	Tumour 20 mm or less; no fixation or nipple retraction. Includes Paget's disease
T_2	Tumour 20–50 mm, or less than 20 mm but with tethering
T_3	Tumour greater than 50 mm but less than 100 mm; or less than 50 mm but with infiltration, ulceration or fixation
T_4	Any tumour with ulceration or infiltration wide of it, or chest wall fixation, or greater than 100 mm in diameter
N_0	Node-negative
N_1	Axillary nodes mobile
N_2	Axillary nodes fixed
N_3	Supraclavicular nodes or oedema of arm
M_0	No distant metastases
M_1	Distant metastases

- Infection at the fracture site.
- Interposition of soft tissue in the fracture gap or wide separation of fragments.

Failure of a fracture to mend is called *non-union*. This may result in prolonged pain (e.g. non-union of the scaphoid) and loss of normal function such as the ability to weight bear (e.g. the tibia).

OSTEOPOROSIS

Osteoporosis is primarily a condition of old age caused by loss of the bone connective tissue matrix. Mineralisation of the matrix is normal. This distinguishes it from the condition, osteomalacia, where the matrix is normal but undermineralised.

The loss of bone mass in osteoporosis weakens the bones so that fractures become more likely –

wrist and hip fractures are common. Weakening of the vertebral bodies causes gradual height reduction and often wedge-shaped compression fractures.

The causes of osteoporosis are:

- menopause (may be preventable with hormone replacement therapy)
- old age
- endocrine disease
- inadequate nutrition.

Osteoporosis is seen radiographically as a loss of bone density (*osteopaenia*) when greater than 30% of the bone mass is lost. Vertebral body height reduction and wedge fractures are typical appearances in the spine.

ARTHRITIS

Arthritis is a disease of the synovial joints. Pain and loss of mobility results from damage to the hyaline cartilage articular surfaces. In the healthy joint, the articular cartilage is smooth, facilitating the sliding of one bone against the other. In arthritis, the cartilage is thinned and loses its smooth surfaces, increasing friction between the articulating bones. Two important forms of arthritis are *osteoarthritis* and *rheumatoid*.

Osteoarthritis affects mainly the elderly and is primarily a condition of the weight-bearing joints, though other joints are also affected. Common presentation includes:

- loss of cartilage thickness
- bony outgrowths called *osteophytes* around the cartilage margins
- thickening of the subchondral bone.

As a result of these changes, those with osteoarthritis may experience pain on movement, stiffness and joint instability. If this becomes severe it may be necessary to perform a total joint replacement (Fig. 21.2).

Rheumatoid arthritis may affect the young as well as the old, though it commonly begins between the ages of 30 and 50. It differs from osteoarthritis in that it is fundamentally an inflammatory condition. Common changes are as follows:

- The synovium lining the joint capsule becomes inflamed and begins to encroach onto the

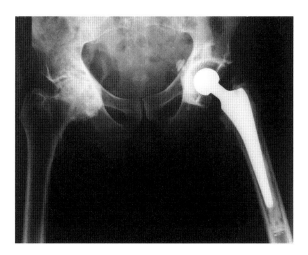

Figure 21.2 Radiograph of the pelvis showing advanced osteoarthritis in the *right* hip joint, with sclerotic bone growth in the femoral head and acetabulum and loss of the joint space. The *left* side has a total hip replacement.

articular surface, causing erosion of the cartilage.
- Eventually the cartilage is completely destroyed and there is a loss of any normal joint space.
- The peripheral joints are commonly affected.
- Loss of normal joint architecture can result in severe deformities, and this is especially evident in the fingers (Fig. 21.3).

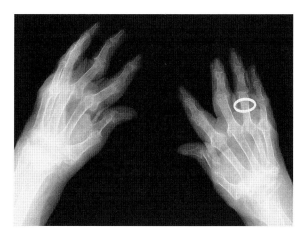

Figure 21.3 Radiograph of the hands showing severe erosions of the metacarpophalangeal and interphalangeal joints, due to rheumatoid arthritis.

- Severe rheumatoid arthritis in the upper cervical spine can cause spinal instability and potential spinal cord damage.

OSTEOMYELITIS

Osteomyelitis is an infection of the bone by bacteria, most often *Staphylococcus aureus*. The infecting organisms gain access to the bone through a wound, such as an open fracture, or via the blood stream. Infection via the blood stream is referred to as *haematogenous* osteomyelitis, the bacteria entering the bone marrow through the nutrient artery.

The bone is painful and the overlying soft tissue swollen. There may also be a generalised fever, as is typical of many infections. If the infection becomes chronic some of the bone may die. There is also the possibility of sinus formation, which drains pus to the skin surface.

Osteomyelitis can be difficult to eradicate. The treatment is by antibiotic therapy and, sometimes, surgical removal of the infected bone.

PAGET'S DISEASE

Paget's is a fairly common disease affecting the elderly, arising from a disordering of normal bone turnover. Affected bones are characterised by an increase in bone synthesis, resulting in a thickened and sclerotic 'cotton wool' appearance radiographically. Paget's usually affects the pelvis, skull and long bones, often progressing from one end towards the centre. Weight-bearing bones affected by Paget's, such as the femur and tibia, can become bowed (Fig. 21.4). When the skull is affected there may be encroachment on the cranial nerve foramina, causing various neurological symptoms including vertigo, blindness and deafness.

BONE TUMOURS

- Primary bone tumours are uncommon.
- The most frequently encountered is osteosarcoma, which usually presents between the ages of 10 and 20:

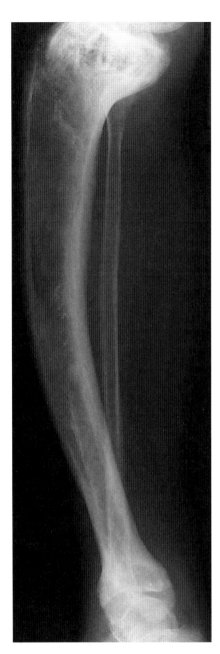

Figure 21.4 Deformity of the weight-bearing long bones occurs due to weakening of the bone structure through Paget's disease.

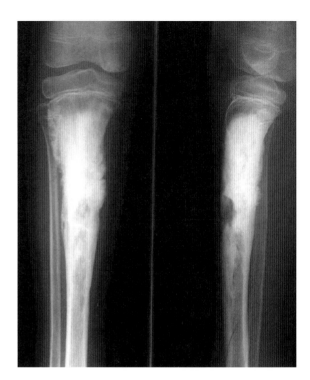

Figure 21.5 Osteosarcoma in the proximal tibia, showing spiculated reactive bone growth under the periosteum.

Secondary bone tumours

- Secondary bone tumours resulting from metastasis from other malignant primary cancers are far more common (Fig. 21.6).
- Cancers typically metastasising to bone are breast, prostate, lung, kidney and thyroid.
- Appear *lytic* (destruction of bone) or *sclerotic* (increased bone density).
- Bone metastases are often painful and may be associated with pathological fractures due to weakening of the bone structure.

CARDIOVASCULAR SYSTEM

Most deaths in Western countries are the result of diseases of the heart and blood vessels. A sufficient supply of blood is essential for the normal function of all of the tissues of the body. When deprived of it they will quickly deplete the oxygen that they require for normal metabolism, leading to cell damage or death.

  – often situated in the large long bones like the tibia, femur and humerus, adjacent to the epiphyseal plate (Fig. 21.5).
  – typical radiographic appearance of patchy bone destruction, sometimes with formation of bone spicules resulting in a sunburst appearance.

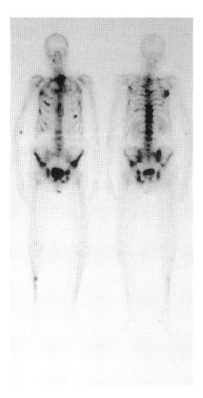

Figure 21.6 Radionuclide bone scan showing areas of increased tracer uptake representing metastases.

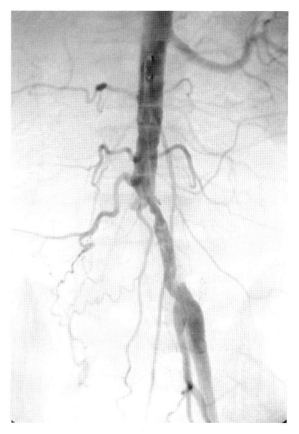

Figure 21.7 Digital subtraction angiogram demonstrating complete occlusion at the origin of the right common iliac artery due to atherosclerosis.

ISCHAEMIA AND INFARCTION

Ischaemia is the reduction or loss of blood supply to a part of the body.

An *infarct* is a region of tissue where the cells have died due to ischaemia.

The main cause of ischaemia and infarction is *atherosclerosis*. This is the gradual accumulation of fatty deposits (*atheroma*) on the inner surface of an artery, which will cause narrowing (*stenosis*) and ultimately block it (*occlusion*) (Fig. 21.7). Atherosclerosis is associated with high levels of cholesterol and other lipids (fats) in the blood, smoking and elevated blood pressure. Arteries that have atherosclerosis are more prone to developing blood clots and this may cause a stenosed vessel to become occluded. Figure 21.8 shows possible complications of atherosclerosis.

Ischaemia and infarction may occur anywhere in the body. They are most immediately life-threatening when they occur in the heart or brain.

THROMBOSIS

One of the normal protective mechanisms of the body is blood clotting, which occurs in response to vascular damage to limit blood loss. A blood clot can also occur pathologically when there is no vascular damage, and this is referred to as a thrombus.

Deep vein thrombosis (DVT)

This occurs in the deep veins of the lower limbs, often as a result of slow blood flow associated

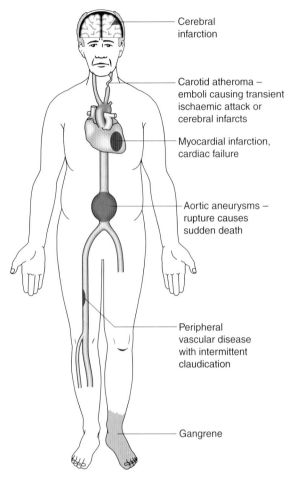

Cerebral infarction

Carotid atheroma – emboli causing transient ischaemic attack or cerebral infarcts

Myocardial infarction, cardiac failure

Aortic aneurysms – rupture causes sudden death

Peripheral vascular disease with intermittent claudication

Gangrene

Figure 21.8 The complications of atherosclerosis.

with immobility; for example on long journeys or postoperatively. The return of blood from the limbs to the heart is impeded by the blockage of the veins and the leg may become red, swollen and tender.

Pulmonary embolism (PE)

This is a due to a mass of material (an *embolus*) lodging in the pulmonary arteries. The embolus is usually thrombus but sometimes fat or other matter. It often occurs secondary to a DVT when some of the clot breaks away from its site of formation in the leg. PE is a serious and potentially fatal condition depending on how much of the lung's arterial blood supply is affected.

ISCHAEMIC HEART DISEASE (IHD)

Ischaemia of the myocardium often results in severe chest pain referred to as *angina pectoris*. It is caused by increased oxygen demand, such as during exertion, in myocardium that is supplied by diseased coronary arteries. The arteries are unable to supply blood rapidly enough to the myocardium because they are stenosed, and the muscle suffers oxygen starvation.

Myocardial infarction (MI) occurs when the myocardium is starved of oxygen long enough for the cells in a particular region to die, usually due to occlusion of a coronary artery. The occlusion may occur suddenly if a thrombus forms on an area of atherosclerotic vessel. If a sufficiently large portion of the heart muscle becomes infarcted the patient may die as the heart will be unable to pump blood adequately, or it may stop – a cardiac arrest. Non-lethal MIs cause severe chest pain and the patient's heart will be damaged. The infarcted muscle will be replaced with scar tissue that lacks the ability to contract and therefore the heart's pumping efficiency is reduced.

Signs and symptoms of MI:

- severe crushing chest pain (in men, frequently absent in women), with sweating and nausea
- shortness of breath
- changes in the electrocardiograph trace
- increased blood levels of cardiac enzymes released from damaged myocardium.

Patients with suspected MI need urgent hospitalisation to receive treatment that minimises the risk of further damage to the heart or death.

HEART FAILURE

When the pumping capacity of the heart does not meet the needs of the body it is said to be in failure. Heart failure may affect the left, right or both ventricles and usually leads to their enlargement and accumulation of fluid in the tissues that feed blood to them (Fig. 21.9).

- Left-sided failure will result in congestion of the lungs with fluid (pulmonary oedema),

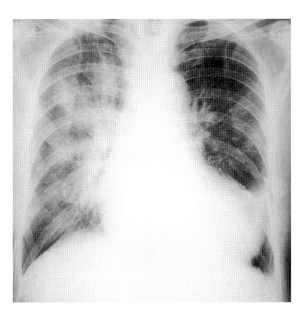

Figure 21.9 Chest radiograph demonstrating enlargement of the heart, and lung oedema due to failure. Enlargement of the heart occurs due to dilatation and ventricular hypertrophy.

because the left ventricle is unable to pump enough blood out of the lungs and into the systemic circulation.

- Right-sided failure causes systemic fluid accumulation for similar reasons. Left-sided failure eventually leads to right failure. When both sides are affected it is usually termed *congestive cardiac failure*.
- Failure of the left ventricle may be due to hypertension, which causes it to have to work hard to expel blood into the systemic circulation, or because of ischaemic heart disease, which damages the myocardium and makes it inefficient at pumping. Patients with heart failure are breathless due to pulmonary oedema and have peripheral oedema, especially in the lower limbs.
- Failure of the right ventricle may be due to mitral valve stenosis or chronic obstructive pulmonary disease and bronchiectasis, which, as lung tissue is destroyed, reduces the available capillary volume causing the vascular resistance to increase. Both of

these diseases result in increased pulmonary pressure, and therefore right heart strain.

HEART VALVE DISEASE

The heart valves should ensure the efficient progress of blood through the heart from atrium to ventricle, and then into the aorta and pulmonary trunk. Diseased valves may either:

- become fused together and impede the flow of blood through them due to stenosis, or
- allow blood to flow back into the chamber it has just left. This is known as *regurgitation* or *incompetence*, and is a result of incomplete closure of the valve leaflets.

These effects are caused by hardening of the valve leaflets as a result of calcification, or scarring from rheumatic fever, a bacterial infection in childhood. The growth of bacterial vegetations on the valves may also worsen valve disorders – this is called *infective endocarditis*.

The greatest clinical significance is attached to disease of the mitral and aortic valves:

- Mitral stenosis – increased resistance to the flow of blood through the valve results in pulmonary hypertension; left atrial and right ventricular hypertrophy; right-sided heart failure.
- Mitral regurgitation – blood refluxes into the left atrium from the left ventricle during systole causing inefficient pumping. The left atrium and ventricle dilate and the muscle becomes thickened to compensate. There may be ultimately left-sided heart failure.
- Aortic stenosis – obstruction to the left ventricular outflow causes left ventricular hypertrophy to overcome the valve's resistance to flow. There is an increased risk of ischaemia and left-sided heart failure.
- Aortic regurgitation – blood refluxes back into the left ventricle from the aorta during diastole. Loss of efficiency in the systolic stroke means that the ventricle must pump a larger volume of blood to maintain adequate supply to the body – the ventricle dilates and hypertrophies. Left-sided heart failure results.

ANEURYSM

An aneurysm is an abnormal enlargement of the diameter of an artery, usually associated with atherosclerosis. The vessel wall may become thin, weakened and more liable to rupture. Common sites for aneurysm are the aorta and other large arteries (Fig. 21.10). Rupture of a large artery is very serious because of the possibility of fatal haemorrhage.

Aneurysms found in the arterial supply of the brain are often congenital. They are usually small in size, but serious in outcome as their rupture will compromise the brain's blood supply and the leaked blood can cause pressure on it.

DIABETES MELLITUS

The hormone insulin causes cells to take up and store glucose and lipids. In diabetes mellitus the levels of glucose and lipids within the blood are elevated because of insufficient insulin, or inability of the cells to respond to it. The high levels of lipids cause an increase in atheroma within the blood vessels and hence reduced blood flow. There are also changes to the capillary vessels, with development of microaneurysms (especially within the retina, renal glomeruli and nerves). Blood flow to certain regions such as the kidneys

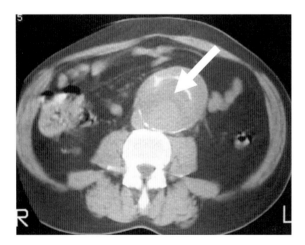

Figure 21.10 This axial computed tomography scan through the abdomen shows gross enlargement of the abdominal aorta due to an aneurysm.

and peripheral vasculature can be severely compromised in diabetes mellitus. Individuals with poorly controlled diabetes are prone to foot ulcers and gangrene, and damage to the kidney tissue and retina. Even in well-controlled diabetes, stroke is twice as likely, and myocardial infarction 3–5 times more likely than in the non-diabetic population.

RESPIRATORY SYSTEM

The respiratory system is responsible for oxygenating the blood and eliminating carbon dioxide. A series of increasingly narrow airways bring air to the alveoli where this gas exchange can occur. Having a very large surface area increases efficiency. Diseases that restrict the airflow in and out of the lungs or that reduce the surface area have a profound effect on respiration.

PNEUMONIA

Pneumonia is the inflammation of the distal airways and alveoli, usually in response to an infection. The infective agent is often bacterial but may also be viral, such as influenza, or fungal (e.g. *Pneumocystis carinii*). It presents as an acute illness with fever, cough and purulent sputum. It is a major cause of death in those over 70 years old.

As part of the inflammatory process, exudate accumulates in the airspaces. This is called consolidation and is evident on the chest radiograph as opacification.

Pneumonia may be classified according to its anatomical distribution:

- Bronchopneumonia
  - patchy consolidation throughout the lungs
  - common in patients debilitated through age (either the very young or old) or serious disease.
- Lobar pneumonia
  - affects diffusely an entire lobe
  - there may be no predisposing factors
  - 90% due to pneumococcus (*Streptococcus pneumoniae*).

CHRONIC OBSTRUCTIVE PULMONARY DISEASE (COPD)

COPD is a term describing the presence of *chronic bronchitis* and *emphysema* simultaneously. A diagnosis of chronic bronchitis is made on clinical grounds when a chronic productive cough exists for at least 3 months of the year over two consecutive years. It has the following features:

- It is usually caused by smoking.
- Inflammation of bronchioles results from irritation of the lining.
- There is hypertrophy of mucus-secreting epithelium causing increased mucus secretion.
- There is increased susceptibility to lung infection.
- Inflammation and infection result in obstruction of airflow through the bronchioles.

Emphysema is also present to a variable degree in COPD. In emphysema:

- Smoking accounts for a large proportion of cases.
- There is a loss of lung surface area due to the fusion of alveoli.
- There is a loss of alveolar elasticity that deprives the airways of their structural support, leading to reduced airflow.

The appearances of COPD on chest radiography are only obvious in severe cases where it is possible to see hyperinflation of the lungs, with flattening of the diaphragm, and increased lucency of the lung fields due to increased X-ray transmission.

BRONCHIECTASIS

Bronchiectasis is characterised by permanent abnormal dilatation of the bronchi (Fig. 21.11). Patients experience a chronic cough, producing large amounts of sputum and having difficulty in breathing (*dyspnoea*). It is caused by severe, recurrent or chronic infection. Associated inflammation leads to scarring and destruction of the airways, which become permanently enlarged.

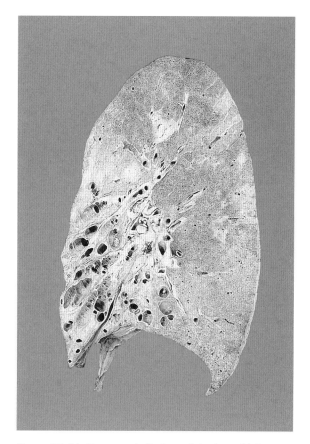

Figure 21.11 Permanent dilation of the bronchi, known as bronchiectasis.

TUBERCULOSIS (TB)

Infection by the bacterium *Mycobacterium tuberculosis* may affect any tissue of the body but is most often found in the lungs, the bacteria normally gaining entry to the body via the airways. Infection is usually through close contact with someone infected with TB in an active stage. Individuals whose immune systems are compromised are at much greater risk of developing infection; those infected with HIV are therefore at greater risk. TB infection often presents with low-grade fever, cough, weight loss, fatigue and night sweats.

The primary focus of infection is normally the mid/upper zone of the lungs where pulmonary lesions known as Ghon complexes form. In this primary stage of infection the disease is usually clinically silent, as the bacteria are walled off within a granuloma. The bacteria may migrate from the initial infection site to the lung apices (secondary tuberculosis) or become widely disseminated throughout the lungs and other organs (miliary tuberculosis).

PNEUMOTHORAX

Normally, the visceral pleura of the lungs adhere to the parietal pleura of the thoracic cavity or the mediastinum by the surface tension created by a thin layer of pleural fluid. In a pneumothorax, air is introduced into the pleural space and the lung in that region no longer adheres to the parietal pleura and falls away. This may occur due to a leak of air from the outer surface of the lung, either spontaneously in healthy individuals, or as a result of pre-existing lung disease.

Depending on its size a pneumothorax will result in tachycardia, difficulty in breathing and pain on the affected side. Whilst small ones will normally spontaneously resolve, larger ones will need the insertion of a chest tube to allow the air within the pleural space to escape.

A tension pneumothorax describes a situation where air is pulled into the pleural space on inspiration that cannot escape on expiration. This is often associated with an injury penetrating the thoracic wall. The result is a steadily increasing compression of the lung on the affected side causing it to collapse, and the mediastinum is pushed away from the midline (Fig. 21.12). This obstructs venous return to the heart and decreases cardiac output. It is a medical emergency that requires urgent placement of a chest drain.

PLEURAL EFFUSION

In certain pathological conditions the amount of serous fluid secreted into the pleural space increases. These include heart failure, bacterial pneumonia, lung cancer and tuberculosis. In the erect position the fluid accumulates at the lung bases and may be identified on the chest radiograph when the volume exceeds 300 ml. If the volume of pleural effusion is very large it will interfere with respiration and must be removed via a chest drain (Fig. 21.13).

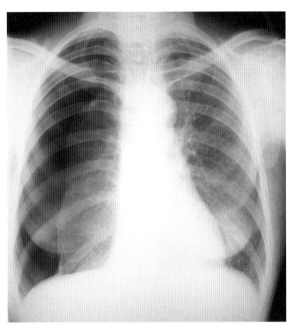

Figure 21.12 Chest radiograph with air in the pleural cavity on the *right*, which has compressed the lung. Note the increased lucency of the thoracic cavity from where the lung tissue has receded.

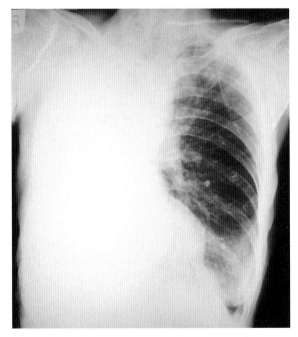

Figure 21.13 Chest radiograph showing a very large pleural effusion on the *right* side of the chest.

LUNG CANCER

Primary lung tumours

Lung cancer is the most common malignant tumour (Fig. 21.14). There are different types of lung cancer, as the tumour may arise from different cell types, though they are usually cells within the bronchi. The prognosis and treatments options are dependent on whether it is a non-small cell lung cancer (85%) or small cell lung cancer (15%).

Typical signs and symptoms are:

* chronic cough
* dyspnoea
* haemoptysis
* weight loss
* mass on chest X-ray
* hoarse voice.

The prognosis is poor for small cell lung cancer because, at the time of presenting, the disease is usually already well advanced and not suitable for surgical resection, which is the procedure offering the best chance of cure. The outlook is slightly better for the non-small cell type, as 20% present when the tumour is still resectable. Primary lung tumours metastasise to the brain, liver and bone. There may be direct invasion of the ribs adjacent to the tumour, and if the primary lesion is situated in the apex (Pancoast tumour), there may be involvement of the brachial nerve plexus, causing severe pain in the shoulder and arm. Another complication is superior vena cava obstruction as a result of compression by the tumour. Restriction of venous return results in marked oedema of the face and upper extremities.

Secondary lung tumours

Carcinoma of the breast, bone, kidney and gastrointestinal tract commonly form lung metastases (Fig. 21.15). They are usually found within the lung parenchyma and may initially be relatively asymptomatic.

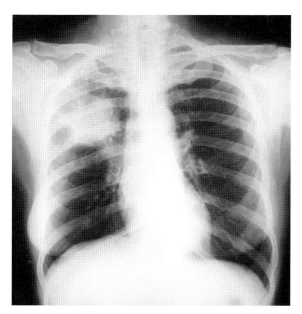

Figure 21.14 Chest radiograph demonstrating a large lung tumour in the *right* upper lobe.

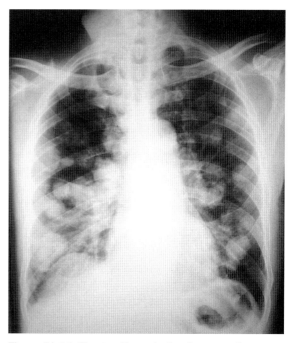

Figure 21.15 Chest radiograph showing extensive metastatic disease within the lungs.

DIGESTIVE SYSTEM

Disorders of the gastrointestinal tract can have profound effects on the sufferer. Diseases may be chronic and disabling, and in some cases life-threatening. The psychological effects of having problem bowels can also be a significant factor in an individual's ability to cope with their disease.

INFLAMMATORY BOWEL DISEASE

Inflammatory bowel disease (IBD) refers to the separate diseases of *ulcerative colitis* and *Crohn's disease*. Both are chronic illnesses that begin most often in childhood or young adulthood. The primary cause is not well understood in either case. They display a pattern of increased disease activity, including acute flare-ups followed by periods of remission. IBD is well-demonstrated by barium contrast studies and will account for a significant proportion of the gastrointestinal work of a radiology department.

Ulcerative colitis

Ulcerative colitis is characterised by inflammation resulting in ulceration of the mucosal lining of the rectum and colon. Occasionally the ulceration may extend sufficiently deeply into the intestinal wall to put it at risk of perforation.

Individuals with ulcerative colitis have abdominal pain, diarrhoea and rectal bleeding. Ulceration forms over a continuous portion of the bowel wall and leads to attempts at healing, with highly vascular granulation tissue. Bleeding occurs from these regions. The ability of the bowel to absorb water from faecal material is grossly impaired, resulting in diarrhoea.

Crohn's disease

Crohn's disease may occur anywhere in the alimentary tract but is most common in the terminal portion of the ileum (Fig. 21.16). Abdominal pain is often present. Deep linear ulcers form, which may extend through the full thickness of the wall,

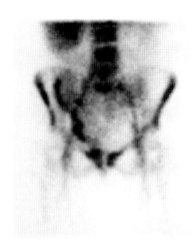

Figure 21.16 Radiolabelled white cell scan. White cells labelled with technetium-99 m migrate to areas of inflammation as well as to bone marrow. This scan shows normal marrow appearances and an intense focus of activity in the terminal ileum.

and this may result in the formation of fistulae between adjacent bowel loops or between the bowel and the skin surface, particularly around the anus. Whereas ulcerative colitis forms a continuous zone of diseased bowel, Crohn's may affect several separate portions, hence the term 'skip lesions'. The bowel develops a thickened and fibrosed wall whilst the lumen becomes stenosed, which may lead to bowel obstruction.

INTESTINAL OBSTRUCTION

Abdominal radiographs are commonly requested for investigating suspected intestinal obstruction. Obstruction may be complete or partial. The bowel proximal to the obstruction accumulates fluid and gas, causing the typical radiographic appearance of dilated bowel loops. Deciding whether the obstruction is in the large or small bowel can be made on the basis of the distribution, diameter and shape of the gas pattern (Fig. 21.17).

Intestinal obstruction is a serious condition because it results in congestion, oedema and eventual death of the proximal bowel. There may be migration of faecal bacteria into the bloodstream from the damaged bowel wall, or it may perforate, resulting in *peritonitis* (a severe infection and inflammation of the peritoneal cavity).

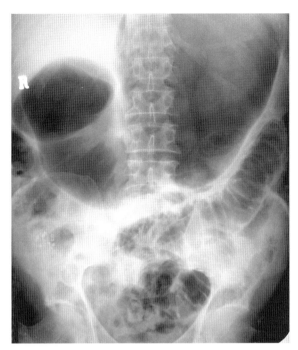

Figure 21.17 Abdominal radiograph showing dilated and gas-filled bowel due to obstruction.

Causes of intestinal obstruction:

- Hernia – the bowel protrudes through an aperture in the abdominal wall. Initially, these may be reducible, but if allowed to persist the bowel becomes congested and swollen. At this point the bowel may become trapped (*strangulated*). Blood flow out of the herniated bowel is obstructed so it may die.
- Volvulus – the bowel becomes twisted around itself, causing a complete obstruction.
- Intussusception – a section of bowel folds into the section of bowel immediately distal to it. It is caused by increased bulkiness of the bowel because of swelling or a polyp, which is then pulled into the distal bowel by peristalsis. The consequences are similar to hernia if the intussusception is not reduced.
- Adhesions – these can occur in the peritoneal cavity following surgery or peritonitis. Fibrosis following healing of

inflamed or damaged peritoneum causes kinks or twists in the bowel that may cause obstruction.
- Tumour – a tumour may become so large that it obstructs the passage of faecal material, or it may form a narrow stricture.
- Paralytic ileus – sometimes the cause of obstruction is due to an absence of motility rather than a mechanical obstruction. In paralytic ileus the muscular wall of the bowel fails to contract and becomes distended.

DIVERTICULAR DISEASE

Diverticula are blind-ended pouches of bowel mucosa on the outside of the bowel wall. It is thought that they form where the muscular wall of the bowel is penetrated by blood vessels and therefore potentially weakened. There is an association with a low-fibre diet and increased age.

As they are open-ended towards the bowel lumen, diverticula are filled with faeces, which can become stagnant and inflamed (Fig. 21.18). The presence of diverticula is called *diverticulosis*; when one or more are inflamed the condition is called *diverticulitis*. This is experienced as abdominal pain and fever. Complications of diverticulitis include abscess formation and perforation.

PEPTIC ULCER DISEASE (PUD)

A peptic ulcer is found in the stomach or duodenum. It may present with upper abdominal pain that is relieved by food, or be clinically silent. This disease is commonly investigated in the radiology department by barium meal, where it will be demonstrated as a cratered area of the mucosal lining. Ulceration of the gastric or duodenal mucosa is dependent on excess gastric acid secretion.

Bleeding from peptic ulcers may result in sufficient blood loss to cause anaemia, and may also be evidenced by digested blood in the stool (*melaena*). Peptic ulcers may be sufficiently severe to perforate the bowel wall, allowing bowel contents and gas to escape into the peritoneal cavity. Erect chest X-rays are often requested in suspected

Figure 21.18 Double contrast barium enema, showing diverticular disease.

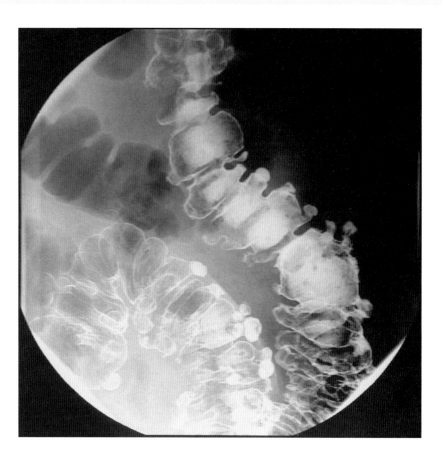

peptic ulcer perforation to identify gas collected beneath the diaphragm, which is indicative of this condition.

COLORECTAL CANCER

There is an association of colorectal cancer with high dietary intake of saturated fats and low intake of dietary fibre, which may explain its high incidence in developed countries. The risk of developing colorectal cancer increases significantly after the age of 40.

The majority of bowel cancers are carcinomas, which are thought to arise from sporadic polyps that develop from the bowel mucosa. Initially these are benign, but there is an increasing association with malignant transformation as they get larger. Approximately 50% are found in the rectum, 30% in the sigmoid and the remainder in the rest of the colon.

Bowel cancers may appear as a fungating mass with an ulcerated centre or as a complete ring of tumour growth. The latter is associated with marked fibrosis that causes the bowel to constrict, forming an annular stricture. This type gives the typical apple core appearance shown by barium enema (Fig. 21.19).

Tumour cells breaking away into the bloodstream are directed expressly to the liver via the hepatic portal system where they will be captured and may develop into secondary deposits. Infiltration of the tumour into the numerous lymphatic channels draining the bowel leads to involvement of the lymph nodes. Cases with liver and lymph node involvement have a poor long-term prognosis; however colorectal cancer has a good chance of cure if it is detected and treated at an early stage. Alterations of bowel habit, especially with evidence of blood in the stool, should always be investigated thoroughly at the earliest opportunity.

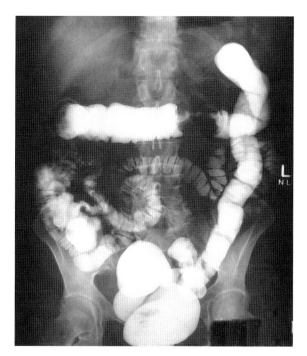

Figure 21.19 Barium enema demonstrating an annular stricture in the transverse colon representing an adenocarcinoma.

URINARY SYSTEM

The kidneys are vital to good health, eliminating unwanted products of metabolism and helping to maintain a stable chemical environment within the body through homeostasis. The purpose of the remainder of the urinary tract is essentially of urine storage or elimination. Disorders of the urinary tract can cause serious and sometimes life-threatening disease.

PYELONEPHRITIS

Pyelonephritis is infection of the kidney tissue. In the acute phase there is pus formation associated with typical symptoms of infection, such as fever, nausea and rigors. If recurrent infections occur, the kidney may become damaged through scar formation, which replaces the functioning tubular tissue. This is most likely to occur in children where there is reflux of urine from the bladder into the ureters due to incompetent ureteral valves.

UROLITHIASIS

Urolithiasis is the formation of stones (*calculi*) within the renal tract. Renal calculi may form anywhere but most often occur in the renal pelvis. Stone formation may result from disturbances of normal physiology, such as change in urine pH, or excessive levels of certain substances within the urine, which are then more likely to precipitate out of solution.

- Around three-quarters of all stones are composed of calcium oxalate. These stones are associated with variable proportions of calcium phosphate and uric acid.
- Around 15% are composed of struvite (magnesium ammonium phosphate). These stones may come to completely fill the pelvicalyceal system, resulting in a 'staghorn' calculus (Fig. 21.20).

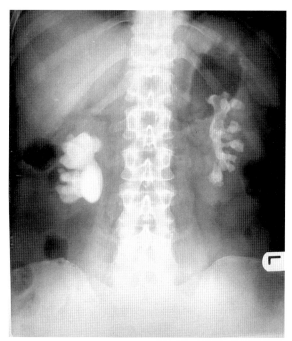

Figure 21.20 Intravenous urogram following intravenously administered iodinated contrast agent showing a dilated *right* renal pelvis and calyces due to obstruction at the pelvi–ureteric junction. The *left* side shows a staghorn calculus completely filling the pelvicalyceal system.

- Approximately 6% are composed of uric acid. These stones are radiolucent and therefore not identified on plain film radiography.

Renal calculi are associated with an increased likelihood of urinary tract infection. Their presence may also cause dull loin pain or *renal colic*, an exceptionally painful condition produced by the passage of the stone along the ureter.

OBSTRUCTIVE UROPATHY

Obstructive uropathy refers to renal tract disease resulting from the obstruction of urinary outflow. The obstruction may be complete or partial and can be caused as a result of calculi, tumours or congenital abnormalities.

Calculi may become lodged within the ureter, causing obstruction of the urine flow out of the kidney. Common sites of calculi obstruction are where the ureter narrows at the pelvi-ureteric junction, the pelvic brim and where it enters the bladder (vesico-ureteric junction). Ureteric obstruction needs to be resolved as soon as possible as the increasing backpressure will cause damage to the kidney. Obstruction results in enlargement of the kidney and dilation of the renal pelvis and calyces (*hydronephrosis*) and of the ureter proximal to the obstruction (*hydroureter*).

Radiology plays an important role in the identification of the cause of obstruction and also in therapeutic procedures. Intravenous urography, unenhanced helical CT and ultrasound are all commonly employed diagnostic procedures.

Some stones are suitable for disintegration using shockwaves – a procedure called lithotripsy. The stones are targeted with fluoroscopic imaging, which guides the shockwave device to the correct position on the flank. If the obstruction is due to a tumour or some other kind of stricture, it may be necessary to employ interventional radiological procedures such as nephrostomy. This refers to percutaneous access to the renal pelvis with placement of an externally sited drain, or positioning of an internally deployed tube, called a stent, to re-establish drainage of the kidney to the bladder.

RENAL TUMOURS

Renal tumours may manifest with obstructive symptoms, and *haematuria* (blood in urine). Radiology plays an important role in their diagnosis and staging.

Renal cell carcinoma (hypernephroma)

This is a tumour arising from the kidney tubular tissue. They may metastasise to bone and lung; spread by local invasion into adjacent organs; and also spread along the renal vein and into the inferior vena cava (IVC), which can result in lower extremity oedema due to the impaired venous return.

Transitional cell carcinoma

The pelvicalyceal system, ureter, bladder and upper part of the urethra are lined with transitional cell epithelium, a specialised type found only in the urinary tract. Transitional cell carcinoma can develop anywhere from this tissue, but most commonly in the bladder.

NERVOUS SYSTEM

Diseases of the nervous system are often profound in their effect on the individual's quality of life. Recent clinical imaging developments have made the diagnosis and treatment of neurological disorders far more effective.

CEREBROVASCULAR EVENT (STROKE)

Stroke results from a severe disruption in blood supply to the brain, resulting in damage to the brain tissue. Neurological effects ensue which may be from very mild through to more severe effects including paralysis, visual and speech disturbances. Strokes affecting the critical centres of the brain result in death. Risk factors are similar to other cardiovascular diseases and include smoking, hypertension, elevated lipid levels, diabetes and old age. Stroke may be due to infarction or haemorrhage.

Infarction

Brain infarction occurs when part of the brain suffers a critical reduction in blood supply to the extent that the affected region dies. This may be caused by:

- thromboembolism within the arterial supply to the brain
- severe reduction in systemic blood flow following cardiac arrest
- vasospasm following subarachnoid haemorrhage

In the case of thromboembolism there is a predisposing condition that promotes the formation of thrombus. This may be atherosclerosis within the internal carotid or cerebral arteries. Alternatively, the thrombus may form in the cardiac chambers in atrial fibrillation, or on the wall of the chamber following myocardial infarction.

Haemorrhage

Bleeding may occur within the brain tissue and is called *intracerebral* haemorrhage, or from the arteries at the base of the brain, including the circle of Willis, which is referred to as *subarachnoid* haemorrhage (SAH).

Intracerebral haemorrhage results in a haematoma that takes up space within the brain matter, causing increased intracranial pressure and distortion of the brain structure. In SAH blood accumulates inside the arachnoid layer of the meninges, giving rise to increased intracranial pressure (Fig. 21.21). As with intracerebral haemorrhage there is distortion of the brain structure. Irritation of the arteries by the free blood may also cause arterial spasm and infarct.

Both types of haemorrhage are closely associated with hypertension, which promotes the formation and rupture of aneurysms.

Transient ischaemic attack (TIA)

TIAs can produce similar symptoms to stroke, but their effect is short-lived and temporary. As the name implies, they result from a transient reduction is blood supply to the brain and the resultant anoxia in vulnerable parts of the brain causes

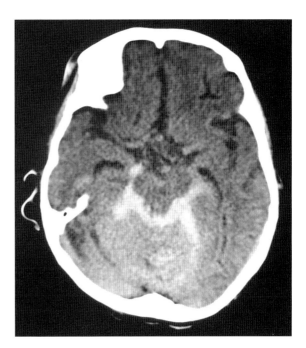

Figure 21.21 Computed tomography of the brain demonstrating high attenuation (*white*) areas within the brain due to the presence of freshly leaked blood from a subarachnoid haemorrhage.

temporary neurological effects. They may occur as a result of temporary thromboembolisation or spasm of the arterial supply to the brain. TIAs often precede full-blown strokes and therefore require speedy medical investigation if experienced.

SPINAL CORD AND NERVE COMPRESSION

Physical compression of the spinal cord and the spinal nerve roots can cause a range of pain and neurological deficit from paraesthesia (tingling) to paralysis. The severity of the effects is dependent on the degree of compression and how much damage is caused to the nerve tissue.

Causes of compression

Intervertebral disc herniation
The intervertebral disc consists of a tough outer ring of dense connective tissue (the annulus fibrosus) surrounding a soft jelly-like centre (the nucleus pulposus). It allows flexibility in the spine and acts as a shock absorber. Sometimes the outer

ring may be damaged and part of the nucleus pulposus herniates through the weakness in the annulus fibrosus. This herniation can cause compression of the spinal cord or the spinal nerve roots. Depending on its severity, the disc may need surgery to remove the parts that are compressing the nerve. This condition is shown very well by magnetic resonance imaging but not radiography.

Cervical spondylosis

Osteophyte formation around the margins of the intervertebral foramina and disc degeneration in the neck is called cervical spondylosis. It can lead to chronic pain and stiffness in the neck that may also radiate to the upper extremities (*radiculopathy*). It is often demonstrated by cervical spine radiography.

Tumour infiltration

Metastases to the vertebral column are usually the cause of the most severe neurological effects (Fig. 21.22). Infiltration of the vertebral bodies leads to severe weakening and collapse. The fragments extrude posteriorly and cause compression of the cord.

Cancers most commonly leading to cord compression:

- Lung
- Breast
- Prostate
- Multiple myeloma
- Non-Hodgkin's lymphoma.

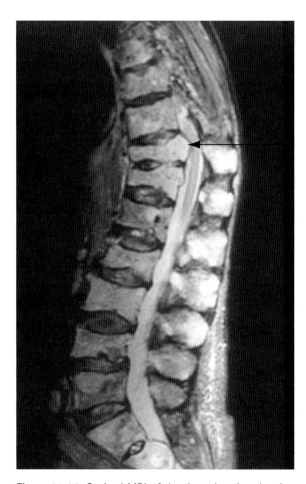

Figure 21.22 Sagittal MRI of the thoracic spine showing collapse due to tumour infiltration of T11 with cord compression.

MENINGITIS

The brain and spinal cord are covered in three layers of membrane, which make up the meninges. Infection of the meninges either by bacteria or viruses causes inflammation called meningitis.

The infection occurs by direct extension from the nasopharynx or via the blood. Bacterial meningitis is the most serious form, and even with the best care about 15% of patients will die. The bacteria responsible for approximately two-thirds of all cases are *Neisseria meningitidis* and *Streptococcus pneumoniae*.

Classical symptoms are:

- headache
- neck stiffness
- fever.

Infection with *Neisseria meningitidis* leads to a specific form of the disease called meningococcal meningitis. It is often accompanied by a generalised septicaemia typified by a non-blanching rash. Immediate treatment of suspected cases with intravenous antibiotics is essential to avoid death or severe after-effects, such as neurological damage and limb loss.

MULTIPLE SCLEROSIS

Multiple sclerosis (MS) is a disabling neurological disorder resulting from damage to the myelin coating of nerve cells in the central nervous system. It usually presents between the ages of 20 and 40. Patients with MS suffer from loss of normal function in certain parts of the body due to disruption of the nerve signals to and from the brain. These symptoms may be episodic, only presenting during a relapse, or permanent. The damaged areas of the nerves form scar tissue called plaques; these are well shown by MRI.

The course of MS is variable, depending on the individual and the age of onset, but usually patients suffer progressive levels of debilitation, with each relapse leaving them in a worse state.

BRAIN TUMOURS

Primary brain tumours

Primary brain tumours may arise from the neuroglial cells. The general term for tumours derived from neuroglial cells is glioma, or more specifically astrocytoma and oligodendroglioma, depending on the cell type of origin.

These tumours may grow slowly or rapidly and spread by local extension into surrounding tissues. They do not metastasise to other organs. The effect they have on the individual is dependent on where they are located in the brain (Fig. 21.23). Tumours in the frontal lobe may affect personality and mood; those in the temporal lobe may affect coordination speech and memory. The precise effect depends on the function of the brain tissue damaged and the size of the tumour. Because they arise from the brain tissue itself, they are referred to as intrinsic tumours.

Extrinsic tumours develop from the tissues covering the brain and spinal cord. A meningioma is a tumour of the meninges. They may grow large and cause considerable distortion and compression of the brain; however, they are usually benign and do not infiltrate the brain tissue. Surgery is usually the first option for removal, and this is often completely curative (Fig. 21.24).

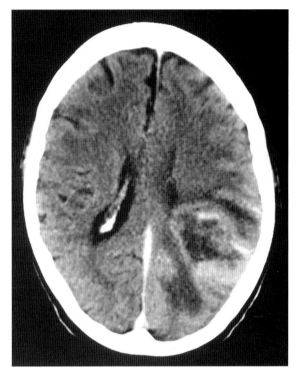

Figure 21.23 Computed tomography showing an enhancing brain tumour within the *left* cerebral hemisphere.

Brain tumours are well shown by CT and MRI, especially when contrast agents are used. In intrinsic tumours the breakdown of the blood–brain barrier allows penetration of the contrast into the tumour, which then shows enhancement.

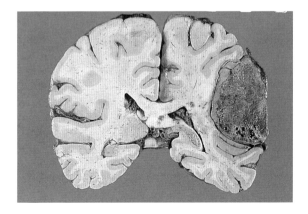

Figure 21.24 Meningioma causing cerebral compression.

Secondary brain tumours

Approximately 50% of intracranial tumours are metastases from a primary in the lungs, breast, stomach, prostate, thyroid or kidney. As with primary tumours, their effect depends on their size and location.

Further reading

Copstead LC, Banasik JL. Pathophysiology, 3rd edn. St Louis: Elsevier Saunders; 2005.

This text covers all aspects of pathology, describing both normal abnormal appearances and including aetiology, pathogenesis, clinical presentation and treatments. It is supported with full colour diagrams and illustrations.

Kumar PJ, Clark ML. Clinical medicine, 6th edn. Edinburgh: Saunders; 2005.

This large textbook covers the entire spectrum of clinical medicine with clear descriptions. There are a large number of tables and diagrams to assist in understanding.

Reid R, Roberts F. Pathology illustrated, 6th edn. Edinburgh: Churchill Livingstone; 2005.

This book provides a very user-friendly text, which is concise and well presented.

Underwood JCE. General and systematic pathology, 4th edn. Edinburgh: Churchill Livingstone; 2004.

This is a detailed and well-structured pathology textbook with all areas covered, from the basic fundamentals through to the pathology of specific systems.

Appendix 1

Trolley settings for radiographic procedures

Karen Dunmall

Prior to performing some radiographic procedures a number of key pieces of equipment are required. These need to be prepared in advance to ensure the smooth running of the examination and optimal patient care. The trolley settings provide an indication of the items that are required for each examination. This is not an exhaustive list for either examination type or equipment required but does provide an overview of the more common examinations and procedures.

ARTERIOGRAM

- 1 × 5 ml syringe
- 4 × 10 ml syringe
- 4 × 20 ml syringe
- Green needle
- Orange needle
- 19 g arterial puncture needle
- Scalpel blade
- 500 ml bag heparinised saline
- Pack of 2 sterile towels
- Sterile covers for C-arm
- One-way tap
- Sharps container
- Skin preparation lotion
- Local anaesthetic (1% lidocaine)
- Contrast medium
- Guide wires
- Catheters

ARTHROGRAM AND JOINT INJECTION

- Biopsy pack
- 2 ml syringe
- 5 ml syringe
- 10 ml syringe
- Green needle
- Orange needle
- Blue needle
- Spinal needle
- Scalpel blade

Extras:
- Skin preparation lotion
- Local anaesthetic (1% lidocaine)
- 0.5% Marcain
- Corticosteroid used to treat arthritis pain and joint inflammation; e.g. Kenalog, Depo-Medrone
- Contrast medium
- Skin dressing
- Sterile gloves and towel

BARIUM ENEMA

For each patient:

- 1 × Bottle of barium sulphate solution
- Plastic tubing and 'puffer'
- Lubricating jelly
- Gauze swabs
- Tape
- Gloves

- 2 ml syringe
- Orange needle
- Steret
- Ampoule of Buscopan or glucagon (smooth muscle relaxant)

BARIUM MEAL

For each patient:

- E-Z-EM barium or Baritop
- Water
- Plastic cup
- Carbex granules and solution
- Straw
- Spoon
- 2 ml syringe
- Orange needle
- Steret
- Ampoule of Buscopan or glucagon (smooth muscle relaxant)

BILIARY STENT AND PERCUTANEOUS TRANSHEPATIC CHOLANGIOGRAM (PTC)

- 1 × 5 ml syringe
- 2 × 10 ml syringe
- 2 × 20 ml syringe
- Green needle
- Orange needle
- Scalpel blade
- 500 ml bag of sodium chloride
- Sterile covers for C-arm
- One-way tap
- Sharps container
- Skin preparation lotion
- Local anaesthetic (1% Lignocaine)
- Sealed tube lubricating jelly
- Transhepatic 'Chiba' needle
- Guide wires
- Biliary catheter
- Biliary stent
- Drainage set (tube, bag connector, bag)

BIOPSY

- 1 × 5 ml syringe
- Green needle

- Orange needle
- Spinal needle
- Scalpel blade
- Skin preparation lotion
- Local anaesthetic (1% lidocaine)
- 2 × 10 ml syringe
- 2 × 20 ml syringe
- T extension set
- Biopsy needle/gun
- Specimen pots/forms
- Sterile ultrasound probe cover
- Sealed tube lubricating jelly
- Sterile gloves and towel
- Skin dressing

CAVERNOSAGRAM

- 2 ml syringe
- 50 ml syringe
- Green butterfly needles
- 50 ml sodium chloride
- Contrast medium
- Tourniquet
- Extension tube
- Kwills
- Tape
- Vasodilator, e.g. alprostadil
- Skin preparation lotion

COLONIC STENT

- 2 × 10 ml syringe
- 2 × 20 ml syringe
- Sodium chloride
- Sterile covers for C-arm
- Skin cleaner
- Guide wire
- Colonic stent
- Colonic stent guide wire
- Large balloon catheter (oesophageal)
- Sealed lubricating jelly
- Contrast medium

CYST ASPIRATION (ULTRASOUND)

- 10 ml syringe
- 20 ml syringe

- Green needle
- Orange needle
- Spinal needle
- Scalpel blade
- Sharps container
- Sterile ultrasound probe cover
- Sealed tube lubricating jelly
- Sterile gloves and towel
- Skin dressing
- Specimen pots

GASTROGRAFIN ENEMA

- Contrast medium (2 × 250 ml Gastrografin, undiluted)
- Empty enema giving bag and Foley catheter OR
- Contrast medium (1 × 500 ml Gastrografin)
- Giving set and Foley catheter
- Lubricating jelly
- Gauze swabs
- Tape
- Gloves

HYSTEROSALPINGOGRAM

Sterile salpingogram set including:

- Speculum
- Uterine cannulas
- 5 ml syringe
- 20 ml syringe
- 50 ml syringe
- Kwill
- Salpingogram catheter
- Extension set
- Sodium chloride 0.9% (Normasol)
- Contrast medium
- Sanitary towel
- Sterile gloves and towel
- Light source for cervical cannulation

MICTURATING CYSTOGRAM

If patient is catheterised:

- Contrast medium, e.g. Urografin 150 (250 ml or 500 ml)

- Giving set
- Connector
- Male / female urine receiver

If patient is uncatheterised:

- Catheterisation pack
- Catheter
- Syringe
- Sterile water (inflate balloon)
- Sodium chloride 0.9% (Normasol)
- Instillagel (anaesthetic antiseptic lubricant)
- Sterile gloves and towel
- 13 nephrostomy drainage (ureteric stenting)
- 1 × 5 ml syringe
- 2 × 10 ml syringe
- 4 × 20 ml syringe
- Green needle
- Orange needle
- Scalpel blade
- 500 ml bag sodium chloride
- Pack of 2 sterile towels
- Sterile covers for C-arm
- Sharps container
- Skin preparation lotion
- Local anaesthetic (1% lidocaine)
- Sealed lubricating jelly
- Contrast medium
- Guide wires
- Catheters
- Selection of ureteric stents
- Locking pigtail drain
- Drain connector
- Drainage bag and holder

NEPHROSTOGRAM

- 50 ml syringe
- Extension set
- Kwill
- Contrast medium
- Gloves

OESOPHAGEAL STENT

- 2 × 10 ml syringe
- 2 × 20 ml syringe
- Sodium chloride
- Sterile covers for C-arm

- Guide wire
- Xylocaine spray
- Lidocaine gel
- Mouth guard
- Oesophageal stent
- Oesophageal stent guide wire
- Large oesophageal balloon catheter
- Sealed lubricating jelly
- Contrast medium
- Suction and oxygen

SIALOGRAM

- Disposal bag
- 10 ml syringe
- Kwill
- Sialogram probes
- Sialogram catheters
- Tongue depressor
- Citric acid or lemon juice
- Cup and receiver
- Mouthwash tablets
- Light source for duct cannulation

SINOGRAM

- Disposal bag
- 20 ml syringe
- Kwill
- Contrast medium
- Selection of catheters
- Extension set
- Sterile gloves and towel
- Tape
- Dressings
- Sodium chloride 0.9%

SMALL BOWEL ENEMA

- Small bowel enema tube
- 5 ml syringe
- 2 × 50 ml syringe

- Large plastic jug
- 1 can cold barium sulphate solution; e.g. Baritop diluted to up to 1500 ml
- Maxalon
- Xylocaine throat spray
- Gloves
- Tape

TRANSHEPATIC (T)–TUBE CHOLANGIOGRAM

- Disposal bag
- Artery forceps
- 20/50 ml syringe
- Kwill
- Extension set
- Connector
- Contrast medium

URETHROGRAM

- Catheter pack
- Sachet of sterile saline
- Sterile lidocaine gel
- 500 ml bottle of Urografin 150
- Giving set
- Sterile gloves
- Sterile hand towel
- Urine bottle

VENOGRAM

- 20 ml syringe
- 50 ml syringe
- Kwills
- Butterfly sets (blue and green)
- Extension set
- Gauze swabs
- Steret
- Tourniquet ×2
- Contrast medium

Appendix 2

Patient pathways in nuclear medicine

Marc Griffiths and Vicki Major

These are simple generic pathways, which may differ from patient to patient depending on imaging modalities available and patient condition. Nuclear medicine involvement in the pathway is found in bold.

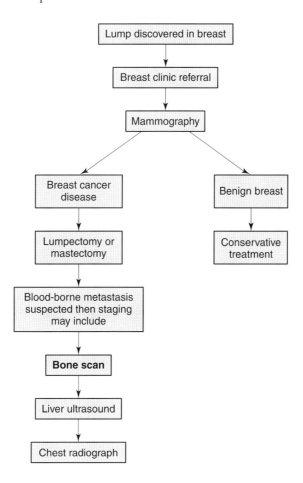

Figure A2.1 Breast cancer.

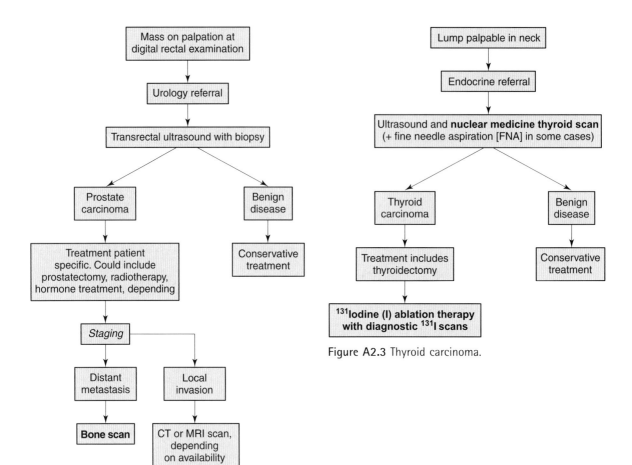

Figure A2.2 Carcinoma of the prostate gland.

Figure A2.3 Thyroid carcinoma.

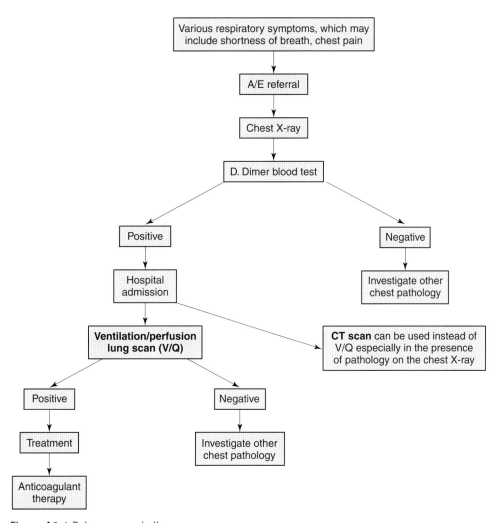

Figure A2.4 Pulmonary embolism.

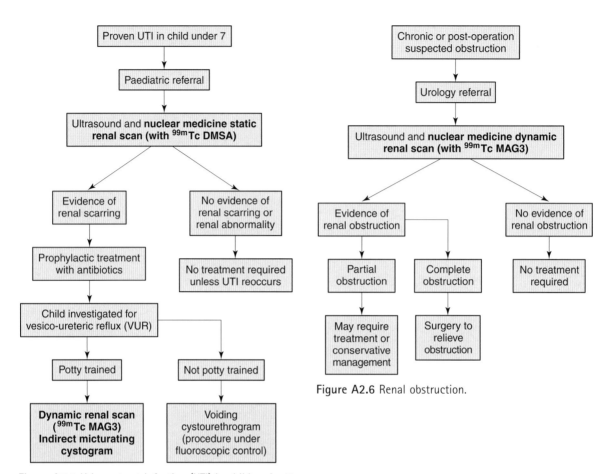

Figure A2.5 Urinary tract infection (UTI) in child under 7.

Figure A2.6 Renal obstruction.

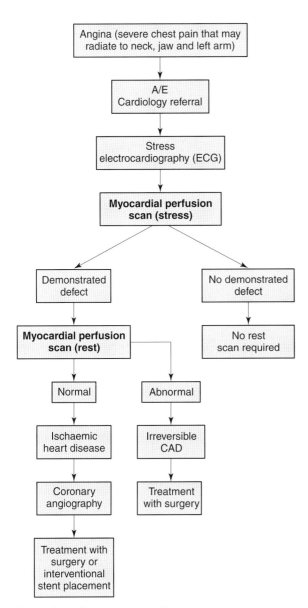

Figure A2.7 Coronary artery disease.

Appendix 3

Computed tomography protocols

Sophia Beale and Catriona Todd

At the core of every CT department are the scanning protocols. These are agreed with the consultant radiologist, lead radiographer and the radiation safety advisor. These protocols must conform to the IR(ME)R (see Ch. 2) regulations and they are designed to give maximum diagnostic information with the least radiation possible.

In this section we give examples of common standard examination protocols. These are actual protocols from a CT department using a 16-slice scanner. However, it may be found that the protocols in other departments may be slightly different, depending on the needs of the department and the type of scanner in use.

Table A3.1 Brain

Patient position		Supine. Use pads and immobilisation straps to keep the head straight				
Preparation		None				
Contrast		If required 50 ml of Niopam 350				
Scout		Lateral				
Scan position 1		Angle to anterior cranial fossa (this avoids irradiating the eyes). The lowest slice should be at the foramen magnum and the top slice at the top of the petrous ridge				
Scan type	Sequential	kV_p	120	*mA*	320
Rotation time	1.0	Dose modulation	No	Total collimation	12 × 0.75
Slice thickness	3 mm	Table feed/rotation	9 mm	MPR	No
		Algorithm	H40	VRT	No
Scan position 2		Same angle as 1st block. Bottom slice should continue on from the top of the 1st block top slice to the top of the cranium				
Scan type	Sequential	kV_p	120	*mA*	360
Rotation time	1.0	Dose modulation	No	Total collimation	12 × 1.5
Slice thickness	9 mm	Table feed/rotation	18 mm	MPR	No
		Algorithm	H40	VRT	No

MPR, multi-planar reformatting; VRT, volume rendering technique

Table A3.2 Sinuses

Patient position	Supine. Use immobilisation pads and strap to keep patient straight				
Preparation	None				
Contrast	None				
Scout	Lateral				
Scan position 1	Lowest slice at the level of the middle of the upper teeth and top slice at the top of the frontal sinuses. Reduce field of view (FOV) to include only the sinuses				
Scan type	Spiral	kV_p	120	mA	100
Rotation time	0.75	Dose modulation	No	Total collimation	16 × 0.75
Slice thickness	2 mm	Table feed/rotation	6.6 mm	MPR	Coronal Sagittal
		Algorithm	H70	VRT	No

MPR, multi-planar reformatting; VRT, volume rendering technique

Table A3.3 Cervical spine

Patient position	Supine. Immobilise the head with pads. For trauma patients do not remove any collars or immobilisation blocks				
Preparation	None				
Contrast	None				
Scout	Lateral				
Scan position 1	Top slice to top of the level indicated by the radiologist and bottom slice to the lowest level indicated by the radiologist				
Scan type	Spiral	kV_p	120	mA	400
Rotation time	0.75	Dose modulation	Yes	Total collimation	16 × 1.5
Slice thickness	2 mm	Table feed/rotation	18 mm	MPR	Axial Obl Coronal Sagittal
		Algorithm	B70	VRT	Yes

MPR, multi-planar reformatting; VRT, volume rendering technique

Table A3.4 Lumbar spine

Patient position	Supine. Arms should be placed behind the head and supported				
Preparation	None				
Contrast	None				
Scout	Lateral				
Scan position 1	Top slice at the uppermost level protocolled by radiologist and lowest slice should be at the lowest level				
Scan type	Spiral	kV_p	120	mA	440
Rotation time	0.75	Dose modulation	Yes	Total collimation	16 × 0.75
Slice thickness	3 mm	Table feed/rotation	9 mm	MPR	Axial Obl Coronal Sagittal
		Algorithm	B70	VRT	If required

MPR, multi-planar reformatting; VRT, volume rendering technique

Table A3.5   Neck

Patient position		Supine. Arms down by side and supported			
Preparation		Insertion of Venflon			
Contrast		80–100 ml Niopam 300 @ 2 ml s^{-1}			
Scout		Lateral			
Scan position 1		Top slice to nasopharynx and lowest slice at the level of the aortic arch			
Scan type	*Spiral*	*kV$_p$*	*120*	*mA*	*200*
Rotation time	0.75	Dose modulation	Yes	Total collimation	16 × 1.5
Slice thickness	3 mm	Table feed/rotation	18 mm	MPR	No
		Algorithm	B60	VRT	No

MPR, multi-planar reformatting; VRT, volume rendering technique

Table A3.6   Chest

Patient position		Supine. Arms should be placed behind the head and supported			
Preparation		Insertion on Venflon			
Contrast		80–100 ml Niopam 300 @ 3 ml s^{-1}			
Scout		AP			
Scan position 1		Top slice at the top of the apex of the lungs. Lowest slice at the level of the lung bases			
Scan type	*Spiral*	*kV$_p$*	*120*	*mA*	*200*
Rotation time	0.5	Dose modulation	Yes	Total collimation	16 × 1.5
Slice thickness	8 mm	Table feed/rotation	22.4 mm	MPR	No
		Algorithm	B50 / B80	VRT	No

MPR, multi-planar reformatting; VRT, volume rendering technique

Table A3.7   Chest high resolution

Patient position		Supine. Arms should be placed behind the head and supported			
Preparation		None			
Contrast		None			
Scout		AP			
Scan position 1		Top slice at the top of the lung apex and bottom slice at the level of lung bases			
Scan type	*Sequence*	*kV$_p$*	*120*	*mA*	*133*
Rotation time	0.75	Dose modulation	Yes	Total collimation	2 × 1
Slice thickness	1 mm	Table feed/rotation	10 mm	MPR	No
		Algorithm	B80	VRT	No

MPR, multi-planar reformatting; VRT, volume rendering technique

Table A3.8 Chest/abdomen

Patient position	Supine. Arms should be placed behind the head and supported			
Preparation	Insert Venflon. −ve or +ve oral contrast 15 minutes before start of the scan			
Contrast	80–100 ml Niopam 300 @ 3 ml s^{-1}			
Scout	AP			
Scan position 1	Top slice at top of lung apex and lowest slice at the bottom of the lung bases			
Scan type	Spiral	kV_p	120	mA	200
Rotation time	0.5	Dose modulation	Yes	Total collimation	16 × 1.5
Slice thickness	8 mm	Table feed/rotation	22.4	MPR	No
		Algorithm	B50/ B80	VRT	No
Scan position 2	Top slice at the top of the liver and lowest slice at the iliac crest			
Scan type	Spiral	kV_p	120	mA	400
Rotation time	0.5	Dose modulation	Yes	Total collimation	6 × 1.5
Slice thickness	8 mm	Table feed/rotation	18 mm	MPR	No
		Algorithm	B50	VRT	No

MPR, multi-planar reformatting; VRT, volume rendering technique

Table A3.9 Chest-abdomen-pelvis

Patient position	Supine. Arms should be placed behind the head and supported			
Preparation	Insert Venflon. −ve or +ve oral preparation			
Contrast	80–100 ml Niopam 300 @ 3 ml s^{-1}			
Scout	AP			
Scan position 1	Top slice at lung apex and lowest slice at level of lung bases			
Scan type	Spiral	kV_p	120	mA	200
Rotation time	0.5	Dose modulation	Yes	Total collimation	16 × 1.5
Slice thickness	8 mm	Table feed/rotation	22.4 mm	MPR	No
		Algorithm	B50 / B80	VRT	No
Scan position 2	Top slice at the top of the liver and bottom slice to bottom of symphysis pubis			
Scan type	Spiral	kV_p	120	mA	400
Rotation time	0.5	Dose modulation	Yes	Total collimation	16 × 1.5
Slice thickness	8 mm	Table feed/rotation	18 mm	MPR	No
		Algorithm	B50	VRT	No

MPR, multi-planar reformatting; VRT, volume rendering technique

Table A3.10   Abdomen-pelvis

Patient position		Supine. Arms should be placed behind the head and supported				
Preparation		Insert Venflon. −ve or +ve oral preparation				
Contrast		80-100 ml Niopam 300 @ 3 ml s^{-1}				
Scout		AP				
Scan position 1		Top slice to the top of the liver and lowest slice to bottom of symphysis pubis				
Scan type	Spiral	kV$_p$	120	mA		400
Rotation time	0.5	Dose modulation	Yes	Total collimation		16 × 1.5
Slice thickness	8 mm	Table feed/rotation	18 mm	MPR		No
		Algorithm	B50 / B80	VRT		No

MPR, multi-planar reformatting; VRT, volume rendering technique

Table A3.11   Kidneys-ureter-bladder (KUB)

Patient position		Supine. Arms should be placed behind the head and supported				
Preparation		None				
Contrast		None				
Scout		AP				
Scan position 1		Top slice above top of the left kidney, lowest slice at bottom of symphysis pubis				
Scan type	Spiral	kV$_p$	120	mA		360
Rotation time	0.5	Dose modulation	Yes	Total collimation		16 × 1.5
Slice thickness	5 mm	Table feed/rotation	18 mm	MPR		No
		Algorithm	B50	VRT		No

MPR, multi-planar reformatting; VRT, volume rendering technique

Table A3.12 Extremity

Patient position	Supine or prone. For elbow and wrist the affected arm should be raised above the head if possible. For ankle and foot imaging then the unaffected limb can be flexed at the knee and bent in order that it is not in the field of view					
Preparation	None					
Contrast	None					
Scout	AP or lateral					
Scan position 1	Top slice to be above the joint under examination or above the top of the fracture. Lowest slice below the joint. For fractures the closest joint should be included					
Scan type	Spiral	kV_p	120	mA	160	
Rotation time	0.75	Dose modulation	Yes	Total collimation	16×0.75	
Slice thickness	3 mm	Table feed/rotation	6.6 mm	MPR	Coronal Sagittal	
		Algorithm	B80	VRT	Yes	

MPR, multi-planar reformatting; VRT, volume rendering technique

Multiple choice questions

AN INTRODUCTION TO ETHICS

Due to the nature of the topic, multiple choice questions are impossible to provide for ethics.

THE LAW AT WORK

1. A classified worker is one who is likely to receive an effective dose of:
   a) more than 2 mSv per year.
   b) more than 0.6 mSv per year.
   c) more than 6 mSv per year.
   d) more than 20 mSv per year.

2. With reference to IR(ME)R:
   a) The regulations are enforced by the Health and Safety Executive.
   b) Only doctors can request an X-ray.
   c) The practitioner is the only person who can authorise an X-ray exposure.
   d) Responsibility for dose optimisation rests with the practitioner.

3. An injury to your back must be reported under RIDDOR if the injury puts you off work for:
   a) 1 day.
   b) 2 days.
   c) 3 days.
   d) more than 3 days.

4. The Data Protection Act
   a) requires that data be accurate and up to date.
   b) only refers to data held on a computer.
   c) does not apply when discussing a patient's healthcare.
   d) defines personal data as that which relates to any individual.

COMMUNICATION

1. Which of the following does NOT indicate active listening?
   a) Look at the person, face them squarely.
   b) Cross arms and legs.
   c) Maintain good eye contact.
   d) Position yourself at the same level (or below) the person.

2. Which of the following is NOT an empathetic response to an aggressive individual complaining about the waiting time?
   a) 'I can see that you are getting angry about the amount of time you have waited.'
   b) 'You have been waiting a long time haven't you. Would you like to me see what's happening?'
   c) 'Lots of staff are off sick and we're very busy!'
   d) 'I'm sorry to have kept you waiting; I can see that it's frustrating you.'

3. If you were in a cubicle asking the patient a question about their examination details, which 'proximity zone' would you be working in?
   a) Social zone.
   b) Intimate zone.
   c) Zone B.
   d) Personal zone.

4. In terms of 'paralanguage', speaking in a voice with a low volume, low pitch and slow pace would indicate that you were:
   a) bored.
   b) surprised.
   c) happy.
   d) confident.

5. An invasion of personal space falls into which of the following categories for barriers to communication?
   a) Environment.
   b) Language.
   c) Physiological.
   d) Psychological.

PATIENT CARE

1. *Neonate* is a term used to describe a baby:
   a) requiring intensive care.
   b) under one year old.
   c) under one week old.
   d) under one month old.

2. A young child is more likely to cooperate during an examination if:
   a) their trust has been gained.
   b) they have not been separated from their parent.
   c) they have been adequately prepared for the examination.
   d) All of the above.

3. Delirium can cause:
   a) disorientation.
   b) gait problems.
   c) raised awareness.
   d) All of the above.

4. A 'progressive deterioration in intellectual functioning' defines which condition?
   a) Delirium.
   b) Anxiety disorder.
   c) Dementia.
   d) Attention deficit disorder.

5. A patient may take responsibility for their own care or treatment if:
   a) they are below the age of 16 and their parent is not present.
   b) they are below the age of 16 and deemed as having sufficient understanding and intelligence.
   c) they are receiving treatment under a private medical scheme.
   d) they are below the age of 15 and terminally ill.

CLINICAL SKILLS FOR PREPARATION OF THE PATIENT AND CLINICAL ENVIRONMENT

1. A bacterium is
   a) a primitive plant cell.
   b) genetic material.
   c) a unicellular organism.
   d) an antibiotic.

2. Meticillin resistant *Staphyloccocus aureus* (MRSA) is a:
   a) virus.
   b) bacterium.
   c) fungus.
   d) protozoan.

3. Which of the following is NOT a means of cross-infection?
   a) Direct contact between individuals.
   b) Transmission of bodily fluids.
   c) Inhalation of droplets/particles in the air.
   d) Hand washing.

4. Which of these cannot be used as part of the sterilization process?
   a) Physical cleaning.
   b) Heat treatment.
   c) Barrier nursing.
   d) Ethylene oxide gas.

5. A spherical shaped bacterium has the suffix:
   a) bacillus.
   b) coccus.
   c) vermicelli.
   d) fusilli.

PROCEDURES IN RADIOGRAPHY

1. Which of the following is not essential information to be recorded on images obtained from mobile radiography?
   a) Time of examination.
   b) Object–film distance (OFD).
   c) Exposure values.
   d) Patient position.

2. Which one of the following would not be used to reduce radiation dose to staff or patients during ward/theatre radiography?
   a) Inverse square law.
   b) Lead-equivalent protection.
   c) A staff member restraining the patient for the examination.
   d) Pulsing mode during fluoroscopy.

3. Which one of the following methods would not be used to reduce the risk of cross-infection between *patient* and *staff* during theatre radiography?
   a) Changing outdoor shoes for theatre footwear.
   b) Handwashing.
   c) Applying sterile covers to X-ray equipment.
   d) Autoclaving.

4. The dress code in theatre serves which of the following purposes:
   a) Keeps uniform clean for wearing the next day.
   b) Enables all health professionals to appear equal.
   c) Calms the surgeon during the operation.
   d) Maintains hygiene and infection control.

5. Which one of the following is not a characteristic of contrast media responsible for causing reactions?
   a) Colour of the phial.
   b) Concentration.
   c) Viscosity.
   d) Osmolarity.

PHYSICS OF RADIOGRAPHY

1. Which components of an atom are found in the nucleus?
   a) Protons and electrons.
   b) Electrons and neutrons.
   c) Neutrons and protons.
   d) Electrons only.

2. The quantity of electrons flowing per second is measured in:
   a) amperes.
   b) joules.
   c) coulombs.
   d) volts.

3. The atomic number of tungsten is:
   a) 110
   b) 74
   c) 184
   d) 75

4. All electromagnetic radiations:
   a) travel through vacuums with a different velocity.
   b) travel in straight lines.
   c) have the same wavelength.
   d) are able to penetrate a brick wall.

5. As the source of X-rays moves closer to the patient the intensity of radiation:
   a) increases.
   b) decreases.
   c) stays the same.
   d) depends on patient size.

THE X–RAY TUBE

1. Oil is used in the X-ray tube assembly to:
   a) aid conduction of heat.
   b) lubricate the rotor bearing.
   c) conduct electricity to the anode.
   d) float the tube insert in.

2) Which of these is the most common material for the vacuum envelope?
    a) Tungsten.
    b) Glass.
    c) Ceramic.
    d) Copper.

3) The line focus principle reduces the:
    a) apparent focal spot size compared to the real.
    b) real focal spot size.
    c) the anode angle.
    d) the image size.

4) Which of these is used to make the anode?
    a) Lead.
    b) Tungsten.
    c) Copper.
    d) Ceramic.

5) Inherent filtration:
    a) is added to the beam.
    b) is not removable from the beam.
    c) is a safety feature to reduce dose.
    d) does not include filtration from the collimator.

PRODUCTION OF X-RAYS

1) What percentage of kinetic energy converts to heat when projectile electrons interact with target atoms?
    a) 1%
    b) 10%
    c) 50%
    d) 99%

2) With a tungsten target, there are no characteristic X-rays in the beam when the kVp is set:
    a) above $90 \, kV_p$
    b) above $80 \, kV_p$
    c) below $70 \, kV_p$
    d) above $70 \, kV_p$

3) If milliamperage (mA) is increased from 100 mA to 200 mA and all other factors remain the same, the X-ray beam will have:
    a) better quality.
    b) twice the penetrating ability.

c) twice the number of X-ray photons.
d) four times more energy.

4) If mA s were doubled, which of the following changes would maintain the radiographic density?
    a) Decrease kV_p by 15%.
    b) Increase kV_p by 15%.
    c) Decrease the FFD by one half.
    d) Double the FFD.

5) An increase in kV_p results in an X-ray beam with:
    a) higher energy X-ray photons.
    b) lower energy X-ray photons.
    c) an increased number of X-ray photons at all energy levels.
    d) a and c only.
    e) b and c only.

EFFECTS OF RADIATION

1. Attenuation of a beam of X-ray photons in matter depends on:
    a) beam size and FFD.
    b) kV and mA s.
    c) density and thickness of material.
    d) collimation and shielding.

2. The thickness of a specific material that will attenuate 50% of the beam of X-ray photons is called the:
    a) linear attenuation coefficient.
    b) exponential coefficient.
    c) total filtration.
    d) half value thickness.

3. Which of the following materials will result in the highest photoelectric absorption?
    a) Muscle.
    b) Fat.
    c) Bone.
    d) Lead.

4. The production of Compton-scattered X-ray photons can be minimised by reducing:
    a) field size.
    b) FFD.

c) OFD.

d) shielding.

5. A stochastic effect of ionising radiation is:
   a) cataract formation.
   b) leukaemia.
   c) skin erythema.
   d) sterilisation.

DIAGNOSTIC EQUIPMENT

1. Why is carbon fibre selected for the table top of an X-ray table?
   a) High attenuation of the material.
   b) Higher absorption of the primary beam.
   c) Cool to the touch.
   d) Reduces dose when undertaking grid radiography.

2. The tube support should:
   a) support the weight of the X-ray tube.
   b) contain interlocks to lock the tube in position.
   c) reduces physical strain on the practitioner.
   d) All of the above.

3. Ceiling suspended tubes are more versatile because:
   a) they have a wider floor coverage.
   b) they can cover a range of examination heights.
   c) they provide a safe working environment as the cables are enclosed.
   d) All of the above.

4. Which of the following is not an item of ancillary equipment?
   a) Cassette.
   b) Cassette holder.
   c) Foam pads.
   d) Stationary grid.

5. The typical range of power ratings for a high voltage generator for general radiography are
   a) 10–60 kW.
   b) 30–55 kW.
   c) 10–60 kV.
   d) 30–55 kV.

FILMS, CASSETTES, INTENSIFYING SCREENS AND PROCESSING

1. The emulsion layer of a film consists of:
   a) calcium tungstate and polyester.
   b) potassium bromide and gadolinium oxysulphide.
   c) gelatin and silver bromides.
   d) polyester and phenidone.

2. Single emulsion films:
   a) are often utilised for imaging of the abdomen.
   b) contain an anticurl/halo backing.
   c) utilise potassium carbonate as the light sensitive salt.
   d) generally produce images of low definition.

3. The fixer solution:
   a) contains hydroquinone.
   b) operates most effectively at a pH level of 7 to 7.5
   c) continues the process of film hardening.
   d) activity is very temperature dependent.

4. Replenishment of processing solution:
   a) is activated by the crossover rollers.
   b) ensures chemicals operate at the correct temperature.
   c) prevents chemicals passing to waste.
   d) maintains solution activity.

5. Intensifying screens:
   a) use ammonium thiosulphate as a phosphor material.
   b) may have an absorptive layer if of low definition type.
   c) ideally demonstrate phosphorescence.
   d) have a waterproof edge seal.

DIGITAL RADIOGRAPHY

1. What does PSP mean?
   a) Phosphorescence stimulated phosphor.
   b) Portable Sony Playstation.
   c) Photostimulable phosphor.
   d) Photomultiplier scanning plate.

2. What is used to read the PSP plate?
   a) White Light.
   b) Heat.
   c) Laser beam.
   d) Electrical charge.

3. Indirect digital radiography (IDR) uses what material coated on its TFT array?
   a) Amorphous silicon.
   b) Barium fluorohalide.
   c) Amorphous selenium.
   d) Caesium iodine.

4. What does PACS stand for?
   a) Patient archive and communications system.
   b) Primary active computer system.
   c) Picture archive and communications system.
   d) Photostimulable active crystal structure.

5. What is used to carry out an erase cycle on a CR plate?
   a) Eraser.
   b) White light source.
   c) Laser.
   d) Heat source.

IMAGE QUALITY

1. If a radiographic image requires 40 mA s to produce the required density and the mA was set at 400 mA, what is the time setting?
   a) 4 s
   b) 0.1 s
   c) 10 s
   d) 0.04 s

2. Which of the following factors does not reduce the contrast of the image?
   a) Collimation.
   b) Compression.
   c) Use of grids.
   d) Air gap technique.

3. A radiographic image which has a few shades of grey is described as having:
   a) high radiographic density.
   b) low radiographic density.
   c) high contrast.
   d) low contrast.

4. Resolution of the images is measured in:
   a) centimetres per second.
   b) cycles per second.
   c) line pairs per millimetre.
   d) line pairs per centimetre.

5. Which of the following factors does not affect the sharpness of the image?
   a) FFD
   b) OFD
   c) FOD
   d) mA s

MAMMOGRAPHY

1. Which is not an anatomical relationship of the breast?
   a) Anterior to the surface of the pectoralis major muscle.
   b) Inferior to the 2nd rib superiorly.
   c) Lateral to the mid-axillary line.
   d) Medial to the medial border of the scapula.

2. Which is not a direct route of lymphatic drainage for the breast?
   a) The axillary nodes.
   b) The internal mammary nodes.
   c) The abdominal lymphatics.
   d) Cervical lymph nodes.

3. Which of the following does NOT need to be included on a mediolateral image of the breast?
   a) Nipple in profile.
   b) Skin edges and glandular tissue edges.
   c) Axillary lymph nodes.
   d) Retroglandular fat tissue.

4. Which of the following symptoms is *highly unlikely* to indicate a malignant tumour in the breast?
   a) Easily moveable rubbery palpable lump.
   b) Puckering of the skin.
   c) Asymmetrical veins on the skin surface.
   d) Bloody nipple discharge.

5. Which of the following technique errors could result in the nipple not being in profile in the craniocaudad projection?
   a) Under-compression of breast tissue prior to exposure.
   b) Overlying fat/axillary tissue.
   c) Breast support table being too high for the patient.
   d) Woman turned too far medially.

NUCLEAR MEDICINE

1. The most commonly used radionuclide used in diagnostic nuclear medicine is:
   a) Iodine 131
   b) Krypton 81 m
   c) Gallium 67
   d) Technetium 99 m

2. Most radiopharmaceuticals are administered:
   a) orally.
   b) intravenously.
   c) subcutaneously.
   d) via aerosol.

3. A Gamma camera is:
   a) a beta radiation monitor.
   b) equipment used to measure bone density.
   c) equipment used to image nuclear medicine patients.
   d) a type of X-ray machine.

4. Technetium emits .... radiation?
   a) alpha.
   b) beta.
   c) gamma.
   d) X.

5. Which of the following is not a Gamma camera component?
   a) Photomultiplier tube.
   b) Sodium iodide crystal.
   c) Anode.
   d) Collimator.

ULTRASOUND

1. Ultrasound is a frequency of sound higher than:
   a) 10 kHz.
   b) 100 kHz.
   c) 20 kHz.
   d) 2000 Hz.

2. What is a side-effect of using ultrasound energy?
   a) Cavitation.
   b) Redness.
   c) Pain.
   d) Numbness.

3. A high frequency transducer is selected to:
   a) image deeper structures.
   b) improve resolution.
   c) widen the field of view.
   d) minimise artefacts.

4. Which of the following are not necessary for patient preparation for an ultrasound scan?
   a) Full bladder.
   b) Informed consent.
   c) Enema.
   d) Fasting.

5. Which of the following areas are not suitable to be examined by ultrasound?
   a) Obstetric.
   b) Urogenital system.
   c) Musculoskeletal.
   d) Gastrointestinal.

COMPUTED TOMOGRAPHY

1. Which of the following is not a component of a modern CT imaging system?
   a) Gantry.
   b) Slip rings.
   c) Image receptor.
   d) Image detectors.

2. What post-processing has been applied to the following image?

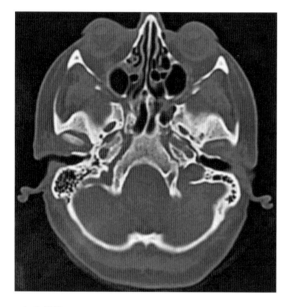

   a) MPR.
   b) VRT.
   c) Bony algorithm.
   d) Pneumo algorithm.

3. According to IR(ME)R what must be documented in the CT logbook?
   a) LMP.
   b) CTDI.
   c) Hospital number.
   d) All of the above.

4. What artefact does the following image illustrate?
   a) Partial volume.
   b) Arcing.
   c) Patient movement.
   d) Metal artefact.

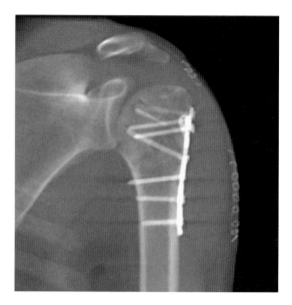

5. Which of the following may NOT be considered a mild contrast reaction?
   a) Bronchospasm.
   b) Vomiting.
   c) Nausea.
   d) Urticaria.

MAGNETIC RESONANCE IMAGING

1. Which of the following are contraindicated for MRI scanning?
   a) Cardiac pacemaker
   b) Intra-orbital metallic foreign body.
   c) Cerebral aneurysm clip.
   d) All of the above.

2. Why do you have to remove metal objects from your pockets before entering an MRI scanner?
   a) Because they will melt.
   b) Because they can be pulled from your pocket at great speed by the magnetic field and cause damage to the scanner and/or the patient.
   c) Because they will produce radiation after the scan.
   d) None of the above.

3. What is the type of contrast agent used in MRI?
   a) Iodine.
   b) Barium.
   c) Gastrografin.
   d) Gadolinium.

4. MRI images are produced by using which of the following combinations?
   a) X-rays and radiowaves.
   b) Magnetism and radiowaves.
   c) Magnetism and X-rays.
   d) Ultrasound and X-rays.

ANATOMY AND PHYSIOLOGY

1. Which of the following is the functional unit of the lung?
   a) Bronchi.
   b) Carina.
   c) Terminal bronchioles.
   d) Alveoli.
   e) Cilia.

2. Which of the following does not make up the paranasal sinuses?
   a) Maxillary.
   b) Spenoidal.
   c) Mastoid.
   d) Ethmoid.
   e) Frontal.

3. Which of the following is an example of a fibrous joint?
   a) Ball and socket.
   b) Hinge.
   c) Pivot.
   d) Suture.
   e) Gliding.

4. What is the name of the cells in the choroid plexus responsible for CSF production?
   a) Goblet cells.
   b) Ependymal.
   c) Cuboidal.
   d) Parenchymal.
   e) Squamous.

5. Which organ is also known as the largest gland in the body?
   a) Parotids.
   b) Spleen.
   c) Thyroid.
   d) Liver.

PATHOLOGY

1. Which of the following statements about cardiovascular disease is false?
   a) It accounts for most deaths in developed Western countries.
   b) It is associated with high blood lipid levels.
   c) It is associated with smoking.
   d) Is always a result of occlusion of a vessel by atheroma.

2. Osteoporosis results from:
   a) increased physical activity.
   b) loss of calcium from the bone connective tissue matrix.
   c) loss of bone connective tissue matrix.
   d) increased calcium intake.

3. A primary bone tumour is which of the following types of cancer?
   a) Glioma.
   b) Sarcoma.
   c) Carcinoma.
   d) Melanoma.

4. Which of the following does not result in spinal cord compression?
   a) Transient ischaemic attack.
   b) Vertebral metastases.
   c) Intervertebral disc herniation.
   d) Vertebral fracture.

5. Which of the following are responsible for the incidence of liver metastases arising from colorectal carcinoma?
   a) Superior mesenteric artery.
   b) Splenic vein.
   c) Hepatic portal vein.
   d) Inferior vena cava.

Short questions

AN INTRODUCTION TO ETHICS

1. After reading the chapter what would be your definition of the word 'ethics'?
2. Which four elements have to be present in order for a dilemma to be an ethical one?
3. What two things are the basis of the theory that is referred to as deontology?
4. What is the main consideration when analysing a dilemma using utilitarian theory?
5. List the four principles as described by Beauchamp and Childress.

THE LAW AT WORK

1. What is meant by the term 'justification' under the Ionising Radiations (Medical Exposure) Regulations 2000?
2. What is the underlying principle of the Manual Handling Operations Regulations 1992?
3. What are your duties as an employee under the Personal Protective Equipment at Work Regulations 1992?

COMMUNICATION

1. List the categories of people with whom you are likely to interact during a typical working day in the radiography department.
2. What emotions do you perceive from the following facial expressions (A–F)?

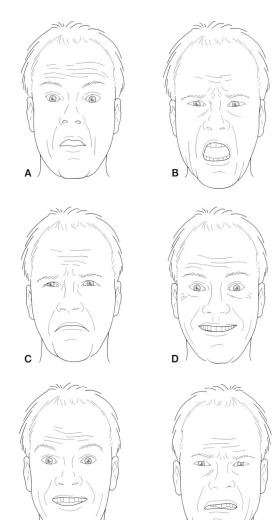

3. What questions should you ask yourself in order to assess a patient's movement capabilities?

4. Look at the following people (A–E); what does the way they are sitting/standing (body posture) tell you about them?

5. Use the questions below to assess the first impressions you may be giving to the service users.
   a. Do you speak first when you see a patient, visitor or family member?
   b. Are you quick to smile genuinely at patient, visitor or family member?
   c. Do you introduce yourself, giving your first and last names clearly?
   d. Do you check how the patient would like to be addressed?
   e. Do you explain your role in a clear understandable way, using jargon free language?
   f. Do you wear a visible and legible identification badge?
   g. Do you clearly inform patients as to what will happen next and check their understanding of the explanation or information given?
   h. Do you ensure your discussions with patients are conducted in an appropriate environment, protecting their rights to confidentiality and privacy at all times?

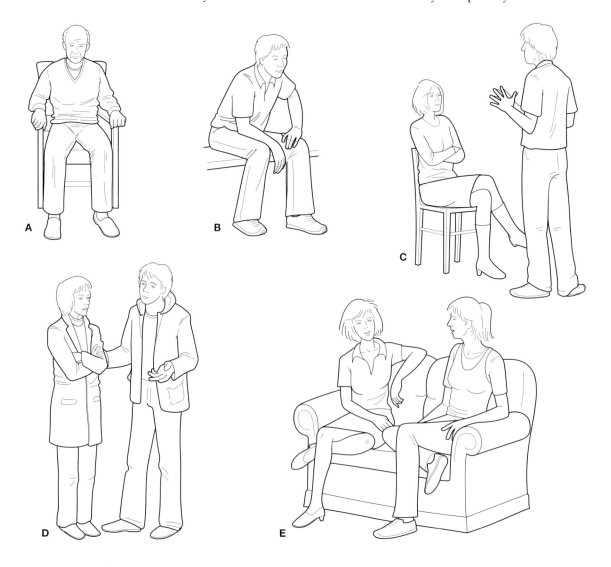

i. Do you maintain eye contact with the patient?
j. Is your clothing neat and professional?
k. Is your clothing, equipment and work area free from inappropriate messages, pictures, etc.?
l. Do patients see you following standard precautions; e.g. infection control?
m. Do you immediately cease any personal conversations when service users approach?
n. Do you respond to requests with genuine interest and kindness?
o. Do you give users your undivided attention and use active listening skills?
p. Do you establish what your patients' needs are before addressing your own needs in carrying out the investigation?
q. When confronted by an angry individual wishing to complain, do you let the person speak without interruption?

PATIENT CARE

1. State four things which should be considered when caring for a patient in a wheelchair.
2. Describe how to deal appropriately with the parent(s) or guardian(s) of a paediatric patient.
3. List three ways in which a potentially aggressive situation may be defused.
4. Explain why a separate paediatric waiting area is beneficial to the child and their parent or guardian.
5. Describe the special considerations which may be given to a patient with a learning disability.

CLINICAL SKILLS FOR PREPARATION OF THE PATIENT AND CLINICAL ENVIRONMENT

1. What is the purpose of hand washing?
2. Explain what you understand by the term 'sterile field'.
3. Identify two ways in which you can gain a positive personal identification from a patient.

PROCEDURES IN RADIOGRAPHY

1. What is the definition of a high dose examination?
2. Briefly explain the difference in usage between an iodine-based and a barium-based contrast agent.
3. State the different imaging procedures which may indicate using the 10 day rule and 28 day rule?
4. Outline the ways in which a radiographer can reduce the dose to staff and other patients on the ward during a mobile chest procedure.
5. What are the clinical indications for carrying out a mobile chest X-ray?

PHYSICS OF RADIOGRAPHY

1. What is electricity?
2. What types of magnetic substances are used in radiography; where would you find them?
3. Describe the differences between elements and compounds.
4. What is resistance?
5. Describe the inverse square law.

THE X-RAY TUBE

1. List the main methods of heat dispersal from the anode of a rotating anode X-ray tube.
2. State the main advantage of modern metal tube housing over glass.
3. Explain the function of the focussing cup.
4. Why is it not possible to use oil to lubricate the bearings of the anode?
5. What material is generally used to make the anode stem and why?

PRODUCTION OF X-RAYS

1. How are X-rays produced in an X-ray tube?
2. Which emission spectrum of which type of radiation interaction is described as 'discrete'?
3. The maximum photon energy in an X-ray beam is determined by what?

4. Beam filtration changes the characteristics of the beam by removing what?
5. Which of the prime exposure factors influences both the quality and quantity of the X-ray photons?

EFFECTS OF RADIATION

1. Explain what is meant by a) attenuation and b) transmission of X-ray photons.
2. Explain how photoelectric absorption of X-ray photons in the body results in a radiographic image.
3. Explain why Compton scatter does not contribute towards image formation in radiographic imaging.
4. Explain why exposure to ionising radiation is hazardous.
5. Explain why effective dose is used to compare radiation exposures to different parts of the body.

DIAGNOSTIC EQUIPMENT

1. What is the function of a dose area product meter?
2. Describe the basic process of traditional fluoroscopy image creation.
3. Outline the four basic areas of equipment care.
4. How does an automatic exposure device work?
5. What is the benefit of a cordless exposure device (CED) in mobile radiography?

FILMS, CASSETTES, INTENSIFYING SCREENS AND PROCESSING

1. Describe the key stages of film processing.
2. Why is an anti-halation/anti-curl layer required for single emulsion film?
3. Describe the process for cleaning an intensifying screen.
4. What is the function of replenishment?
5. If the processor temperature is not maintained at a constant level, what will happen?

DIGITAL RADIOGRAPHY

1. Describe the benefit of the greater exposure latitude found in digital radiography when compared to conventional radiography.
2. How is the latent image retrieved from the PSP?
3. What is the difference between direct and indirect digital radiography (DR)?
4. List three advantages of an amorphous selenium detector?
5. What is PACS used for?

IMAGE QUALITY

1. List the factors that affect the density on a radiograph.
2. List the factors that affect the contrast on a radiograph.
3. Illustrate the optimum geometric positioning to obtain an optimum image.
4. List the factors which influence unsharpness on the image.
5. Describe the factors that increase the magnification of the patient on the image.

MAMMOGRAPHY

1. State two ways in which the breast compression plate is designed to be fit for purpose.
2. State two ways in which the mammography equipment is designed to limit radiation dose to patients.
3. Why is it necessary to use low kV_p when imaging the breast?
4. Outline the reason for carrying out screening mammography between 50 and 64+ years.
5. Outline the difference in technique for a mediolateral oblique between a hyposthenic and hypersthenic woman.

NUCLEAR MEDICINE

1. Which physical properties make technetium-99m suitable for diagnostic nuclear medicine imaging?

2. Explain the importance of patient comfort during a bone scan. Explain how patient comfort can be achieved.
3. Explain why nuclear medicine imaging complements anatomical imaging.
4. Explain how the radiation dose can be minimised in nuclear medicine.
5. Describe the different types of renal nuclear medicine imaging.

ULTRASOUND

1. What are the advantages of using ultrasound?
2. What is the purpose of the gel during the ultrasound scan?
3. What is the role of Doppler in ultrasound?
4. How is an ultrasound scan useful in pregnancy?
5. What are the occupational hazards for the operator using ultrasound?

COMPUTED TOMOGRAPHY

1. Which cross-sectional anatomy would you expect to see on a CT image scanned at the level of L2?
2. List five checks you should make prior to scanning a patient in CT.
3. State the process of image production during a CT scan from X-ray source to final image. Use a flow diagram to help you explain.
4. What are the advantages of a 16-slice scanner over a single slice scanner?
5. Define the following terms:

   a. partial volume artefact
   b. motion artefact.

MAGNETIC RESONANCE IMAGING

1. Discuss the major contraindications against having an MRI scan.
2. Describe how an MRI scanner works.
3. What is the name of the contrast agent used in MRI and what does it look like on an image?
4. Discuss how fat and water look different on a T1 weighted and T2 weighted scan.
5. When is a superconducting MRI magnet on (creating a magnetic field)?

ANATOMY AND PHYSIOLOGY

1. What is the role of glucocorticoid hormones in the body?
2. Describe two differences between the male and female urethra.
3. What is the function of the cardiac sphincter?
4. Why do arteries have thicker wall layers than veins?
5. What are the paranasal sinuses?

PATHOLOGY

1. Describe the possible appearance of intestinal obstruction on a plain radiograph of the abdomen.
2. Which conditions can result in pleural effusion?
3. In ureteric urolithiasis, what are the common sites for stones to become lodged?
4. Explain how inflammatory bowel disease may be imaged using a radionuclide technique.
5. What are some of the signs and symptoms of myocardial infarction?

Answers to multiple choice questions

THE LAW AT WORK

1(c), 2(c), 3(d), 4(a)

COMMUNICATION

1(b), 2(c), 3(d), 4(a), 5(d)

PATIENT CARE

1(d), 2(d), 3(a), 4(c), 5(b)

CLINICAL SKILLS FOR PREPARATION OF THE PATIENT AND CLINICAL ENVIRONMENT

1(c), 2(b), 3(d), 4(c), 5(b)

PROCEDURES IN RADIOGRAPHY

1(b), 2(c), 3(d), 4(d), 5(a)

PHYSICS OF RADIOGRAPHY

1(c), 2(c), 3(b), 4(b), 5(a)

THE X-RAY TUBE

1(a), 2(b), 3(a), 4(b), 5(b)

PRODUCTION OF X-RAYS

1(d), 2(c), 3(a), 4(c), 5(d)

EFFECTS OF RADIATION

1(c), 2(d), 3(d), 4(a), 5(b)

DIAGNOSTIC EQUIPMENT

1(d), 2(d), 3(d), 4(a), 5(b)

FILMS, INTENSIFYING SCREENS AND PROCESSING

1(c), 2(b), 3(c), 4(d), 5(d)

DIGITAL IMAGING

1(c), 2(c), 3(a), 4(c), 5(b)

IMAGE QUALITY

1(b), 2(b), 3(d), 4(c), 5(d)

MAMMOGRAPHY

1(d), 2(d), 3(c), 4(a), 5(c)

NUCLEAR MEDICINE

1(d), 2(b), 3(c), 4(c), 5(c)

ULTRASOUND

1(c), 2(a), 3(b), 4(c), 5(d)

COMPUTED TOMOGRAPHY

1(c), 2(c), 3(b), 4(d), 5(a)

MAGNETIC RESONANCE IMAGING

1(d), 2(b), 3(d), 4(b)

ANATOMY AND PHYSIOLOGY

1(d), 2(c), 3(d), 4(b), 5(d)

PATHOLOGY

1(d), 2(c), 3(b), 4(a), 5(c)

Answers to short questions

AN INTRODUCTION TO ETHICS

1. The actual definition is 'the study of the moral value of human conduct' but you may want to regard ethics as a framework that assists us when dealing with ethical dilemmas, or even the study of right and wrong.
2. Moral agent, action, subject and consequence.
3. Rights and duties.
4. The consequences of the action.
5. Beneficence, nonmaleficence, autonomy and justice.

THE LAW AT WORK

1. Justification is undertaken by a practitioner. For an exposure to be justified, the benefit to the patient from the diagnostic information obtained should outweigh the detriment of the exposure.
2. Avoid manual handling where there is a risk of injury.
3. To use any equipment provided in accordance with instructions and training. To return that equipment to its proper location. To report any defects in the equipment to the employer.

COMMUNICATION

1. Patients, nursing staff, radiologists, radiographers, clerical staff, ancillary staff and portering staff. This list is not exhaustive.

2. Fear; anger; sadness; happiness; surprise; disgust.
3. Considerations should include:
   a. Is the person demonstrating any physical incapacity, e.g. do they have a walking stick?
   b. What are their facial features indicating?
   c. Are they in pain?
   d. What is their body posture indicating?
4. You may be able to infer the following:
   a. Gripping the chair could indicate the man is tense and nervous or in pain.
   b. This man is leaning forwards, which could indicate he is interested and listening.
   c. The woman's arms are folded, which could indicate she is closed to the man's ideas. Also he is standing over her, indicating he considers he is in a position of superiority.
   d. Both are standing in equal positions; however, one man has his arms folded and no eye contact, indicating he is closed to the other's communication.
   e. These women are mirroring each others' body language, indicating they are comfortable with each other in close contact.
5. If you have responded negatively to any of the statements, please reflect on how these aspects may be affecting your communications with others and use the information within the chapter to help you modify your behaviours. Verbal behaviour: 1, 3, 4, 5, 7, 14. Non verbal: 2, 6, 8, 9, 10, 11, 12, 13, 15, 16, 17.

PATIENT CARE

1. Answer should include any four of the following:
   a. Why the patient is using the wheelchair.
   b. The patient may require help changing.
   c. More time may be needed for the examination.
   d. Whether the patient needs pushing in the chair or whether they prefer to propel themselves.
   e. The patient may still be able to mobilise, despite being in a wheelchair.
   f. Moving and handling guidelines must be followed.
2. Answer may include the following points:
   a. Reassure the parent, being careful not to falsely reassure.
   b. Remain patient and calm at all times and ensure you are firm yet polite.
   c. Do not separate the parent and child unless absolutely necessary if this is likely to cause distress.
   d. Involve parents in the care of the child, informing them what you are doing and why.
3. Answer may include three of the following:
   a. Clear communication.
   b. Informing the patient about what is happening.
   c. Appropriate body language.
   d. Appropriate facial expressions.
   e. Calm, non-confrontational voice.
   f. Minimise waiting times.
4. Answer should include:
   a. A separate waiting area may prove less stressful for parents as they do not have to worry about other patients.
   b. The child can be more easily distracted with toys and books whilst waiting.
   c. A quieter area, avoiding the hustle and bustle of a busy waiting area can help calm the child prior to their examination.
5. Answer should include:
   a. It may be useful to involve a friend, carer or relative in the examination as they may know how best to gain cooperation from the patient.

   b. Talk directly to the patient so they feel included.
   c. Talk to the patient using language appropriate for his level of understanding.
   d. Avoid asking the patient too many questions or providing too many choices.
   e. Be patient and be prepared to repeat instructions several times.
   f. A patient may respond to a demonstration of what is required rather than a verbal explanation.

CLINICAL SKILLS FOR PREPARATION OF THE PATIENT AND CLINICAL ENVIRONMENT

1. The purpose is to reduce the risk of transmission of microorganisms via hands of staff.
2. A sterile field can be defined as a region for work within which it is deemed to be sterile. All items and materials placed onto the sterile field must also be sterile.
3. For checking patient identification use open questions:
   'What is your name?'
   'What is your date of birth?'
   You could include the address but that is not as reliable as the above.

PROCEDURES IN RADIOGRAPHY

1. These are examinations that are defined as procedures that carry the potential fetal dose greater than 10 mGy (e.g. abdominal/pelvic CT, barium enema).
2. A barium based contrast agent is composed of a suspension of large insoluble particles which have good coating properties utilised in the visualisation of the lining of the gastrointestinal tract. Iodine based contrast agents are used to visualise the circulatory system or any other cavity where there is a need for water solubility. It can also be used in cases of suspicion of perforation or aspiration.
3. Plain film abdomen, pelvis, lumbar/sacral spine may be undertaken within the 28 days if

the patient verifies that there is no possibility of pregnancy. For high dose examinations (e.g. Abdominal/pelvic CT, barium enema) patients should be booked an appointment within the first 10 days of the menstrual cycle.
4. By using lead-equivalent rubber aprons for main staff (e.g. the radiographer and anyone who might be assisting in positioning). For the members of staff and patients who can move from the immediate vicinity, distance is the suggested method of dose reduction. For the radiographer a combination of distance and lead protection is used.
5. The patient is unable to come down to the department due to ill health or infection risk (barrier nursed). For theatre the patients are usually unconscious from a general anaesthetic or sedated in the case of epidural anaesthesia.

PHYSICS OF RADIOGRAPHY

1. Electricity is moving electric charges; for example electrons moving through a wire.
2. Ferromagnets are used in radiography. They are found in transformers, relays and MRI equipment.
3. Elements are made up of atoms of one type of material; for example copper or hydrogen. Compounds are made up of different elements; examples of this are water, which contains hydrogen and oxygen, and silver bromide containing silver and bromine.
4. Resistance is the force that tries to slow or stop the movement of electrons. It is measured in ohms and depends on the shape, type of substance and temperature of the material.
5. As the distance increases, the intensity decreases.

THE X-RAY TUBE

1. The heat dispersal methods are:
   a. Anode to glass envelope – radiation.
   b. Glass envelope to oil – conduction.
   c. Oil to tube housing – conduction.
   d. Tube housing to room – convection.
2. They have longer life and are less likely to fail.

3. The focussing cup reduces the spread of electrons due to like charges repelling as the electrons travel from cathode to anode.
4. Due to the vacuum in the envelope and the high temperatures, oil would vaporise destroying the vacuum.
5. Molybdenum is used to make the stem as it has a low thermal conductivity, which prevents heat travelling down the stem to the rotor bearings, combined with a high physical strength to withstand the forces involved in rapidly accelerating the anode to its operational speed.

PRODUCTION OF X-RAYS

1. X-rays are produced when high-speed projectile electrons interact with the X-ray tube target.
2. Characteristic radiation is graphically illustrated in the form of a line spectrum. The energy of a characteristic photon depends on the differences between the electron binding energies of a particular target material. As a result, the spectrum produced by characteristic X-rays is referred to as discrete or distinct.
3. Maximum energy is realised if all the kinetic energy of a projectile electron is converted into a single X-ray photon. The maximum voltage (kV_p) determines the maximum photon energy in an X-ray beam.
4. Inherent and added filtration reduces the quantity of low energy X-rays that are not beneficial to the radiographic image. Beam filtration increases the average energy of the X-ray beam and results in reduced patient skin dose.
5. The prime exposure factors are kV_p, mA and exposure time. Changes in kV_p affect both the quality and quantity of photons in the X-ray beam. Changes in mA, exposure time or mA s only affect the quantity of photons in the X-ray beam.

EFFECTS OF RADIATION

1. Attenuation is the transfer of X-ray photon energy to the matter through which it passes,

by photoelectric absorption or Compton scatter type interactions. Transmission is the direct passage of X-ray photons through matter, without any interactions. Attenuation is the inverse of transmission: if 10% of the beam of X-ray photons is attenuated then 90% of the beam will be transmitted.

2. X-ray photons are absorbed by photoelectric absorption to a varying extent in different body tissues, depending on their density and proton number. So many more X-ray photons will be absorbed in dense bone with a proton number of approximately 12 compared to muscle with a much lower density and proton number of approximately 7.6. Where the X-ray photons have been absorbed in bone and removed from the beam, the image will appear white; where some X-ray photons are absorbed in the soft tissue and some transmitted, the image will appear grey; in areas where there is very low density air, such as the lungs, there will be virtually zero absorption so all the X-ray photons will be transmitted and the image will be black.

3. Compton scatter occurs alongside photoelectric absorption and is a process of partial absorption and partial scatter. The absorption is not dependent on proton number in the same way as photoelectric absorption, so it does not contribute towards differential absorption. The scattered X-ray photon may reach the image receptor, but at a variable angle, not necessarily from the direction of a low density/low proton number structure. In this way, scattered photons may contribute towards image blackening in areas that should be lighter and results in an overall decreased image contrast. To increase image quality, the production of Compton scatter can be reduced by reducing the volume of patient irradiated; i.e. by good collimation to the area of interest. Scattered photons reaching the image receptor can be reduced by the use of a radiation grid.

4. Ionising radiation, such as X-ray photons, result in the release of secondary electrons carrying kinetic energy following either photoelectric absorption or Compton scatter.

These secondary electrons transfer their kinetic energy by ionisation and excitation of surrounding atoms. These processes may cause breakage of chemical bonds between atoms, such as those in the DNA of a cell, which may result in a detrimental effect such as the delayed induction of cancer.

5. Effective dose takes into account the potential for damage from different radiations to different parts of the body, compared to a whole body dose. Some organs within the body are relatively resistant to the stochastic effects of ionising radiation whilst the remainder are more sensitive. So an absorbed dose of radiation to one part of the body may be potentially more damaging than the same dose to another part of the body. Tissue weighting factors are applied to the absorbed dose to take this into account and enable comparison of the radiation detriment.

DIAGNOSTIC EQUIPMENT

1. A DAP meter records the entrance dose to the patient, allowing the dose to be measured.
2. The X-ray tube produces the incident X-ray beam; the X-ray is transmitted through the patient; the image intensification unit converts X-rays into a light signal and amplifies them; the monitor displays an electronic signal.
3. Routine daily checks for wear and tear, mechanical fault recording, physical inspection of ancillary equipment, quality control checks of all equipment.
4. An AED contains chambers, which are selected depending on the examination. Once the chamber has received the exposure set it will terminate the exposure. This provides an optimum image.
5. A CED will allow a distance of up to 11 m to be achieved between the primary beam and the operator. This improves radiation safety to the operator, especially in confined spaces where the device can function around corners.

FILMS, CASSETTES, INTENSIFYING SCREENS AND PROCESSING

1. Film entry, developer, fixer, wash, dry.
2. It educes the cross-over effect and prevents the curling of the film due to uneven absorption of fluid in the processor.
3. Using a manufacturer recommended screen cleaner and a lint free cloth. Cleaning should be either from the centre out or from top to bottom. Once completed, the cassette should be stood on end like a book to dry.
4. Replenishment is required to ensure a continuous replacement of chemicals, thus ensuring optimum processing conditions.
5. If the processor temperature is not constant, the films will be either over- or underdeveloped, depending on whether the temperature is too high or too low.

DIGITAL RADIOGRAPHY

1. Digital radiography utilises the whole of the characteristic curve to form the image, allowing areas of under- or overexposure to be viewed. Conventional film is unable to use a wide exposure latitude, as shown in the characteristic curve where exposures in the foot and shoulder areas cannot produce an acceptable image (i.e. foot area – image too faint, shoulder area – film overexposed and blackened).
2. Answer should include:
   a. Placed in a CR reader.
   b. Laser scans.
   c. Electrons gain energy and leave traps and decay.
   d. As they move down in energy, light is emitted.
   e. Light is collected and amplified and then digitised.
3. Direct DR – incoming photons are transformed directly into an electronic signal; indirect DR – produces an analogue signal which is then converted to a digital signal.
4. Advantages include: better spatial resolution; only one energy conversion is required; it has

a simple design; and each individual pixel does not require a photo diode.
5. PACS is used for image acquisition, display, storage and retrieval in most hospitals and clinical environments.

IMAGE QUALITY

1. The factors involved are: mA s; kV_p; source–image distance (SID); grids; film–screen speed; collimation; tube filtration; processing.
2. The factors involved are: kV_p; subject contrast; collimation; film–screen combination; grids; air gap; processing; VDU characteristics; contrast agents.
3. The patient and cassette or image receptor should be in contact or as close as possible.
4. Movement; the resolution of the imaging system; the geometry of the imaging system.
5. The patient distance from the receptor; the angle of the patient in relation to the receptor.

MAMMOGRAPHY

1. Smooth with rounded edges for patient safety and comfort; made of clear Perspex to see compressed breast tissue and AED position.
2. The presence of a predetermined collimation area; the automatic optimisation of parameters (GE units) and combinations of target material/filter.
3. In mammography the lowest kV_p should be selected so as to give the highest subject contrast, as the absorption coefficient of soft tissue falls rapidly with an increasing kV at low energies. This is due to the attenuation of the X-ray beam by various tissues being dependent on the cube of the proton number of the structure (Z^3); e.g. adipose tissue Z = 6, fibrous/glandular tissue Z = 7. A low kV_p aids to amplify the differences in density to allow the different tissues to be identified.
4. Screening mammography is carried out between the ages of 50 and 64+ because this correlates to the menopausal/post-menopausal

phase of the breast when there is a more noticeable increase in fat deposition and glandular tissue reduction, thus aiding visualisation of lesions.

5. A hypersthenic woman would require an angle of less than 45°, potentially 40°, on the breast support table whilst a hyposthenic woman would benefit from greater than 45°, potentially 50–55°.

NUCLEAR MEDICINE

1. Technetium-99m is cheap and easy to produce; it is a pure Gamma emitter; it has a half-life of 6 hours; binds readily to pharmaceuticals and has a 140 keV energy level.
2. A bone scan lasts about 30 minutes. The patient can not move during scan or the whole scan needs to be performed again. The patient has to lie flat; you need to explain the procedure to the patient, put a pillow under her head, a pad under the knees and support her arms.
3. Nuclear medicine images show the function of a system in the body. They do not show any anatomical landmarks. If anatomical scans such as CT scanning are viewed in conjunction with physiological nuclear medicine scans then the area of physiological significance, such as a metastasis, can be located more accurately.
4. The most effective way of minimising dose is distance. Apply the inverse square law. Also use syringe shields, lead glass and lead shields when drawing up and administering radiopharmaceuticals. Avoid spillage of radionuclides. Give the patient clear instructions.
5. Static renal scans use technetium-99m DMSA – the radiopharmaceutical demonstrates the renal tissue; the patient is imaged 3 hours post administration. A dynamic renal scan is called a renogram – the patient is scanned immediately post administration of the radiopharmaceutical and this demonstrates activity in the kidney over time. A renogram demonstrates the collecting system and excretion of the kidneys.

ULTRASOUND

1. No radiation risk; non-invasive; no special preparation required; an immediate report is produced; it is painless; it is cost effective.
2. Coupling gel: reduces air bubbles; improves transmission of ultrasound; reduces friction.
3. Doppler is used to:
   a. assess vascularity of a lesion/cyst.
   b. calculate velocities.
   c. detect stenosis.
   d. assess haemodynamics.
4. It can date the pregnancy; detect fetal abnormalities; monitor fetal growth; exclude multiple pregnancies; assess placental site and amniotic fluid volumes.
5. Repetitive strain injury (RSI); vision fatigue; upper limb disorders; it may be stressful due to having to break bad news.

COMPUTED TOMOGRAPHY

1. Colon, liver, kidney, aorta, liver and IVC (inferior vena cava).
2. Answer to include any five of the following:
   a. Name.
   b. Date of birth.
   c. Allergies.
   d. Preparation.
   e. Pregnancy status.
   f. Address.
   g. Artefacts removal.
3. X-rays are attenuated by the patient; unattenuated X-rays hit the image detectors; data are converted to numerical data; numerical data are converted to gray scale image; the gray scale image is displayed on the monitor.
4. Any five correct answers from: speed, decreased motion artefact, increased image quality, decreased partial volume, better MPRs, more accurate assessment of the patient, decreased dose, increased resolution in images of vasculature, increased patient throughput, etc.
5. a) An artefact cause by too large a volume of tissue differences within a voxel.
   b) Caused by patient movement, usually breathing.

MAGNETIC RESONANCE IMAGING

1. There are many implants that would be contraindicated in MRI imaging but the main major ones are: cardiac pacemakers, cochlear implants, aneurysm clips, neurostimulators, some heart valves and intra-orbital foreign bodies.
2. When a patient is put into an MRI scanner the body's hydrogen protons become aligned to the main magnetic field. An RF pulse or another magnetic gradient is applied which flips the protons over. When the RF pulse or additional magnetic gradient is removed, the protons relax back to the main magnetic field and emit a small signal. A radiofrequency coil picks up this signal.
3. The contrast we use in MRI is gadolinium and it looks white on a T1 weighted scan.
4. Fat looks bright/white on a T1 weighted scan and water looks dark/black. On a T2 weighted scan fat is dark/black and water is bright/white.
5. 24 h a day, 7 days a week and 365 days a year.

ANATOMY AND PHYSIOLOGY

1. They play a role in metabolism, regulate glucose levels in the body and are involved with growth and development as well as with anti-inflammatory and immune responses.
2. The male urethra is longer than the female one; the male urethra functions as a passage for excretion of urine and ejaculation of sperm whereas the female urethra functions as a passage for urine only.
3. The cardiac sphincter functions as a valve to allow food to pass from the oesophagus into

the stomach and prevents food from the stomach from being regurgitated back into the oesophagus.
4. The arteries have thicker wall layers to withstand the high pressure at which the heart pumps blood into them.
5. These are a series of blind air-filled sacs which give the voice its rich, full-bodied tone.

PATHOLOGY

1. The obstruction prevents passage of bowel gas, which accumulates in the section proximal to the obstruction. This results in radiolucent areas on the film which may show the typical appearance of colonic haustrations or small intestinal circular folds, depending on the site of the obstruction.
2. Conditions include heart failure, bacterial pneumonia, lung cancer and tuberculosis.
3. Common sites of calculi obstruction are where the ureter narrows at the pelvi-ureteric junction, the pelvic brim and where it enters the bladder (vesico-ureteric junction).
4. Inflammatory bowel diseases, such as Crohn's and ulcerative colitis, are associated with increased infiltration of white cells as part of the inflammatory response. By intravenously injecting a technetium-99m radiolabelled portion of a patient's white cells it is possible to localise areas of inflamed bowel and assess its severity.
5. Severe crushing chest pain (although often not found in women), with sweating and nausea; shortness of breath; changes in the electrocardiograph trace; increased blood levels of cardiac enzymes released from damaged myocardium.

Index

NB: Page numbers in **bold** refer to boxes, figures and tables